Primer of Intraoperative
Neurophysiologic Monitoring

Primer of Intraoperative Neurophysiologic Monitoring

Edited by

Garfield B. Russell, M.D., FRCPC
*Associate Professor of Anesthesia and Director of
Neuroanesthesia, Pennsylvania State University College of
Medicine; Staff Anesthesiologist, Department of Anesthesia,
The Milton S. Hershey Medical Center, Hershey, Pennsylvania*

Lawrence D. Rodichok, M.D.
*Associate Professor of Medicine and Neurology, Pennsylvania
State University College of Medicine; Director, Clinical
Neurophysiology Laboratories, The Milton S. Hershey
Medical Center, Hershey, Pennsylvania*

With 26 contributing authors

Butterworth–Heinemann

Boston   Oxford   Melbourne   Singapore   Toronto   Munich   New Delhi   Tokyo

Library of Congress Cataloging-in-Publication Data

Primer of intraoperative neurophysiologic monitoring / [edited by]
    Garfield B. Russell, Lawrence D. Rodichok.
        p.   cm.
    Includes bibliographical references and index.
    ISBN 0-7506-9553-6 (alk. paper)
    1. Neurophysiologic Monitoring.   I. Russell, Garfield B.
  II. Rodichok, Lawrence D.
    [DNLM: 1. Intraoperative monitoring--methods.
  2. Electrodiagnosis--methods.   3. Evoked Potentials--physiology.
  WO 181 P953 1995]
  RD52.N48P75   1995
  617'.91'0028--dc20
  DNLM/DLC
  for Library of Congress   95-12875
                                          CIP

British Library Cataloguing-in-Publication Data

A catalogue record for this book is available from the British Library.

The publisher offers discounts on bulk orders of this book.
For information, please write:

Manager of Special Sales
Butterworth–Heinemann
313 Washington Street
Newton, MA 02158–1626

10 9 8 7 6 5 4 3 2 1

Printed in the United States of America

Contents

Contributing Authors

Gregory C. Allen, M.D., FRCPC
Assistant Professor of Anesthesia, Pennsylvania State University College of Medicine; Attending Anesthesiologist, Department of Anesthesia, The Milton S. Hershey Medical Center, Hershey, Pennsylvania

David P. Archer, M.D., M.Sc., FRCPC
Associate Professor of Anaesthesia and Clinical Neurosciences, Departments of Anaesthesia and Clinical Neurosciences, University of Calgary; Associate Professor of Anaesthesia, Foothills Hospital at the University of Calgary, Calgary, Alberta, Canada

Julien F. Biebuyck, M.B., D. Phil.
Eric A. Walker Professor and Chairman, Department of Anesthesia, Pennsylvania State University College of Medicine, Hershey, Pennsylvania

Terri W. Blackburn, M.D.
Fellow, Department of Anesthesia, Pennsylvania State University College of Medicine; Instructor, Department of Anesthesia, The Milton S. Hershey Medical Center, Hershey, Pennsylvania

Arthur Cronin, M.D.
Resident, Department of Anesthesiology, Pennsylvania State University College of Medicine and The Milton S. Hershey Medical Center, Hershey, Pennsylvania

Andrea C. Erwin, B.A., R. EP T.
Technical Administrator, Clinical Neurohysiology Laboratory, Department of Medicine, Duke University Medical Center, Durham, North Carolina

C. William Erwin, M.D.
Professor of Psychiatry and Associate Professor of Medicine (Neurology), Duke University School of Medicine, Durham, North Carolina

Debra J. Forney
Neurophysiology Technologist, Operating Room Monitoring, Department of Medicine Ancillary, The Milton S. Hershey Medical Center, Hershey, Pennsylvania

Robert Gieski
Neurophysiology Technologist, Operating Room Monitoring, Neurophysiology Laboratory of the Department of Medicine, The Milton S. Hershey Medical Center, Hershey, Pennsylvania

John M. Graybeal, C.R.T.T
Research Assistant in Neuroanesthesia, Department of Anesthesia, Pennsylvania State University College of Medicine, Hershey, Pennsylvania

Jeffry L. Jones, M.D.
Assistant Professor of Anesthesia, Pennsylvania State University College of Medicine; Staff Anesthesiologist, The Milton S. Hershey Medical Center, Hershey, Pennsylvania

John C. Keifer, M.D.
Assistant Professor of Anesthesia, Pennsylvania State College of Medicine; Anesthesiologist, Department of Anesthesia, The Milton S. Hershey Medical Center, Hershey, Pennsylvania

Francis G. King, M.D., FRCPC
Chairman, Department of Anesthesia, Memorial University of Newfoundland and Department of Anesthesia, Health Sciences Center, St. John's, Newfoundland, Canada

W. Andrew Kofke, M.D.
Associate Professor of Anesthesiology/Critical Care Medicine and Neurologic Surgery, University of Pittsburgh Medical Center, Pittsburgh, Pennsylvania

Francis E. LeBlanc, M.D., Ph.D,. FRCSC
Professor of Surgery and Neurosurgery, Department of Clinical Neurosciences, University of Calgary; Director, Epilepsy Research Unit, Department of Clinical Neurosciences, Foothills Hospital, Calgary, Alberta, Canada

Ralph A.W. Lehman, M.D.
Professor of Surgery (Neurosurgery), Pennsylvania State University College of Medicine and University Hospital, Hershey, Pennsylvania

Wayne K. Marshall, M.D.
Associate Professor, Department of Anesthesia, Pennsylvania State
University College of Medicine; Chief, Division of Pain Management,
Department of Anesthesia, The Milton S. Hershey Medical Center,
Hershey, Pennsylvania

Patrick M. McQuillan, M.D.
Assistant Professor of Anesthesia, Pennsylvania State University College of
Medicine; Staff Anesthesiologist, The Milton S. Hershey Medical Center,
Hershey, Pennsylvania

Nanette Newberg, M.S.
Adjunct Faculty, College of Health, University of Utah; Intraoperative
Monitoring, Department of Rehabilitation, Primary Children's Medical
Center, Salt Lake City, Utah

Lawrence D. Rodichok, M.D.
Associate Professor of Medicine and Neurology, Pennsylvania State
Univesity College of Medicine; Director, Clinical Neurophysiology
Laboratories, The Milton S. Hershey Medical Center, Hershey,
Pennsylvania

Garfield B. Russell, M.D.
Associate Professor of Anesthesia and Director of Neuroanesthesia,
Pennsylvania State University College of Medicine; Staff Anesthesiologist,
Department of Anesthesia, The Milton S. Hershey Medical Center,
Hershey, Pennsylvania

Mary C. Schwentker, B.S.
Senior Research Technician, Department of Anesthesia, Pennsylvania State
University College of Medicine, Hershey, Pennsylvania

Lee S. Segal, M.D.
Assistant Professor of Orthopedic Surgery and Pediatrics, Pennsylvania
State University College of Medicine and The Milton S. Hershey Medical
Center, Hershey, Pennsylvania

David A. Wiegand, M.D.
Associate Professor of Otolaryngology/Head and Neck Surgery,
Pennsylvania State University College of Medicine and The Milton S.
Hershey Medical Center, Hershey, Pennsylvania

Joyce I. Winters, R. EEG T.
Supervisor, Neurophysiology Laboratory, Department of Medicine, The
Milton S. Hershey Medical Center, Hershey, Pennsylvania

Preface

The use of intraoperative neurophysiologic monitoring has become part of the standard of care for many surgical procedures, particularly at most major academic centers. We receive regular inquiries from large and small community hospitals as they attempt to bring these techniques to their centers, often at the request of surgical or anesthesia staffs. The general techniques used in intraoperative neurophysiologic monitoring—electroencephalography and sensory evoked potentials—are commonly used by neurologists. Auditory evoked responses are used by audiologists. Anesthesiologists have varying exposure to these studies as well. However, the application of these techniques to the operating room setting has been developed by a rather unique group of neurophysiologists—a group that includes anesthesiologists, audiologists, and neurologists. The technical and interpretative modifications that have evolved have taken intraoperative neurophysiologic monitoring beyond the scope of standard training in any of these disciplines. This book is an effort to bring together the neurophysiologic, anesthetic, and surgical aspects of such monitoring. A successful program will require the cooperation of each discipline.

The initial chapters are intended to review the anatomic and physiologic principles involved in monitoring the brain and spinal cord. Subsequent chapters cover the basic neurophysiologic testing techniques. Each is intended to review the standards of practice in the diagnostic laboratory as well as their modification and standards in the intraoperative setting.

The field of intraoperative neurophysiologic monitoring is new and only very general standards have been suggested by the American EEG Society. These are included in individual chapters. The recently formed American Society of Neurophysiologic Monitoring has been the most active and organized group of practitioners and technologists.

Standards of "normality" are generally not given since these are not entirely relevant in the operating room. Rather, each patient serves as his or her own control. Most often, a postinduction, preincision study is used for this purpose. Each center must establish for itself how much variability in latency and/or amplitude it considers acceptable thereafter. This must be based on correlations with clinical outcome.

Very few instruments are specifically designed for intraoperative monitoring. Those that are used have often been adapted from the diagnostic laboratory. Modifications have often been made in both software and hardware.

Certainly, each instrument must conform to the safety standards of the institution and the American EEG Society for use in the operating room environment.

Successful monitoring depends on a number of critical assumptions. First, one must be monitoring the appropriate pathway(s) and in a fashion that will lead to the earliest possible detection of a significant change. Second, one must have adequate information concerning variables that may affect the responses being monitored. Finally, there must be effective communication at all times among the neurophysiologic monitoring team, the anesthesiologist, and the surgeon. All communications must be fully documented in the monitoring record. We find it very useful to conduct regular meetings of all involved, including the surgeons requesting monitoring, to review representative cases and to discuss other issues as they arise.

Garfield B. Russell, M.D., FRCPC
Lawrence D. Rodichok, M.D.

Acknowledgments

Our experience with intraoperative monitoring would not have been possible without the dedication of our technologists, especially Mary C. Schwentker, B.S. We are also indebted to Debra Forney, Robert Gieski, and Joyce Winters, R.EEG.T, for their commitment to excellence in a very difficult environment. All members of our Department of Anesthesia have been helpful and cooperative, especially Dr. Wayne Marshall, who helped develop the program. Dr. Julien Biebuyck, Professor and Chairman of the Department, has been consistently supportive of our efforts. Dr. Jeffrey Owen, current president of the American Society of Neurophysiologic Monitoring, has been especially generous in sharing his considerable experience and expertise.

We thank Bonnie Merlino for secretarial assistance and, in particular, Cynthia Carroll for her administrative and secretarial efforts.

Garfield B. Russell, M.D., FRCPC
Lawrence D. Rodichok, M.D.

Thank you to Claude Hender, who opened my eyes to science; Dr. Melvin Parsons, who, by example, taught that there was more to being a true physician than being a doctor; Dr. Michael Snider, who made it clear that being a clinician and a scientist are not mutually exclusive; Dr. Julien Biebuyck, for leadership by example and action; Floss, Britt, Wes, and Lea, who make it all possible; and Wesley and Winnie Russell, who gave freedom to grow, develop, and change.

Garfield B. Russell, M.D., FRCPC

Introduction: The Marriage of Neuroscience, Neurophysiology, and the Neurosurgical Patient

Julien F. Biebuyck, M.B., D.Phil.

"Prediction is difficult, especially if it concerns the future."
—Francis Crick

The explosive growth of new information in neuroscience still leaves us fundamentally ignorant of how brain cells work together—to achieve recognition, evaluation of sensory input, selection, and coordination of response. While molecular and cellular studies forge ahead, there is a resurgence of interest in integrative systems level research. This augurs well for clinical scientists, whose important role is to apply basic studies to integrative neurophysiologic research in the human.

The only way to understand how the human brain works is to study the human brain, especially in attempting to understand higher cognitive functions including consciousness, altered consciousness, sleep, memory, and intelligence. Undoubtedly the preservation of some of these higher cognitive functions is one of the main objectives of a team of neurologists, neurophysiologists, neuroanesthesiologists, and neurosurgeons as it approaches a patient with a central nervous system problem. Despite recent advances in noninvasive studies, the vast majority of our knowledge of neuroscience is still based on neuroanatomic studies of dead animals or neurophysiologic studies of anesthetized animals who are not conscious. Neuroscientists have traditionally avoided studies of conscious animals. The study of "consciousness" was also avoided because the problem was considered too complex and "philosophical" and thus not easily amenable to experimental study (Figure 1).

The brain uses similar electric signals to process all the information it receives and analyzes. The origins of the nerve fibers and their destinations within the brain determine the content of the information they transmit. Nerve cells use these signals to transmit information via electric currents generated across their surface membranes. These currents flow through the intracellular and external fluids and result primarily from the movements of charges carried by sodium, potassium, calcium, and chloride ions.

1

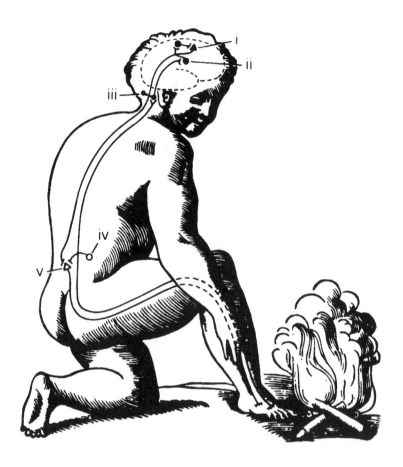

Figure 1 The philosopher René Descartes (1596-1650) had profound interests in physiology. In De Homine he gave the first illustration of a neural pathway in his model of reflexive behavior in the human. The message from the sensory nerve receptors reaches the spinal cord (at iv) and continues along a nerve to the brain (i, ii, and iii). It is also transmitted in the spinal cord to a nerve to muscle (v). *Reprinted with permission from MI Posner, ME Raichle. Images of the Mind. New York: Scientific American Library, 1994.*

Individual neurons encode complex information and concepts into similar electric signals. The nervous system receives information from various transducers in the body; these transducers turn chemical or physical influences, such as light, sound, or pressure, into electromechanical signals. Some transducers respond to signals that come from *outside* the body, as the photoreceptors of the eyes do when they respond to light. Other transducers respond to activity that is largely *inside* the body, such as changes in pH and blood gas tensions. The gray matter of the cortex (2–5 mm thick) contains mainly neurons and accessory cells (glia). The human cortex contains some tens of billions of neurons. A typical neuron responds to the many sources of electric impulses that impinge on its cell body and branches (dendrites) in different ways; inputs may excite, inhibit, or modulate the activity of the neuron. If the neuron becomes sufficiently excited it fires, sending an electrical spike down its axon, which connects with many other neurons. The neuron requires energy to sustain these activities and to synthesize transmittal, but its main function is to receive signals and send them out. At rest a neuron usually sends spikes down its axon at a relatively slow, irregular, "background" rate, often between 1 and 5 Hz (1 Hz is one spike per second). When the neuron receives many excitatory signals, its rate of firing increases to 50–100 Hz or more. Neurons can send signals of only one type down their axons; there are no "negative" spikes. A spike travels down the axon until it reaches a synapse, where transmission of the impulse is chemical, not electrical.

The oldest method for studying brain waves—the electroencephalograph (EEG)—involves placing one or more electrodes directly onto the scalp. There is plenty of electrical activity inside the brain, but the electrical properties of the skull act as a barrier to picking it up. A single electrode responds to the electric fields produced by many tens of millions of nerve cells, so the contribution of an individual cell or group of cells is overwhelmed. The great advantage of an EEG is that its discrimination in time is in the range of a millisecond or so. Thus the rising and falling of brain waves can be followed quite well. What is less clear is what the waves signify. The waves in an awake brain are clearly very different from the waves seen in slow-wave sleep. In rapid eye movement (REM) sleep the brain waves are very similar to those in an awake brain (hence "paradoxical sleep").

In the 1950s and 1960s scientists began recording the electrical activity of individual cells in the brains of awake, behaving animals. This work confirmed an already familiar principle of brain organization: there is a specific region of the brain specialized for processing information from each of the senses. An EEG can be recorded immediately after some perceptual input, such as the sound of a sharp click in one ear. The response of the stimulus is usually very small compared to the electrical background signals. The event has thus to be repeated many times, and all the signals averaged, lined up from the beginning of each event. This often provides a fairly reproducible trace of the typical brain waves associated with that brain activity.

Neurons in the brain are surrounded by neurologic cells. Glial cells behave passively in response to electric current, and unlike neurons, their membranes do not generate conducted impulses. However, glial membrane potentials are depolarized by the potassium released into intercellular spaces during neuronal impulse conduction. This potassium-mediated glial depolarization creates potential changes that can be recorded from the surface of the tissue. As a result glial cells contribute to the EEG. The potential changes recorded by the EEG represent the summed electrical activity of the underlying mass of neurons and glial cells. Therefore, any method that separates the contribution of various elements, such as neurons and glia, is of potential interest.

Scans can produce better spatial localization than the EEG does. Scanners may respond to some aspect of the *static structure* of the brain, or they may detect *activity*. Computed tomography (CT) uses x-rays to scan. Magnetic resonance imaging (MRI) gives high-resolution pictures by recording the density of protons (the nuclei of hydrogen atoms). Both these methods can define *structural* changes in the brain. Positron emission tomography (PET) can record local *activity* of the brain averaged over a minute or more. The technique depends on the intravascular injection of a radiolabeled atom with a short half-life, such as ^{15}O, which emits a positron when it decays. When any part of the brain is more active than usual its blood flow increases. The map produced by the computer corresponds, in effect, to the level of blood flow to each brain region in the scan.

PET scans have limitations, apart from their expense. Spatial resolution is not very good (at present near 8 mm). They also have very poor time resolution—an appreciable fraction of a minute is required to obtain a good signal, whereas the EEG works in the millisecond range. New methods are being developed to combine PET and MRI scans and to develop new MRI methods to detect metabolic activities in the brain.

PET scanning has been used to apply functional imaging to the human brain to study language, that most profoundly human of all abilities. PET has contributed to our understanding of the brain mechanisms that underlie the processing of single words. Cognitive science explores the characteristics of intelligent systems, whether in nature or computers. Cognitive neuroscience draws on the new methods of inquiry and imaging that allow the human brain to be studied during life in ways that were never before possible.

Development of imaging techniques as research tools may mean that nontraditional scientists such as philosophers and experts in the arts will play a greater role in our future understanding of the brain. Many of our most creative thinkers have a strong tendency to convert almost everything into pictures in their minds. New research opportunities require special talents and abilities in areas where many nonmathematicians and nonphysicists have their strengths—in visualization of scientific concepts and in the analysis and manipulation of complex, three-dimensional information graphically displayed.

Techniques like PET and MRI have the potential to tell us where activity is occurring in the brain while it performs various tasks. What these techniques do not tell us is the duration of activity in the active areas and their sequence of activation. Neurons communicate only in milliseconds, but it takes about 40 seconds to obtain the necessary data to construct a PET image of blood flow in the human brain. Thus, PET cannot capture the much faster fluctuations in neuronal activity. Functional measurements with MRI are faster but still slower than the electrical events by which neurons communicate. Thus, study of the electrical activity produced by neurons in close proximity to an electrode still gives the most immediate information (Figure 2).

In this century new imaging technologies represent the most dramatic progress in medical, particularly neurologic, diagnostic procedures.

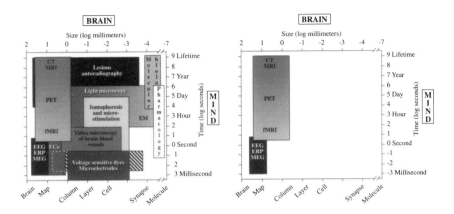

Figure 2 An array of techniques to examine the brain. The brain can be viewed at various levels of spatial resolution ranging from a molecule to the entire brain. Mind events can be envisioned as occurring over times as brief as a few milliseconds—the time it takes one neuron to communicate with another—or as long as a lifetime. The potential contribution of each technique is graphically summarized by putting the spatial resolution on the horizontal axis and the temporal resolution on the vertical axis. The spatial and temporal precision of the techniques can then be compared. In the left graph are all the research techniques available; in the right graph, all the techniques that cannot be applied to human subjects have been eliminated. *Reprinted with permission from MI Posner, ME Raichle. Images of the Mind. New York: Scientific American Library, 1994.*

1895	X-rays
1940s	Nuclear medicine
1950s	Ultrasound techniques, including Doppler sonography
1970s	Computerized tomography
1980s	Magnetic resonance tomography applied to patients
1990s	Positron emission tomography, digital imaging methods, and sonography applied to patients

We place the date of the clinical application of neurophysiology to 1933, when the first report was published on EEG recordings in humans.

Although we have powerful new instruments and improved capabilities for analyzing signals (such as surface potentials), even the most sophisticated or comprehensive analysis can be useless unless the structures and mechanisms of neural function are considered. This book establishes useful links between physiology and clinical practice. Evoked potential measurements represent a promising technology; they are not an end in themselves. They can and should be used to gain *de novo* information, not merely to confirm facts known from anatomic studies or clinical testing. It should become evident that by building on the physiologic foundation one can make more astute clinical diagnoses. Clinical scien-

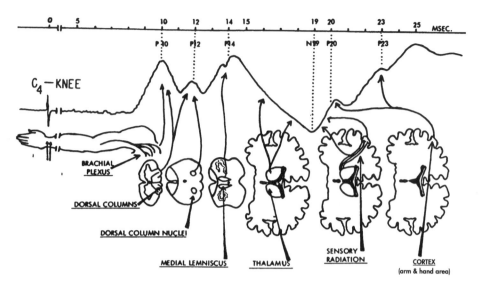

Figure 3 Tentative sites of origin of short-latency somatosensory evoked potentials (SSEPs). Some of the likely generators contributing to early components of the SSEP. *Reprinted with permission from WC Weiderholt, E Meyer-Harding, B Budnick, KL McKeown. Stimulating and recording methods used in obtaining short-latency somatosensory evoked potentials (SEPs) in patients with central and peripheral neurologic disorders. Ann N Y Acad Sci 1982;388:349-358.*

tists can also perform invaluable research by properly applying evoked potential studies to patients. Their data may define the territory and generate questions for scientists who can investigate their cellular and behavioral mechanisms of the nervous system using technologies other than evoked potentials.

An understanding of the neural origins of scalp-recorded event-related potentials (ERP) is essential to their full use as clinical tools. Thus, investigation of human ERP requires, first, the identification of the gross anatomic location of the sources of each ERP component, and second, the definition of the specific cellular processes that generate a particular surface-recorded potential (Figure 3).

There is a compelling need to monitor the central nervous system during surgery as reliably as the cardiovascular system. Raudzens posed the following questions in 1982:

"Can evoked potentials be reliably recorded in the operating room without added risk or inconvenience?

Do intraoperative changes in evoked potentials correlate with postoperative (neural) deficits?

Can intraoperative evoked potential changes be used to prevent postoperative neural deficits?"

Our interest today has not altered—we are interested in a predictive index of neurologic outcome, and the same three questions may be applied to each neural monitoring method in turn.

There is increasing interest in the use of evoked response techniques to evaluate patients with nervous system trauma. Combinations of visual evoked potentials, somatosensory evoked potentials, auditory evoked potentials, and auditory brain stem responses are being used to seek correlations with abnormalities and clinical outcomes. Multimodality evoked potentials obtained in the first few days after head injury have been shown to correlate with final outcome 6 months or more later. Somatosensory evoked potentials can provide information on the functional status of the cervical spine, brain stem and cerebral hemispheres. The proximity of the brain stem auditory pathway to pontomedullary respiratory centers has suggested that brainstem auditory evoked potentials might also help elucidate the pathogenesis of certain adult and infant sleep apnea syndromes.

This book reflects the impact of newer diagnostic techniques on clinical neurology, neurosurgery, and neuroanesthesia. These new approaches have accelerated and enabled the development of new therapeutic techniques, both invasive and noninvasive. The greater understanding that these new monitoring techniques have brought to underlying neurologic events has been important for clinicians and medical school faculty, whose teaching of neuroscience knowledge and translation of that knowledge into clinical approaches is made easier by the ability to teach principles as well as facts.

KEY REFERENCES

Bodis-Wollner I. Evoked potentials. Ann N Y Acad Sci 1982;388:xi–xii.

Greenberg RP, Newlson PG, Becker DP. The somatosensory evoked potential in patients with severe head injury: outcome prediction and monitoring of brain function. Ann N Y Acad Sci 1982;388:683–688.

Kuffler SW, Nichols JG. From Neuron to Brain: A Cellular Approach to the Function of the Nervous System. Sunderland, MA: Sinauer, 1976.

Peterson SE, Fiez JA. The processing of single words studied with positron emission tomography. Annu Rev Neurosci 1993;16:509–530.

Raudzens PA. Intraoperative monitoring of evoked potentials. Ann N Y Acad Sci 1982;388:308–326.

Vaughan HG Jr. The neural origins of human event-related potentials. Ann N Y Acad Sci 1982;388:125.

West TG. In the Mind's Eye. Buffalo, NY: Prometheus, 1991.

RECOMMENDED READING

Bullock TH. Integrative systems research on the brain: resurgence and new opportunities. Annu Rev Neurosci 1993;16:1–15.

Crick F. The Astonishing Hypothesis. The Scientific Search for the Soul. New York: Charles Scribners' Sons, 1994.

Posner MI, Raichle ME. Images of the Mind. New York: Scientific American Library, 1994.

1

Intraoperative Neurophysiologic Monitoring: A Historical Perspective

John M. Graybeal, C.R.T.T.

The recognition of bioelectricity dates back to the early Greeks. Both Aristotle and Plato knew of the numbing powers of a primitive electric fish, the "torpedo." From *narke*, the Greek term for this electrical effect, are derived the terms *narcosis, narcolepsy,* and *narcotic.* The electrical current from these fish was used to treat such diseases as gout, headache, paralysis, and even "mental illness." Use of these fish continued into the seventeenth century, when machines capable of controlled production of electricity, such as Guericke's electrostatic sulfur sphere, were developed. Interest in the use of electricity in medicine continued into the middle of the twentieth century, as demonstrated in Reynolds and Sjoberg's 1969 book *Neuroelectric Research: Electroneuroprosthesis, Electroanesthesia and Nonconvulsive Electrotherapy.*

EARLY BIOELECTRICITY

The eighteenth century saw the use of electricity grow in the fields of medicine and physiology. Benjamin Franklin, Luigi Galvani, and Allesandro Giuseppe Antonio Anastasia Volta are just a few of the preeminent scientists who investigated its use. In 1752, Franklin is reported to have treated a young woman with a 10-year history of convulsions by administering electric shocks. Over the course of 3 1/2 months of treatment both by Franklin and by self-electrification, she was reported to have developed an excellent state of health.

Galvani used an in vitro preparation with a frog's sciatic nerve to demonstrate animal electricity. He noted that every time an electric charge was applied to the nerve the frog's leg muscles twitched. He also attempted to use atmospheric electricity, conducted through a kite, to stimulate the frog's nerve. In his 1791 publication *Commentary on the Effect of Electricity on Muscle Motion,* he concluded that nerves must contain some form of intrinsic electricity. This conclusion led to great controversy with Volta, the inventor of the first electric battery, who contended that this phenomenon could be produced by the potential between two dissimilar metal strips placed in contact with both the nerve and the muscle. These two scientists debated animal versus chemical electricity until their deaths.

Early Recordings of Neurophysiologic Events

Du Bois-Reymond, in 1848, was the first to demonstrate what is now known as the **demarcation potential**. Also using the frog model, he extended his study of the "nerve current" (*Nervenstrom*) into the spinal cord and brain. This was probably the first attempt to look for electrical currents in the brain. He is also credited with being the first to demonstrate the **action potential** of nerves and the **electromyogram** in humans. Using himself as a test subject, Du Bois-Reymond was able to demonstrate with short tetanizing currents that the resultant "negative variation" was distinct from the variations that produced the electrotonic state.

The 1870s was a decade of significant progress in neuroelectrophysiology. No less than three major contributions occurred during this time. First, Fritsch and Hitzig, in 1870, used direct stimulation of the canine cerebral cortex to recruit localized muscle groups. Second, Ferrier furthered these studies and in 1873 lectured on the localization of function in the brain. Despite the use of ether and chloroform throughout Ferrier's studies, he was the subject of considerable attention from antivivisectionists of that time. This work led to the eventual mapping of the mammalian motor cortex. Third, in 1874, Bartholow reported the first use in humans of electrical stimulation of the brain and extremity movement of the contralateral side.

In 1875, Richard Caton published an abstract in the *British Medical Journal* entitled "The electric currents of the brain." He reported that "feeble currents of varying direction pass through the multiplier when the electrodes are placed on two points of the external of the skull." He also reported that "impressions through the senses were found to influence the currents of certain areas." He noted that a large current over the region of a rabbit's brain (found by Ferrier to be related to the movement of the eyelids) was markedly influenced by shining a light into the opposite eye.[1] Caton was the first to describe the baseline electric activity now referred to as the electroencephalogram (EEG). He described a variable baseline activity. He was also the first to demonstrate the visual evoked potential.

Von Marxow and Beck both repeated Caton's experiments looking for somatosensory evoked potentials. In experiments in 1883, Von Marxow noted that the evoked potentials observed prior to administering anesthesia were abolished by anesthesia, proving that anesthesia abolished the sensation, not merely its memory. Beck, in 1890, demonstrated both the background electric activity and the evoked potential in anesthetized and curarized dogs, showing that these electric signals were not related to movement itself.

Although the scientific foundation was laid in the nineteenth century, crossover into human studies and eventual clinical utilization took several decades. Hans Berger (1877–1941) is credited with the first reported recording of the human EEG, primarily 10-Hz alpha waves. These recordings were done without an amplifier. Berger was able to do these first in humans with large surgical skull defects, which allowed placement of needle electrodes on or near the cortex. After obtaining an amplifier in 1931, he was able to make similar transcranial recordings.

Early Intraoperative Recordings

Clinical neurophysiology monitoring in the operating room dates back to the late 1930s. Drs. Wilder Penfield and Herbert Jasper collaborated at the Montreal Neurological Institute. They recorded intraoperative EEGs from the exposed cortex of patients undergoing surgical exploration for localization and treatment of focal epilepsy. In addition to being credited with the first use of EEG recordings intraoperatively, they organized the "EEG ski meetings," the first, in 1939, being the initial conference on EEG use during brain surgery. Dr. Jasper was instrumental in the formation of the American EEG Society in 1946, serving as its first president.

DEVELOPMENT OF MODERN RECORDING EQUIPMENT

The most interesting point common to all of these early investigators is the technical level of recording equipment available to them.

Early neurophysiologists were not blessed with the technically sophisticated signal processing and recording equipment available today. The first "instrument" for recording action potentials from peripheral nerves was the "rheoscopic frog." This preparation (usually hind legs) could reportedly detect weaker currents than the galvanometers of that period. This system was used well into the nineteenth century. In 1820, Oersted demonstrated the electromagnetic effect that was the basis for the galvanometer. This type of galvanometer was also used by Du Bois-Reymond in 1848 (see above). Various forms of the galvanometer were used into the twentieth century.

Development of Recording Equipment for Evoked Potentials

Braun (1890) invented the cathode-ray oscillograph. This device produced a display with increased fidelity resulting from thousands of superimposed repetitions. Recording of spontaneously occurring events was impossible because of the number of repetitions required. The ability to photograph the "spots of lights" on the oscillograph, developed in the early 1930s, allowed investigators to produce permanent records and to begin investigations into the high-frequency activity of the nervous system. Erlanger and Gasser were awarded the Nobel Prize in 1944 for studies in which they used this type of oscillograph recording system to record action potentials and show that they are the sums of potentials from fibers of different size, type, and conduction velocity.

An electromechanical signal-averaging system using vacuum tubes and analog technology, described by Dawson in 1951, was the first device capable of distinguishing a small regular signal from a large irregular background signal.

This averaging computer separated the cortically detected evoked potential from the background electroencephalogram by storing small-time epoch signals in a storage capacitor. Activity synchronous with the stimulation rate tended to accumulate over time, while all nonsynchronous signals tended to cancel.

Work at the Massachusetts Institute of Technology in the mid 1950s was directed to auto- and cross-correlation studies of the EEG. Barlow (1987) reported an averaging system for brain evoked potentials that produced good waveforms using settings of 0.5 msec and averaging 200 responses. This averaging response computer (ARC), as the system was called, is a digital computer capable of response averaging and amplitude and time interval histogram calculations. Sances et al. commented in 1980 that the visual evoked potentials recorded in cats and humans using this system were of as good quality as any produced by modern equipment.

Development of Recording Equipment for Electroencephalograms

Berger, in 1929, used a string galvanometer to measure the EEG in humans. Although these recordings revolutionized electrophysiology, it soon became clear that several problems existed with the recording equipment used. The equipment was able to measure the electric potential between only two points at one time (single channel). Making a permanent record required a photograph of each record.

Development of the differential amplifier, attributed to Matthews in 1934, allowed recording from several channels at the same time. In addition to this benefit, another unexpected benefit was produced by use of the differential amplifier. Electrostatic pickup was greatly reduced, thereby reducing 50- to 60-Hz interference. Improvements in the differential amplifier have almost completely eliminated the need for patient shielding in a grounded Faraday cage. This technology was incorporated by both Grass and Offner to manufacture the first multichannel EEG recording machines.

The time and associated expense required to produce photographic records of the EEG signal were unacceptable. The "Crystallograph," developed in 1936, used a piezoelectric crystal to move an ink pen across a paper tape and produce a continuous written record of the EEG. The first device of this type responded to frequencies to over 200 Hz with over 1-cm excursions.

The next major advance did not occur until 1956; this was the development of transistors. EEG machines may have been the first scientific machines to be transistorized. Introduction of transistorized EEGs improved the reliability of the equipment and the records they produced.

Development of Processing Equipment for Electroencephalograms

Investigators in the 1930s sought to develop analysis systems that would provide more information than was available from visual observation of the EEG record. In 1938, Gibbs and Grass obtained a Fourier frequency spectrum for the EEG by continuously replaying a section of the EEG record several times through a filter. Parr and Walker build an on-line spectrum analysis system in 1943. This was the foundation for a variety of the computer-processed EEG systems of today, including compressed spectral array (introduced by Bickford in 1971 as a clinical tool to view the EEG record), density spectral array, and others.

INTRAOPERATIVE NEUROPHYSIOLOGIC MONITORING

While initial use of neurophysiologic monitoring dates to the early 1900s, debate continues concerning its appropriate use in the operating room and intensive care unit. The advent of small, relatively portable, affordable equipment has allowed use of these technologies in the operating room. The routine use of neurophysiologic monitoring intraoperatively is a field in constant development. In a review of intraoperative evoked potential monitoring, Grundy referred to the controversies and limitations surrounding this new technology.[2] That review was written in 1983. A 1992 statement from the Scoliosis Research Society concluded "that the use of intraoperative spinal cord neurophysiological monitoring during procedures including instrumentation is not investigational. [The Scoliosis Research Society] considers neurophysiological monitoring a viable alternative as well as an adjunct to the use of the wake-up test during spinal surgery."[3] The debate continues, although with increasing numbers of controlled studies and good case reports, neurophysiologic monitoring is becoming not only accepted but expected. Recording standards have been developed and are constantly being revised. Health care reform and outcome-based decisions may well increase the importance of quality monitoring technology in general and specifically increase the frequency and variety of uses for neurophysiologic monitoring techniques.

KEY REFERENCES

1. Caton R. The electric currents of the brain. Br Med J 1875;2:278.
2. Grundy BL. Intraoperative monitoring of sensory-evoked potentials. Anesthesiology 1983;58:83.
3. Scoliosis Research Society. Somatosensory evoked potential monitoring of neurologic cord function during spinal surgery. A position statement. Park Ridge, IL: Scoliosis Research Society, 1992.

RECOMMENDED READINGS

Bartholow R. Experimental investigations into the functions of the human brain. Am J Med Sci 1874;67:305.

Grass AM. The electroencephalographic heritage until 1960. Am J EEG Tech 1984;24:133. *A collection of thoughts on and figures depicting the early development of EEG recordings by one of the principles of the field.*

Hoff HE, Geddes LA. The rheotome and its prehistory: A study in the historical interrelation of electrophysiology and electromechanics. Bull Hist Med 1957;31:327.

Jasper HH. History of the early development of electroencephalography and clinical neurophysiology at the Montreal Neurological Institute: The first 25 years, 1939–1964. Can J Neurol Sci 1991;18:533.

Larson SJ, Sances A. Evoked potentials in man. Neurosurgical applications. Am J Surg 1966;111:857.

Offner FF. Bioelectric potentials—their source, recording, and significance. IEEE Trans Biomed Eng 1984;31:863.

Sances A, Myklebust J, Larson SJ, Cusick JF. The evoked potential and early studies of bioelectricity. J Clin Eng 1980;5:27. *This article discusses the early accounts of bioelectricity and evoked potential instrumentation.*

Schoenberg BS. Richard Caton and the electrical activity of the brain. Mayo Clin Proc 1974;49:474. *A discussion of bioelectricity prior to the 1870s. Included are a thorough discussion of Caton's life along with figures showing the equipment and experimental techniques of the time.*

2

Functional Neuroanatomy For Neurophysiologic Monitoring

Arthur Cronin, M.D.
John C. Keifer, M.D.

This chapter is an outline, beginning with the scalp and ending with the peripheral nerves, of the anatomy fundamental for both understanding and performing neurophysiologic monitoring. The depth of detail is sufficient to provide a simple description of the pathways of the commonly recorded evoked potentials and a description of the optimal positions for stimulating lead placement. Knowing these pathways is essential. For example, to obtain useful information during cerebral aneurysm clipping, one must deduce the brain tissue at risk from the location of the aneurysm, and then stimulate the appropriate peripheral nerve corresponding to this area.

SCALP, CALVARIA, AND MENINGES

The outermost protection for the brain is the thick, mobile, and highly vascularized **scalp**. The scalp includes three fused outer layers of skin, subcutaneous tissue, and the tough fibrous **galea** (helmet). Under the galea is a layer of loose, mobile connective tissue that overlies the innermost layer, the **pericranium**, which is the periosteum for the cranial vault. The **cranial vault** comprises the **frontal bones** anteriorly, the **parietal bones** laterally, the **occipital bones** posteriorly, and both the **temporal bones and greater wing** of the **sphenoid bones** inferolaterally. The **calvaria** is the superior portion of the vault. Bone thickness varies throughout the vault, with the frontal calvaria being 6–8 mm thick, including solid **outer** and **inner tables** separated by a cancellous vascular **diploe**. Beneath the bone there are three tissue layers enveloping the brain. The outermost, the **dura mater**, is the strongest and thickest. The **arachnoid** ("spider's web") is a gossamer-thin membrane that underlies the dura and encloses the **subarachnoid space**. Within the subarachnoid space are **cerebrospinal fluid** (CSF), "bridging" veins traveling from the cortex to dural venous sinuses, and larger blood vessels supplying the brain. The innermost membrane, the **pia mater**, is also very delicate and intimately follows the contour of the cortex. Composed of two layers, the pia is highly vascular and sheaths blood vessels as they enter the brain.

15

THE BRAIN
Lobar Organization and Cortical Topography

The brain is organized into five lobes—the **frontal, parietal, temporal, occipital,** and **insula.** The location of each lobe corresponds roughly to the overlying like-named bone, except for the insula, which is located deep to the frontal, parietal, and temporal lobes. Within each lobe is a characteristic pattern of ridges (**gyri**) and grooves (**sulci**), which provide a rough guide to the functional organization of the cortex. The frontal lobe includes the **primary motor cortex** in the **precentral gyrus** as well as the **motor speech area (Broca's area)** in the **inferior frontal gyrus,** usually on the left side. The **primary somatosensory cortex** is located in the **postcentral gyrus** of the parietal lobe. The **receptive speech area** is located in the **supramarginal** and **angular gyri** of the parietal lobe, but it also includes adjoining regions of the temporal and occipital lobes. The temporal lobe is the major terminus for input from the olfactory and auditory systems and is involved in integrating receptive language function. In addition, the temporal lobe is associated with the functions of memory and learning. The occipital lobe performs predominantly visual functions.

Functional Anatomy

Anatomically each functional area of the cortex is exquisitely organized. For example, the primary motor and sensory cortex can be described as a **homunculus,** with each body part represented by a cortical region. The size of this cortical region depends on the neural complexity of the body parts, the face and hands occupying disproportionately large areas. This organization is useful during neurophysiologic monitoring because it permits accurate prediction of which evoked potentials would monitor to specific brain areas (e.g., the tibial nerve in the leg for medial cortical injury or the median nerve in the arm for more lateral cortical injury).

Blood Supply

The anterior pair of **internal carotid arteries** and the posterior pair of **vertebral arteries** supply the **circle of Willis,** from which arises the blood supply to the brain (Figure 2.1). The posterior circulation, the vertebral-basilar circulation, is formed by the junction of the vertebral arteries, which enter the cranium through the foramen magnum and form a single midline **basilar artery** at the ventral pontomedullary junction. Branches from the vertebral-basilar system supply the spinal cord, brain stem, and cerebellum. At the upper border of the pons the basilar artery bifurcates into two **posterior cerebral arteries,** which supply the thalamus, hypothalamus, and the inferior and posterior regions of the cerebral hemispheres, including the medial temporal and occipital lobes. Anteriorly, each internal carotid artery bifurcates to form the **anterior cerebral artery** and the larger **middle cerebral artery.** The anterior cerebral artery sends a

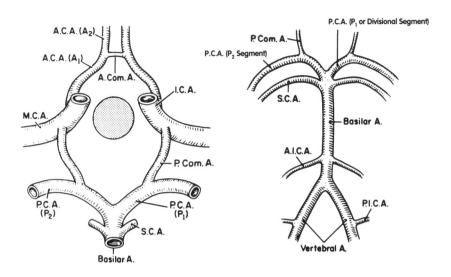

Figure 2.1 Normal circle of Willis (left). I.C.A. = internal carotid artery; A.Com.A. = anterior communicating artery; A.C.A. (A$_1$) = precommunicating segment of the anterior cerebral artery; A.C.A. (A$_2$) = postcommunicating segment of the anterior cerebral artery; M.C.A. = middle cerebral artery; P.C.A. (P$_1$) = precommunicating segment of the posterior cerebral artery; P.C.A. (P$_2$) = postcommunicating segment of the posterior cerebral artery; P.Com.A. = posterior communicating artery; S.C.A. = superior cerebellar artery. Vertebral and basilar arteries and their major branches (right). P.I.C.A. = posterior inferior cerebellar artery; A.I.C.A. = anterior inferior cerebellar artery; S.C.A.= superior cerebellar artery; P.C.A. = posterior cerebral artery; (P$_1$) = precommunicating segment and (P$_2$) = postcommunicating segment; P.Com.A. = posterior communicating artery. *Reprinted with permission from AL Day. Arterial Distributions and Variants. In JH Wood (ed), Cerebral Blood Flow: Physiological and Clinical Aspects. New York: McGraw-Hill, 1987.*

few perforating branches into the anterior deep structures of the brain, but the main trunk of the artery runs anteriorly and medially through the **interhemispheric fissure**. This trunk supplies the medial cortex of the frontal and parietal lobes, including the leg area. The middle cerebral artery also gives off several important perforating branches, the **striate arteries**, before it reaches the **lateral fissure** where, on the surface of the insula, it divides into the many branches supplying the lateral cortex.

Critical to an understanding of the cerebral circulation is knowledge of the collateral circulation; ideally, the circulation provides an alternate blood supply if an arterial blockage occurs. The circle of Willis is the major source of collateral blood flow, but there are several additional sources. For example, ischemia from occlusion of the internal carotid artery can be reduced by external carotid artery flow through branches of the facial artery. Shunting from the facial artery to the ophthalmic artery leads to the circle of Willis. The three major cortical arteries anastomose through superficial pial branches, and the major cerebellar arteries have a similar anastomosis. However, the perforating arteries, such as the striate arteries, are "end arteries" without any alternate blood supply.

The Ventricular System

Within the brain are four ependyma-lined cavities containing the **choroid plexus,** which produces CSF (see Chapter 21). CSF from the **lateral ventricle** in each hemisphere flows medially through **the interventricular foramina of Monro** into the single **third ventricle.** The third ventricle empties via the **cerebral aqueduct** into the **fourth ventricle,** which lies between the pons and cerebellum. From the fourth ventricle the CSF has three exits: laterally through the two **foramina of Luschka,** or medially through the **foramen of Magendie.** The CSF circulates in the subarachnoid space, bathing the spinal cord and brain. Absorption of CSF occurs in the **arachnoid granulations,** which protrude into the **superior sagittal sinus,** a venous channel between the dura and the cranium that drains into the internal jugular vein.

The Brain Stem

The brain stem is perhaps the most complicated area in neuroanatomy and neurophysiology. Not only is it a bridge between the spinal cord and the cerebrum and cerebellum, but it also contains integrated networks critical for the regulation of consciousness, respiration, and cardiovascular control. Additionally, the brain stem contains nuclei for the cranial nerves. Assessment of the functional integrity of the cranial nerve–brain stem–cortex pathway is useful when working around the facial nerve or the auditory nerve, such as during resection of cerebellopontine angle tumors.

Considering the tortuous courses of the auditory tracts, it is not surprising that the brain stem auditory evoked response is a complicated signal. Sound is transformed by the cochlea into neuronal action potentials, which are carried by the **cochlear nerve** through the **internal auditory canal** to the **ventral cochlear nucleus** in the **inferior cerebellar peduncle** (Figure 2.2). The tonotopic organization, based on frequency as translated by the **organ of Corti** in the cochlea, is maintained throughout the pathway. In the ventral cochlear nucleus the nerve fibers bifurcate, sending one branch to the **dorsal cochlear nucleus** (also in the inferior cerebellar peduncle) and leaving the other branch in the ventral cochlear nucleus. Fibers from the ventral cochlear nucleus form the **trapezoid body,** which crosses the midline of the pons, and then ascend in the **lateral lemniscus** to the inferior colliculus. From the **inferior colliculus,** fibers project to the medial geniculate body. Fibers from the **medial geniculate body** form the **auditory radiation** through the **internal capsule** to the cortex of the superior temporal gyrus. Fibers from the dorsal cochlear nucleus, instead of crossing in the trapezoid body, cross the midline in the **dorsal acoustic stria** and join the other fibers in the lateral lem-

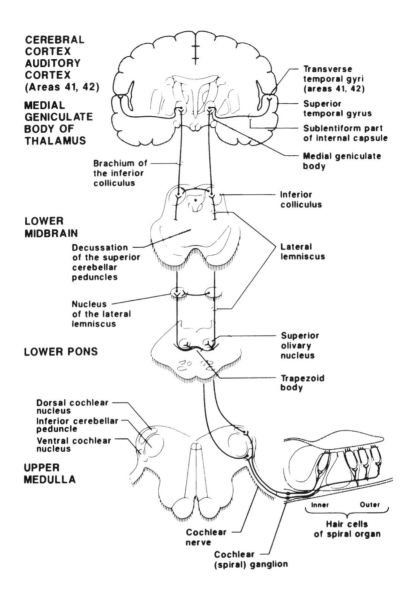

Figure 2.2 Schematic representation of the auditory pathways along which brain stem responses are conducted. *Reprinted with permission from C Watson (ed), Basic Human Neuroanatomy—An Introductory Atlas. Boston: Little, Brown, 1991.*

niscus. Each nucleus serves as a center where influences from other nuclei are integrated. While most fibers follow this course, some fibers ascend through the lateral leminiscus without first crossing the midline, and some fibers from the inferior colliculus cross to the contralateral medial geniculate body.

The Vertebral Column

The vertebral column is composed of a stack of 33 vertebrae, including seven cervical, 12 thoracic, five lumbar, five fused sacral, and four fused coccygeal. Each nonfused vertebra has a unique shape. However, all share the following features: the **body,** which supports weight; the **arch,** which is formed by two **pedicles** and two **lamina;** two **transverse processes,** which project laterally; and one **spinous process,** which projects dorsally. Articulation with superior and inferior vertebrae is through the **intervertebral disc,** which separates the bodies, and by the **facet joints** on the superior and inferior articulation surfaces of the vertebral arches. Exceptions to this general description are the cervical vertebrae, which have a **foramen transversarium** in each transverse process for the passage of the vertebral arteries, and the first and second cervical vertebrae. The first cervical vertebra, the **atlas,** is ring-shaped without any body or spinous process. The second cervical vertebra, the **axis,** has a superior projection from its body (the **dens**), which fits between the spinal cord and the anterior arch of the atlas and functions as the pivot point for head rotation. Between vertebrae are the bilateral **intervertebral foramina,** which are posterior to the body and anterior to the facet joint. The spinal nerves and blood vessels enter and leave the vertebral canal through these foramina at each level. Connecting the vertebrae are several ligaments. The most superficial is **the supraspinous ligament,** which connects the tips of the spinous processes. The **interspinous ligament** joins the entire length of the spinous process of adjacent vertebrae, and the **ligamentum flavum** joins the posterior arches of adjacent vertebrae. The vertebral arches enclose the **vertebral canal,** which includes the meninges, blood vessels, CSF, spinal nerves, and spinal cord.

THE SPINAL CORD
Topography

The spinal cord and 31 pairs of spinal nerves functionally link the brain to the rest of the body. In the adult the spinal cord is 0.5 m long, ending at the body of L1 in a collection of nerve roots called the **cauda equina.** The diameter of the cord is 1 cm, increasing to 1.5 cm at the **cervical** (C3-T2) and **lumbar** (L1-S2) **enlargements.** Like the brain, the spinal cord includes white matter and gray matter, which correspond to fiber tracts and cell bodies, respectively. However, unlike the brain, the gray matter in the spinal cord is surrounded by the white fiber tracts. In a transverse slice of the cord the gray matter forms an H shape with two **ventral horns** and two **dorsal horns** connected by **the gray commissure.** The surrounding white matter is divided into **anterior, posterior,** and **lateral funiculi.** Enveloping the cord are the three meninges and the CSF. Spinal nerves and blood vessels pass through the intervertebral foramen at each level. The spinal nerves are composed of a **ventral root** and a **dorsal root**. The ventral root is actually a group of root filaments, which emerge from the **ventrolateral sulcus,** and the dorsal root is also a group of filaments, which enter the spinal cord at the **dorsolateral sulcus.** Before joining the ventral root in the intervertebral foramen, each dorsal root contains a swelling, the **dorsal root ganglion,** which contains the cell bodies of these neurons. The cell bodies for the fibers in the ventral root are in the ventral horns.

Ascending Spinal Tracts

Sensory input reaches the dorsal horn of the spinal cord through the dorsal roots of the spinal nerves. Pain and temperature sensation cross the spinal cord from the dorsal horn to the ventrolateral white matter. These fibers compose the **lateral spinothalamic tract** (Figure 2.3). Because spinal nerves contribute fibers sequentially, there is a rough somatotopic organization. The sacral regions are lateral and the cervical regions medial as the tract ascends through the brain stem and continues with most of the fibers to terminate in the thalamus. Touch and proprioception are carried together in the **dorsal columns**. Fibers enter the dorsal columns directly from the dorsal roots and ascend ipsilaterally to the **gracile** and **cuneate nuclei** in the medulla. Axons from these nuclei cross to the other side of the brain stem and form the **medial lemniscus,** which terminates in the thalamus. This sensory pathway—(1)ascending in the ipsilateral dorsal column to the gracile and cuneate nuclei in the medulla, (2) crossing midline in the pontine medial lemniscus and ascending to the contralateral cortex through the internal capsule—is the dominant contributor to the cortical sensory evoked potential. Unlike the two pathways above, the **anterior spinothalamic tract** does not arise directly from a neuron located in the dorsal root ganglion. Instead it arises from neurons in the posterior horn, crosses the spinal cord in the **anterior white commissure,** and ascends contralaterally in the anterior funiculus through the brain stem to the thalamus. This pathway carries light touch sensation; however, injury to this pathway produces minimal clinical deficit since the posterior columns also carry touch sensation. There are also other ascending tracts, particularly to the cerebellum.

Descending Tracts

The main descending fiber tract is the **corticospinal tract,** which arises predominantly from the precentral gyrus but also from the somatosensory cortex (Figure 2.4). The fibers descend to the **pyramid** of the medulla, where 90% cross the midline in the **pyramidal decussation** before continuing in the lateral funiculus of the spinal cord. They terminate on interneurons in **the intermediate gray matter** or directly on motor neurons whose axons emerge from the spinal cord as the ventral root. The 10% uncrossed corticospinal fibers descend as **the ventral corticospinal tract** in the ventral funiculus. The remainder of the descending tracts arise from the brain stem. The **rubrospinal tract** arises from the **red nucleus**

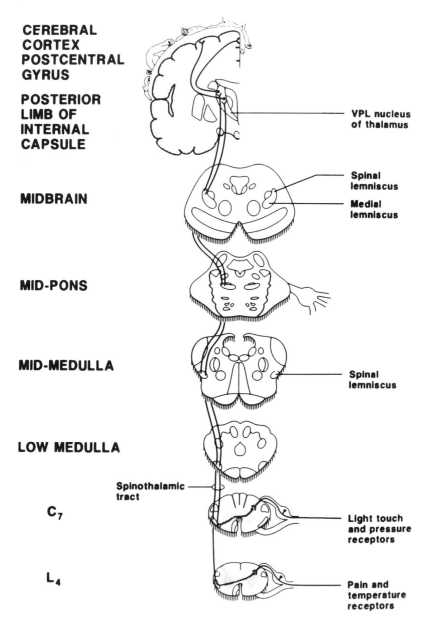

Figure 2.3 The spinothalamic tracts. *Reprinted with permission from C Watson (ed), Basic Human Neuroanatomy—An Introductory Atlas. Boston: Little, Brown, 1991.*

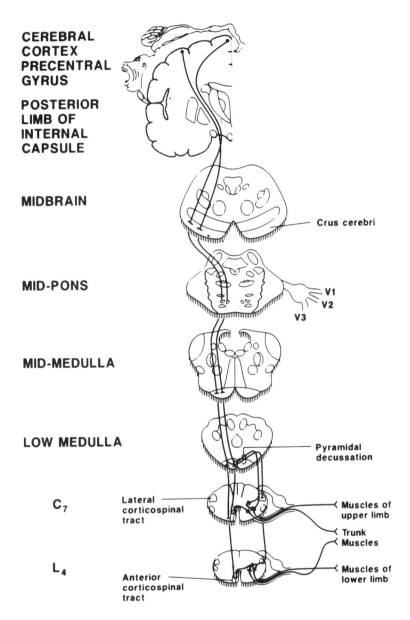

CEREBRAL CORTEX PRECENTRAL GYRUS

POSTERIOR LIMB OF INTERNAL CAPSULE

MIDBRAIN

Crus cerebri

MID-PONS

V1
V2
V3

MID-MEDULLA

LOW MEDULLA

Pyramidal decussation

C_7

Lateral corticospinal tract

Muscles of upper limb

Trunk Muscles

L_4

Anterior corticospinal tract

Muscles of lower limb

Figure 2.4   The corticospinal tracts. *Reprinted with permission from C Watson (ed), Basic Human Neuroanatomy—An Introductory Atlas. Boston: Little, Brown, 1991.*

in the **midbrain** and accompanies the corticospinal tracts. Its major function is control of flexor muscle tone. Fibers from the **lateral vestibular nucleus** form the **lateral vestibulospinal tract** in the ventral funiculus of the spinal cord. These fibers descend uncrossed to terminate in the ventral horn and mediate much of the cerebellar influence on motor control, particularly extensor muscle tone. The **reticulospinal fibers** arise from the **medial reticular formation** and descend in the ventrolateral and dorsolateral funiculi. In addition to control of movement, these fibers are involved in cardiovascular and respiratory control.

Blood Supply

The blood supply to the spinal cord is from the **anterior spinal artery,** which supplies the ventral two-thirds of the cord, and two **posterior spinal arteries,** which supply the dorsal one-third of the cord. The anterior spinal artery arises from two small branches of the vertebral arteries and runs in the ventral median fissure. There it receives additional blood supply from **anterior radicular arteries** throughout the length of the spinal cord. Radicular arteries arise from the vertebral, deep cervical, ascending cervical, posterior intercostal, lumbar, and lateral sacral arteries. Branches from these arteries follow the spinal nerves through the intervertebral foramina and bifurcate into anterior and posterior radicular arteries supplying not only the spinal arteries but also the meninges and vertebrae. Below the superior cervical region the spinal artery depends on the radicular arteries for blood supply. The midthoracic region has the fewest radicular arteries, so it is a watershed area at risk for ischemia during hypotension. The **great radicular artery**, otherwise known as the **artery of Adamkiewicz,** usually arises from a lower thoracic or superior lumbar artery and is much larger than the other radicular arteries. It provides the major contribution to the caudal two-thirds of the anterior spinal artery. The two posterior spinal arteries arise from small branches of the vertebral or **posterior inferior cerebellar arteries.** They then descend along the posterior cord, receiving additional supply from posterior radicular arteries. There is extensive collateralization between the posterior and anterior spinal arteries. However, because of the physical separation between motor and sensory components of the spinal cord, and because of the heterogenicity of blood supply, monitoring of one function (such as sensation with somatosensory evoked potentials [SSEPs]) does not necessarily reflect the status of the entire spinal cord. Therefore it is possible to have ischemia of the motor pathway without effects on the ascending sensory pathways in the posterior columns.

PERIPHERAL NERVES

Thirty-one pairs of spinal nerves exit through the intervertebral foramina and either enter a nerve plexus, such as the **brachial plexus** or the **lumbosacral plexus,** or continue individually to innervate a segment or dermatome. After leaving a plexus the individual nerves, containing motor and sensory fibers, typically run as part of a neurovascular bundle to the muscle or dermatome that they innervate. Measurement of both somatosensory and motor evoked potentials requires either stimulation or recording from these peripheral nerves at sites where the nerve is close to the skin and can be reliably located.

Brachial Plexus

The brachial plexus contains the innervation for the upper extremity and the shoulder. Its accessibility depends on body habitus, but is usually possible at **Erb's point**, which is just lateral to the insertion of the sternocleidomastoid muscle into the clavicle. Branches from the brachial plexus include the median nerve and the ulnar nerve.

Median Nerve
A branch of the brachial plexus, the median nerve is formed from C5–T1 spinal nerve roots. In the antecubital fossa the median nerve is just medial to the biceps muscle and the brachial artery. In this location it is accessible for recording and stimulation. In the forearm it runs deeply, innervating most of the anterior muscles and providing sensation to the lateral palm, palmar surface of the thumb, and the lateral two-and-a-half fingers. It is most commonly stimulated on the volar surfaces of the wrist deep and lateral to the palmaris longus tendon.

Ulnar Nerve
The ulnar nerve is also a branch of the brachial plexus and receives contributions from C7–T1. It is easily palpable at the elbow just posterior to the medial epicondyle of the humerus. It is stimulated either here in the ulnar groove or on the medial aspect of the volar surface of the wrist medial to the ulnar artery and lateral to the tendon of the flexor carpi ulnaris. The ulnar's sensory distribution is the medial part of the hand, and the motor distribution includes the hypothenar muscles, the adductor pollicis muscle, and all the interossei muscles.

The Lumbrosacral Plexus

The lumbrosacral plexus contains the innervation to the lower extremity, pelvic muscles, and sphincters. It is not accessible to direct stimulation.

Sciatic Nerve
The sciatic nerve emerges from the lumbrosacral plexus with contributions from L4–S3, which make it 2 cm in diameter and the largest nerve in the body. It is most accessible just inferior to the gluteus maximus muscle in the midposterior thigh just deep to the biceps femoris muscle. The sciatic nerve is really two nerves, the tibial and the common peroneal, both of which are useful for neurophysiologic monitoring.

Common Peroneal Nerve   The common peroneal nerve arises from the sciatic nerve at the superior angle of the popliteal fossa. It runs inferolaterally, passing superficial to the lateral head of the gastrocnemius muscle and the head of the fibula before entering the lateral compartment of the leg and lying deep to the peroneus longus muscle. For much of its course in the lateral popliteal fossa, and as it winds around the fibula, this nerve is easily located.

Tibial Nerve   The tibial nerve, which is the other component of the sciatic nerve, can be located either in the middle of the popliteal fossa or at the ankle between the medial malleolus and calcaneous. At the ankle the posterior tibial artery is a palpable landmark for the tibial nerve, which lies immediately posteromedial to the artery.

KEY REFERENCES

Carpenter MB. Core Text of Neuroanatomy. Baltimore: Williams & Wilkins, 1991. *Comprehensive yet concise neuroanatomy text.*

Heimer L. The Human Brain and Spinal Cord. New York: Springer-Verlag, 1983. *Functional neuroanatomy and dissection guide with clinical implications. Elegantly written and illustrated.*

Moore KL. Clinically Oriented Anatomy (2nd ed). Baltimore: Williams & Wilkins, 1985. *Readable, clear, well-illustrated, and comprehensive anatomy text; does not include detailed description of central nervous system.*

Netter FH. Atlas of Human Anatomy. Summit, NJ: Ciba-Geigy, 1990. *Atlas of large, detailed, and well-labeled color illustrations and diagrams.*

3

Functional Neurophysiology

Francis G. King, M.D., F.R.C.P.C.

CEREBRAL METABOLISM, OXYGENATION, AND REGULATION OF FUNCTION

Normal cerebral function depends on a continuous supply of oxygen and glucose. The brain has a relatively high metabolic rate, consuming about 20% of total body oxygen, or approximately 50 ml of O_2 per minute for the average adult male. The value **for cerebral metabolic rate of oxygen consumption (CMRO$_2$)** is expressed as milliliters of oxygen consumed per 100 g of brain tissue per minute. The CMRO$_2$ averages **3.0–3.5 ml/100 g/minute** in humans. About 40% of the energy consumed by the brain is used to maintain its cellular integrity. This basal metabolic requirement is needed to (1) maintain the ionic gradients across cell membranes, (2) carry out biosynthesis, (3) provide for axonal transport, and (4) ensure basic homeostatic cellular functions of the brain. The remaining 60% of energy consumed by the brain is used to maintain the synaptic activity in the working brain as it carries out sensory, motor, and higher cortical functions.

Cerebral Metabolism

Under normal conditions, aerobic metabolism of glucose accounts for 95% of brain energy. The complete metabolism of 1 mole of glucose to CO_2 and water yields 38 moles of high-energy substrate adenosine triphosphate (ATP). About 5% of glucose may be anaerobically metabolized to lactic acid. This inefficient method of energy production yields only 2 moles of ATP, as glucose undergoes anaerobic glycolysis to pyruvate and lactate. Anaerobic glycolysis aggravates normal cellular function as it lowers intracellular pH secondary to hydrogen ion production. Under abnormal conditions the brain may use alternate sources of energy. During periods of starvation, the brain may use ketone bodies (acetoacetate and beta-hydroxybutyrate) to provide up to two-thirds of its metabolic needs. The brain may also metabolize lactate when levels are high.

CMRO$_2$ can be reduced by anesthetic agents. The intravenous agents have variable effects on CMRO$_2$, with barbiturates and etomidate producing the greatest decrease. At very large doses, barbiturates may reduce CMRO$_2$ by 50%.

Propofol, benzodiazepines, and lidocaine may decrease $CMRO_2$ by 20–30%. Narcotics have a minimal effect, while ketamine may initially produce an increase in $CMRO_2$. The volatile anesthetic gases produce a dose-dependent reduction in $CMRO_2$. Isoflurane effects the greatest reduction of up to 50%. Enflurane may increase $CMRO_2$ if it precipitates electrical seizure activity. N_2O has minimal effect on $CMRO_2$. Sevoflurane and desoflurane decrease $CMRO_2$ to a similar degree as isoflurane.

Hypothermia reduces $CMRO_2$ by about 5% for each 1°C drop in body temperature. At 28°C $CMRO_2$ is decreased by 50%. At 22°C cerebral activity has been reported as minimal. Profound hypothermia can be used to dramatically reduce $CMRO_2$ and afford prolonged periods of brain protection. At 17°C the brain may be protected for periods of 35–60 minutes of total circulatory arrest. The **Q10**, or ratio of two values for $CMRO_2$ at two different temperatures, 10°C apart, does vary as temperature falls. In fact the decrease in $CMRO_2$ in relation to decreasing temperature can be represented by a sigmoid rather than linear line. Decreases in temperature, even mild decreases of 2–3°C, also decrease excitatory amino acid release from ischemic neurons.

Normal cerebral function is disrupted when there is a decrease in cerebral arterial oxygen tension to approximately 50–60 mm Hg. This also occurs with mild hypoglycemia. The brain does not tolerate severe hypoxemia or severe hypoglycemia for even short periods. Because of its high oxygen consumption, even a brief 10- to 15-second interruption of cerebral blood flow may result in a loss of consciousness. A prolonged interruption of blood supply for 3–8 minutes can cause irreversible cellular damage as the energy stores of ATP, adenosine 5-diphosphate, adenosine monophosphate, and phosphocreatine are depleted. Acute sustained hypoglycemia can be as devastating to the brain as hypoxemia. Hyperglycemia can further exacerbate global hypoxic brain injury by accelerating cerebral acidosis and cellular injury.

Global $CMRO_2$ remains constant over a narrow range in normal brain. It may be affected by age; it is 25% higher in young children than adults and decreased by 10% in the elderly. The decreased $CMRO_2$ in the elderly may be due to neuronal loss with aging. In children, the increased $CMRO_2$ may be due to developmental or hormonal differences. Regional $CMRO_2$ and global $CMRO_2$ are not the same. Regional $CMRO_2$ is continually changing with the regional activity of the brain. Stimulated areas of the brain show increased metabolism and increased cerebral blood flow (CBF). Unstimulated regions of brain show a decreased metabolic rate and a decreased CBF. This relationship between CBF and $CMRO_2$ is referred to as **coupling.**

CEREBRAL BLOOD FLOW AND AUTOREGULATION
Cerebral Blood Flow Measurement

The **Kety-Schmidt technique** for measuring CBF was introduced almost 50 years ago. This technique has provided much of the information known about

CBF. It is based on the Fick principle and involves the arterial and venous measurement of an inert indicator gas such as nitrous oxide or xenon[133]. Cerebral arterial measurements of the indicator gas are obtained from the vertebral or carotid artery, while the cerebral venous samples are taken from the internal jugular vein. This method yields the average global CBF. Because of the sampling technique involved, glucose, lactate, and O_2 measurements may be made to calculate the $CMRO_2$. Less invasive methods of CBF measurement use external scintillation detectors to measure the washout of a radioactive indicator.

More sophisticated techniques for measuring CBF have the advantage of being relatively noninvasive and can measure both global and regional CBF. These techniques use cyclotron-produced short-lived radioisotopes of oxygen or metabolic substrates. The regional activity of these positron-emitting isotopes can be measured **by positron emission tomography (PET)** scans. Using this technique it is possible to measure CBF, regional blood flow, $CMRO_2$, and a number of other parameters that can be used to study the hemodynamic and metabolic status of the brain. Since regional CBF and CMR are coupled to neuronal activity, PET measurements may also be used for functional brain mapping. Areas of the brain that are metabolically active during specific sensory, motor, or cognitive activities are revealed. Methods have been developed to integrate this information anatomically through use of a computerized brain atlas program. More recently, this information has been further integrated into **computed tomography and high-resolution magnetic resonance imaging.**

The **transcranial doppler** is another method that has been used in an attempt to measure CBF (see Chapter 22). Unfortunately, it cannot quantitatively assess CBF but does provide a method to monitor blood velocity and associated changes in CBF for specific cerebral arteries. It has been used to measure blood flow velocity in the middle cerebral artery during carotid artery surgery. It may also help detect cerebral vasospasm with subarachnoid hemorrhage or after cerebral aneurysm clipping.

Cerebral Blood Flow

The normal brain receives about 15% of the total cardiac output. CBF is expressed as milliliters of blood flow per 100 g of brain tissue per minute. **Normal CBF is 46–65 ml/100 g/minute** (or 750 ml/minute for the normal 1,400-g brain). Global CBF remains fairly constant, whereas **regional CBF is quite variable and coupled to regional metabolic activity.** White matter has a CBF of 20 ml/100 g/minute. Gray matter has a CBF of 80 ml/100 g/minute. Increases in regional metabolic activity result in increases in local metabolites such as CO_2, lactate, and hydrogen ions. These products of metabolism act on the vascular endothelium promoting vasodilation and increased regional blood flow.

Slowing of the electroencephalogram (EEG) has been reported to occur when CBF decreases below 20 ml/100 g/minute. Evoked potentials are suppressed when perfusion is less than 15 ml/100 g/minute. At 6 ml/100 g/minute

Table 3.1 Clinical Correlates With Cerebral Perfusion Pressure (CPP) and Cerebral Blood Flow (CBF)

CPP (mm Hg)	CBF (ml/100 g/min)	Clinical Finding
100	50	Normal
50	>20–25	Slowing EEG; cerebral impairment
25–40	15–20	EEG may be flat
<25	<10	Irreversible brain damage

there is massive efflux of K^+ with onset of a metabolic cascade resulting in cellular death (Table 3.1).

Autoregulation of Cerebral Blood Flow

CBF is held constant over a wide range of arterial blood pressure (BP). This **autoregulation** of CBF operates within a mean BP of 60–160 mm Hg (Figure 3.1). As mean BP falls below 60 mm Hg, CBF is reduced proportionately. As mean BP is increased above 160 mm Hg, CBF is also increased. The cerebrovascular resistance varies directly with blood pressure to maintain flow. The mechanism is not clear but is probably a result of an intrinsic response to the smooth muscle cells of the cerebral arteries. These muscles constrict as pressure within the arteries increases and vasodilate as pressure decreases. In chronically hypertensive patients, autoregulation is shifted to the right, with an increase in the lower and upper range of autoregulation.

In the normal brain, inadequate CBF can occur below a mean blood pressure of 60 mm Hg. Below this level, CBF becomes pressure-dependent, and evidence of cerebral impairment and slowing of the EEG may be seen. In normotensive individuals, a mean pressure of about 40 mm Hg produces signs of cerebral ischemia. Mean pressures above 160 mm Hg can cause disruption of the blood-brain barrier, leading to brain edema and hemorrhage. Pathologic states and pharmacologic interventions may modify or abolish normal autoregulation. Autoregulation is easily altered by trauma, hypoxia, lactic acid, and pharmacologic agents such as volatile anesthetic agents, sodium nitroprusside, or nitroglycerine.

Inhalation agents have a particularly important effect on autoregulation of CBF. Volatile anesthetics impair autoregulation in a dose-dependent manner. At an equivalent minimal alveolar concentration, halothane causes the greatest increase of CBF, up to 200%. Enflurane increases CBF by 40%, followed by isoflurane at 20%. This effect can be somewhat counteracted by hyperventilation. Nitrous oxide can also cause an increase in CBF. Of note with these agents is the **uncoupling** of CBF from $CMRO_2$.

Cerebral Perfusion Pressure

Cerebral perfusion pressure (CPP) is the effective pressure that results in blood flow in the brain. It is a calculated value that reflects the difference

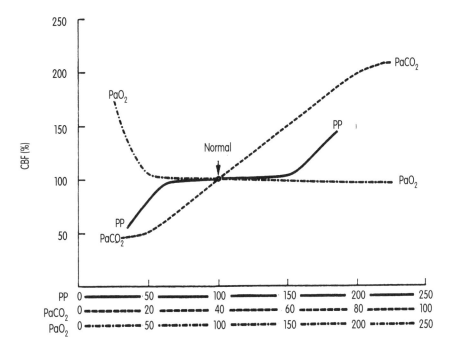

Figure 3.1 Factors that affect cerebral blood flow: cerebral perfusion pressure (PP), $PaCO_2$, and PaO_2 (mm Hg). *Reprinted with permission from JD Michenfelder. Anesthesia and the Brain. New York, Churchill Livingstone: 1988.*

between the mean systemic arterial blood pressure (MAP) providing the driving force for blood flow into the brain, and the pressure preventing blood flow into the brain—that is, **the intracranial pressure (ICP)** or cerebral venous pressure (VP), whichever is higher. That is,

$$CPP = MAP - ICP \text{ (or VP if higher)}$$

For example, the CPP for a normal awake individual with a blood pressure of 120/70 and a normal ICP of 10 mm Hg would be

$$CPP = 87 - 10 = 77 \text{ mm Hg}$$

Autoregulation of CBF is best referred to in terms of CPP rather than MAP, particularly when operating at the lower limits of autoregulation. CPP primarily depends on mean blood pressure when ICP is within normal limits. However, when ICP is abnormally elevated, CPP becomes much more important. A mean BP of 60 mm Hg is the lower limit of normal autoregulation of CBF. A CPP of 50 mm Hg is the corresponding lower limit of normal autoregulation. However, an abnormal elevation of ICP to 20 mm Hg produces a CPP of (60 – 20) 40 mm Hg at this lower limit of autoregulation. CPP below 50 mm Hg can cause cerebral impairment and slowing of the EEG. CPP between 25 and 40 can be associated with undetected EEG activity with scalp electrodes (Table 3.1).

Effect of Carbon Dioxide on Cerebral Blood Flow

Carbon dioxide readily crosses the blood-brain barrier and affects the hydrogen ion concentration in the cerebral spinal fluid (CSF) around and inside cell walls of the arterioles.

$$CO_2 + H_2O \leftrightarrow H_2CO_3 \leftrightarrow H^+ + HCO_3^-$$

Increased hydrogen ion concentration causes vasodilatation of the cerebral vasculature, while decreased concentration causes vasoconstriction. The change in pH inside those cells most likely causes vascular tone alterations by changing the intracellular concentration of ionized calcium.

$PaCO_2$ over a range of 20–80 mm Hg and CBF have a direct positive correlation (see Figure 3.1). CBF changes about 4% for each mm Hg change in $PaCO_2$. A $PaCO_2$ of 80 mm Hg may cause CBF to increase to twice normal. This results in maximum vasodilation of the cerebral vasculature. A $PaCO_2$ of 20 mm Hg decreases CBF to one half the normal flow. Below a $PaCO_2$ of 20–22 mm Hg cerebral ischemia may occur, not only because of vasoconstriction and decreased flow, but also because of the leftward shift of the O_2 dissociation curve and decreased release of O_2 to tissue secondary to respiratory alkalosis.

A chronic elevation of $PaCO_2$ results in CBF returning toward baseline levels over approximately 24 hours. CBF may return to normal in 6–8 hours with acute sustained changes in $PaCO_2$. The CSF pH gradually returns to normal by adjusting CSF bicarbonate concentration to compensate for the elevated hydrogen ion concentration.

Normal CO_2 reactivity is a hallmark of normal cerebral vessels. However, most diseases affecting cerebral vasculature can attenuate or abolish normal CO_2 reactivity. Decreased $PaCO_2$ causes healthy vessels to constrict, thereby increasing blood flow to diseased areas. This increased blood flow may be of benefit to an area of brain that is ischemic but has the potential to increase bleeding or edema in an area of tumor or hemorrhage. Increasing $PaCO_2$ may cause healthy vessels to dilate and divert or steal blood away from diseased vessels. Increasing $PaCO_2$ may also cause an increase in brain edema by increasing CBF and cerebral blood volume.

Effects of Oxygen on Cerebral Blood Flow

Oxygen has little effect on CBF until PaO_2 falls below 50 mm Hg. At these hypoxic levels there is a dramatic increase in CBF (see Figure 3.1). The mechanism for this vasodilation is not a direct effect of the low oxygen levels on the cerebral vasculature but of the acidosis that develops secondary to the hypoxia. Extreme hyperoxia (usually a PaO_2 >350 mm Hg) can cause vasoconstriction.

The Sympathetic Nervous System and Cerebral Blood Flow

The sympathetic and parasympathetic nervous systems provide innervation to the cerebral blood vessels. The sympathetic nerves arise from the superior cervical ganglion and the parasympathetic from the hypothalamus and reticular formation, terminating in the visceral efferent neurons of cranial nerves III, VII, IX, and X. Stimulation of the sympathetic system can cause vasoconstriction of the large cerebral vessels and may have some role in cerebral vasospasm. However, maximum stimulation of the sympathetic nerves reduces CBF by only 5–10%. The sympathetic response to hemorrhagic shock causes an increase in vasoconstriction in the brain through stimulation of the sympathetic nerves as well as through release of sympathomimetic agents such as adrenaline and noradrenaline. This can result in decreased CBF and signs of brain ischemia. This differs from **induced hypotension** in which sympathetic tone is not increased and intravascular volume is maintained. Therefore, low levels of systemic blood pressure may be well tolerated during pharmacologically induced hypotension.

CEREBROSPINAL FLUID FORMATION, FUNCTION, AND DYNAMICS

Normal CSF is a clear, colorless liquid with a specific gravity of 1.005 and a pH of 7.33. It has less than 5 lymphocytes/ml and no red cells. The total volume of CSF in the subarachnoid space is approximately 120 ml. CSF is produced at a rate of 0.5 ml/minute, with its total volume being replaced every 4 hours.

CSF is formed by the choroid plexus in the lateral and third ventricles of the brain. The actual mechanism of CSF secretion is related to the metabolism of the epithelial lining of the choroid plexus. There is strong support for the idea that CSF is secreted rather than a product of passive ultrafiltration. CSF secreted in the lateral ventricles passes into the third ventricle through the foramina of Monro and then along the aqueduct of Sylvius into the fourth ventricle (Figure 3.2). From the fourth ventricle CSF passes through the two lateral foramina of Luschka and a midline foramen of Magendie to enter the cisterna magna. The cisterna is continuous with the subarachnoid space that surrounds the entire brain and spinal cord. The CSF is then returned to the blood via the arachnoid villi that project into the large sagittal venous sinus.

Intracranial Pressure

The volume of the rigid cranial vault is fixed. Of this volume, 80% is brain, 12% is blood, and the remaining 8% is CSF. Intracranial pressure rises if there is any increase in one component without an equivalent decrease in another. The change in **intracranial pressure** in relationship to changes in intracranial volume is referred to as intracranial compliance. Normal CSF pressure is 10 mm Hg. Increases in volume are well compensated until the intracranial pressure exceeds 20 mm Hg. At that point any further increases in volume produce a pre-

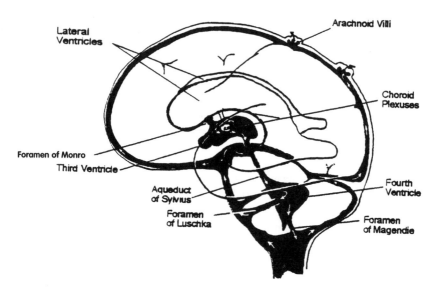

Figure 3.2 Circulation of cerebral spinal fluid. *Reprinted with permission from AC Guyton. Textbook of Medical Physiology (8th ed). Philadelphia: Saunders, 1991.*

cipitous rise in intracranial pressure. Clinically, intracranial compliance can be determined in patients with intraventricular catheters in place. Intracranial pressure increases of more than 4 mm Hg following injection of 1 ml of saline indicate decreased compliance. A sustained elevation of intracranial pressure can lead to brain ischemia, infarction, or herniation of the brain.

A change in CSF volume is the major compensatory component for ICP control within this system. Initially there is displacement of CSF from the cranial vault into the spinal compartment. There may also be an increase in CSF absorption or a decrease in CSF production. A decrease in cerebral blood volume, primarily through decreasing the venous blood volume, also provides another compensatory mechanism.

Factors Affecting Cerebrospinal Fluid Secretion

CSF production can be reduced by **carbonic anhydrase inhibitors,** such as **acetazolamide.** The associated inhibition of HCO_3^- affects Na^+ and fluid production at the choroid plexus, resulting in decreased CSF production. **Furosemide, ethycrinic acid, spironolactone,** and **vasopressin** all decrease CSF formation. This is probably secondary to their effect on Na^+ transport. Adrenal **corticosteroids** are thought to inhibit CSF formation by inhibition of Na^+/K^+-activated adenosinetriphosphatase. Digoxin decreases CSF production in animal models. However, toxic blood levels would be required to affect secretion of CSF in humans.

THE BLOOD-BRAIN BARRIER

The endothelial cells of brain capillaries have tight junctions, which restrict extracellular passage of substances between them. This **blood-brain barrier** allows lipid-soluble substances, water, carbon dioxide, and oxygen to freely enter the brain while impeding the flow of ionized particles and larger molecules. For example, mannitol is a large molecule that penetrates poorly. Substances that do not cross the blood-brain barrier may be actively transported across the capillary endothelial cells by carrier-mediated processes.

Changes in serum concentrations of Na+, K+, Cl−, or glucose may result in an electrolyte or concentration gradient across the blood-brain barrier. Net movement of water into or out of the brain reestablishes equilibrium over a short period. Rapid correction of serum electrolyte or glucose abnormalities can cause rapid fluid shifts within the brain, leading to cerebral edema. Mannitol is a large enough molecule that it does not normally cross the blood-brain barrier. Because of its osmotic activity in the serum, it can be used to decrease brain volume by decreasing brain water content. The blood-brain barrier can become disrupted by severe hypertension, infection, tumor, trauma, shock, radiation, or ischemia.

CEREBRAL ELECTRICAL ACTIVITY

Electrical Activity of Neurons

Sodium and potassium ions contribute to the resting membrane potential of neurons. The difference in intra- and extracellular concentrations of potassium and sodium produces a resting membrane potential of −70 mV. The ions move across the cell membrane through sodium and potassium channels. These channels are made up of proteins that form a hydrophilic pore in the cell membrane, which allows the ions to pass through. Each channel is highly selective for either sodium or potassium. During rest, most sodium channels are closed, while more of the potassium channels are open. The opening and closing of the ion channels control the conductance of the cell membrane for that ion. Depolarization of the cell membrane produces an action potential with a peak voltage of about +20 mV. The summation effect of individual action potentials causes the cell depolarization to exceed a membrane threshold and depolarization to spread. The action potential is propagated over long distances along the neuronal axons. When it reaches the distal end of the axon it causes **voltage-dependent calcium channels** to open and allows calcium to enter the terminal vesicles. The terminal vesicles then fuse with the terminal membrane, releasing neurotransmitters into the synaptic cleft. The neurotransmitter diffuses across to the postsynaptic neuron, where it combines with its receptor, causing a change in the membrane potential of the postsynaptic neuron.

Synaptic Transmission

Different neurotransmitters may cause inhibition or excitation of the postsynaptic neuron. **Gamma-amino-butyric acid (GABA)** is the major inhibitory neurotransmitter in the brain. It hyperpolarizes the postsynaptic membrane, making it less likely to reach the threshold necessary to generate an action potential. Two major GABA receptors have been identified—**GABA$_a$** and **GABA$_b$**. The GABA$_a$ receptor has a slower onset with a more prolonged activation than the GABA$_b$ receptor. Benzodiazepines and barbiturates enhance the inhibitory effect of the GABA$_a$ receptors. The GABA$_a$ receptor opens chloride channels, whereas GABA$_b$ receptors open potassium channels or close calcium channels. The gain of chloride ions in the cell, or loss of potassium or calcium ions out of the cell, produces a resting membrane potential that is more negative and more difficult to depolarize. Some neurons may contain both types of receptors, providing both a rapid-onset and a short-duration effect. Glycine is the major inhibitory neurotransmitter in the spinal cord.

Glutamate is the major neurotransmitter that causes excitation of postsynaptic neurons in the brain. By depolarizing the neurons, it makes them more likely to fire action potentials. Three types of glutamate receptors have been identified: (1) alpha-amino-3-hydroxy-5-methyl isoxazole-4-propionic acid (**AMPA**), (2) **kainate**, and (3) N-methyl-D-aspartate receptor (**NMDA**). The AMPA and kainate receptor channels are responsible for the normal excitatory responses seen with glutamate. The NMDA receptor is important in changing a neuron's long-term excitability over a period of hours to days.

Several different neurotransmitters are involved in the fine control of interneuronal communication. The concentration of a neurotransmitter in the synaptic cleft may be controlled by neurotransmitters that act on presynaptic terminals to regulate the amount of neurotransmitter that the terminal releases. **Neuromodulators** are compounds that when released into the synaptic cleft alter the effect of other excitatory or inhibitory inputs to that neuron. The same compound may be a neuromodulator at one synapse and a neurotransmitter at another. **Cotransmitters** may be released from the same presynaptic terminal to produce a synergistic action on the postsynaptic terminal. Neurotransmitters may also work through intracellular **second messengers**, which then activate intracellular enzyme systems to produce a change in intracellular activity.

Electroencephalogram

The EEG can be used to monitor the electrical activity of the brain. (For a full description of the EEG, see Chapters 5 and 6.) The EEG waves recorded from the surface of the scalp are a result of a large number of neurons simultaneously emitting an electrical potential. It is the summated excitatory and inhibitory postsynaptic potentials arising from the dendrites of the superficial cortex that produce these detectable voltages. These voltages, or brain waves, may range from 0–300 μV and have frequencies of 1–50 or more cycles per second or Hertz.

The traditional EEG is a plot of voltage against time. Interpretation of EEG waveforms is based on pattern recognition and quantitation of the waveforms. The EEG patterns are described as continuous, rhythmical, or transient, as well as by the temporal relationship to activity or background interference.

Frequency is defined as the number of times per second the wave crosses the zero voltage line. Amplitude is the electrical height of the wave. The frequency bands are divided into delta (0–3 Hz), theta (4–7 Hz), alpha (8–13 Hz), and beta (>13 Hz) rhythms. Generally, the average frequency increases with higher degrees of cerebral activity. Beta waves would be seen during periods of intense mental activity, whereas delta waves would be seen during sleep.

Anesthetic agents can have a wide variety of effects on EEGs, making interpretation difficult for the untrained physician. The complexity of the equipment and difficulty in interpretation has limited EEG use in the operating room in the past. Induction of anesthesia initially produces an excitatory phase with an increase in fast-wave (beta) activity. With increasing depth of anesthesia, EEG frequency decreases to levels of activity where slower waves (theta and delta activity) predominate. Deep anesthesia produces a burst suppression pattern on the EEG, followed by an isoelectric pattern.

Changes in normal physiologic parameters may also affect EEGs. Hyperventilation that leads to a decrease in $PaCO_2$ can cause EEG slowing. Increasing $PaCO_2$ may cause increased frequency of EEGs. Severe elevation of $PaCO_2$, on the other hand, produces a decrease in frequency and amplitude of the EEG. A PaO_2 of less than 50–60 mm Hg may cause an initial EEG activation, followed by slowing and eventually electrical silence as the PaO_2 falls to dangerously hypoxic levels. Hypothermia (<35°C) causes a progressive slowing of cerebral activity and slowing of the EEG.

Computerized Electroencephalogram Processing

Cerebral monitoring in the operating room has become a practical reality with the introduction of computerized processing of the EEG. These computerized EEG monitors convert analog EEG voltages into digital numbers at a high sampling rate of 100–300 times per second. Each data sample is grouped into "epochs" of 2–4 seconds for analysis. Using various algorithms, this information is converted to a plot of amplitude on the y-axis against frequency on the x-axis. Successive segments of EEG data are stacked one on top of the other, creating a pseudo-three-dimensional display, with time and amplitude presented on the y-axis.

Sensory Evoked Potentials

Sensory or electrical stimulation of a peripheral sensory organ produces an evoked potential (EP), which can be recorded at various positions along the sensory pathway to the sensory cortex. These EPs may be classified according to the mode of stimulation (i.e., somatosensory). (For a full description of somatosensory evoked potentials, see Chapter 17.) The amplitude of these EPs is very low (0.1–20 µV) and subject to interference from background electrophysiologic activity. Special **signal averaging** is required to produce a quality signal for analysis. The waveforms are described in terms of their **polarity, amplitude,** and **post-stimulus latency.** This form of monitoring has been used intraoperatively to monitor the integrity of the sensory pathway during surgical procedures on the spine, such as scoliosis repair. The halogenated anesthetic agents decrease the amplitude and increase latency of cortical EP, particularly if used in concentrations of more than 0.5 MAC. Brain stem responses seem to be less affected by the choice of anesthetic agent than cortical responses. Boluses of intravenous agents should be avoided because they can alter the pattern of the somatosensory EP during critical times of intraoperative monitoring. Physiologic factors such as temperature, blood pressure, and arterial tensions of oxygen and carbon dioxide affect somatosensory EPs and should be controlled during intraoperative recording.

SPINAL CORD NEUROPHYSIOLOGY

Cerebrospinal Fluid Circulation

The circulation of CSF in the spinal subarachnoid space differs from that in the cranial space. The cranial and spinal subarachnoid spaces are joined at the cisterna magna. CSF produced in the ventricles of the brain appears in the cisterna magna within minutes. CSF fluid flows out of the cisterna magna and into the cranial and subarachnoid space. During immobility there is very little flow of CSF along the spinal cord. Even with changes in pressure gradients due to changes in posture or arterial and respiratory pulsations, the spinal CSF circulation remains sluggish. About 10–15% of the total CSF is absorbed in the spinal subarachnoid space through spinal arachnoid villi in the spinal nerve roots.

Spinal Cord Blood Flow

Our knowledge of the blood circulation to the spinal cord in humans is limited. Most of the information available is derived from animal studies. Spinal cord blood flow is affected by the same factors that affect cerebral blood flow. Spinal cord perfusion pressure is equal to mean systemic blood pressure minus cerebrospinal fluid pressure. Autoregulation is maintained between spinal cord perfusion pressures of 50–130 mm Hg. Hypercarbia produces an increased blood flow in the spinal cord, while hypocarbia decreases blood flow. Information from primate studies suggests that the gray matter blood flow is about 60 ml/100 g/minute and white matter blood flow is 10 ml/100 g/minute.

The spinal cord is supplied by the **anterior** and **posterior spinal arteries**. The anterior spinal artery, derived from the vertebral arteries at the level of the foramen magnum, supplies the anterior two-thirds of the spinal cord. The two posterior spinal arteries, derived from the posterior inferior cerebellar arteries, supply the posterior one-third of the spinal cord. Anterior and posterior radicular arteries arise from the vertebral, deep cervical, intercostal, and lumbar arteries to join with the anterior and posterior spinal arteries. The largest of these radicular arteries (the **artery of Adamkiewicz**) joins the anterior spinal artery between T8 and T12 and is the major blood supply to the lower two thirds of the spinal cord.

RECOMMENDED READING

Barash PG, Cullen BF, Stoelting RK. Clinical Anesthesia (2nd ed). Philadelphia: Lippincott, 1989. Pp 32, 871–918.

Blitt CD. Monitoring in Anesthesia and Critical Care Medicine (2nd ed). London: Churchill Livingstone, 1990. Pp 17–18, 431–524.

Cottrell JE, Turndorf H. Anesthesia and Neurosurgery (2nd ed). St. Louis: Mosby, 1986. Pp 1–81.

Guyton AC. Basic Neuroscience. Philadelphia: Saunders, 1991. Pp 5–7, 57–101.

Guyton AC. Textbook of Medical Physiology. Philadelphia: Saunders, 1991;61.

Kalkman CJ, Been HD, Ongerboer de Visser BW. Intraoperative monitoring of spinal cord function. A review. Acta Orthop Scand 1993;64(1):114–123.

Michenfelder JD. Anesthesia and the Brain. New York: Churchill Livingstone, 1988. Pp 1–48.

Morgan GE, Mikhail MS. Clinical Anesthesiology. Norwalk, CT: Appleton & Lange, 1992. Pp 25, 419–430.

Steinmetz H, Huang Y, Seitz RJ et al. Individual integration of positron emission tomography and high-resolution magnetic resonance imaging. J Cereb Blood Flow Metab 1992;12:919–926.

Willatts SM, Walters FJM. Anaesthesia and Intensive Care for the Neurosurgical Patient. London: Blackwell Scientific, 1986. Pp 1–111.

4

Neuropathophysiology: The Basics

Garfield B. Russell, M.D., FRCPC

Although the brain and spinal cord are contiguous parts of the nervous system, they differ in cell distribution, blood supply, and functional capabilities. The autoregulation of blood flow is slightly different (see Chapter 3). Mechanisms of ischemia differ; the spinal cord has a much more precarious blood supply with multiple sources and without the interconnection of blood sources provided by the circle of Willis to the brain. However, the basic neuronal homeostatic disruptions and biochemical changes after injury are similar. For that reason, as the pathophysiology of neuronal injury is discussed, the brain and spinal cord are viewed as part of a single entity.

INJURY AND NEURONAL RESPONSES

Whatever the initial mechanisms of neuronal and glial injury (whether penetrating trauma, tissue ischemia from arterial clamping or decreased perfusion pressure, or overdistraction of the spinal cord during scoliosis repair), a final common pathophysiologic pathway is followed. Tissue **homeostatic function is disturbed**. Electrical activity is altered and energy substrates are depleted. The end result can be a loss of cellular function and structural integrity.

Altered Cellular Homeostasis

Neural tissue has **high baseline energy consumption with limited energy reserves**. This makes it vulnerable to injury with oxygen or glucose deprivation. As energy deprivation develops, cells try to maintain functional levels of high-energy phosphates (adenosine triphosphate [ATP], adenosine diphosphate [ADP], adenosine monophosphate [AMP]). Small stores of phosphocreatine (PCr) are used, glycolysis increases, and energy-consuming spontaneous electrical activity rapidly stops.

Energy Substrate Conservation

ATP is 90% unbound with 80% free in the cytosol. ATP is vital for the maintenance of normal cellular function (Table 4.1). The intracellular levels of high-energy phosphates are controlled by the following buffering reactions:

$$(1) \quad PCr + ADP + H^+ \leftrightarrow ATP + Cr$$

$$(2) \quad 2\ ADP \leftrightarrow ATP + AMP$$

$$(3) \quad 2\ ATP \leftrightarrow ATP + AMP$$

ATP levels sufficient for maintenance of homeostatic function are maintained longer in neonates than adults but still for only very short intervals despite four- to fivefold increases in glycolytic rates.

In the brain, 70% of ATP is used to maintain transmembrane ionic gradients. Depletion of energy substrates and degeneration of the rate of supply leads to a cascade of cellular metabolic dysfunction.

Energy Substrate Depletion
The end results of this cascade of biochemical and structural dysfunction are multiple end products that result in cellular injury. Specific disruptions of cellular function occur and contribute to overall nervous system dysfunction.

Acidosis Perioperative brain ischemia is usually focal rather than global. Intracellular and extracellular pH can vary significantly. However, both extracellular and intracellular **acidosis** occur at cerebral blood flow rates (40–50% of baseline) below which ionic homeostasis is lost. Tissue hypoxia and ischemia interfere with ATP, H_2O, and CO_2 production from pyruvate. As a result, pyruvate is primarily reduced to lactate. Cellular acidosis severity (intracellular pH may fall as low as 6.2–6.4) correlates with glucose and glycogen availability at ischemia. Depletion of ATP results in anaerobic metabolism of available substrates and lactate and H^+ production.

Ionic Homeostasis Disruption Transmembrane loss of normal ionic gradients occurs when cerebral blood flow temporarily decreases from the normal 50 ml/100 g/minute to 10–12 ml/100 g/minute. Permanent decreases have **higher critical perfusion thresholds** of 17–18 ml/100 g/minute. Cellular energy metabolism and both the passive and active ion flux across normal membranes are coupled. During ischemia with ATP decreases to less than 50% of normal, ion gradients are lost as the **ion pumps fail.**

Ischemia results in **cell depolarization** with loss of the intracellular –60 mV potential leading to disruption of a delicate ion balance (Figure 4.1).

Table 4.1 Neural Functions of High-Energy Phosphates

1. Ionic gradient development and stabilization
2. Electrical gradient development and stabilization
3. Neurotransmitter release and uptake
4. Neurosecretion control and substance synthesis
5. Biosynthesis of necessary compounds for function

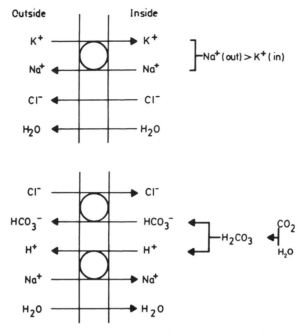

Figure 4.1 Ionic fluxes showing mechanisms for maintenance of normal cellular volume. The Na$^+$-K$^+$ pump shown in the top panel allows outward movement of water. Inward water movement can occur by reuptake of Na$^+$ via Na$^+$-H$^+$ antiporter coupled to Cl$^-$-HCO$_3^-$ exchange. *Reprinted with permission from BK Siesjo, T Wieloch. Cerebral mechanisms in ischaemia: neurochemical basis for therapy. Br J Anaesth 1985;57:57.*

Ionic flux then depends primarily on passive concentration gradients. Na$^+$, Ca^{2+}, and Cl$^-$ enter cells and K$^+$ leaves. Initially, **extracellular K$^+$ rises** slowly, **pH falls,** and Ca^{2+} stays the same. There is then rapid K$^+$ exit and cellular accumulation of Na$^+$, Ca^{2+}, and Cl$^-$ with associated inward water movement and **cell edema.**

Intracellular movement of Ca^{2+} into ischemic cells **through voltage-dependent and agonist-operated membrane channels** is associated with (1) **release of Ca^{2+}** from intracellular stores in endoplasmic reticulum and mitochondria, (2) **altered cellular sequestration,** and (3) **reduced protein-binding** with calmodulin and calcibindin (Figure 4.2). However, the functions of calcium on enzymes as an inhibitor (hexokinase) and activator (phospholipases A and C) are sustained and can become part of the biochemical cascade leading to cell death.

The Ischemic Cascade

The **increase of intracellular Ca^{2+}** is associated with hyperactivity of lipases, endonucleases, protein kinases, and proteases (Figure 4.3). Activation of phospholipases A2 and C by Ca^{2+} and receptor agonists leads to hydrolysis of phospholipids to lysophospholipids and free fatty acids, such as arachidonic acid. More Ca^{2+} is released from intracellular sites. The lysophospholipids and

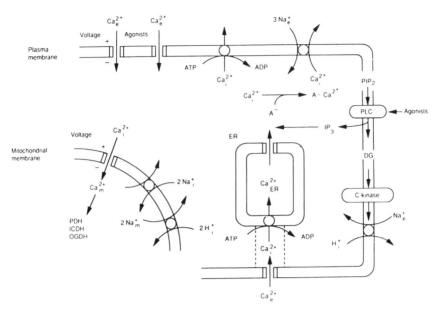

Figure 4.2 Calcium homeostatic processes. Cytosolic Ca^{2+} concentration is a balance between influx, efflux, binding, sequestration, and release. A pump-leak relationship may also be present in intracellular membranes. ADP = adenine diphosphate; PIP_2 = phosphatidylinositol biphosphate; PDH, ICDH, OGDH = dehydrogenases; ER = endoplasmic reticulum; PLC = phospholipase C; DG = diglycerides. Subscripts: i = intracellular; e = extracellular; m = mitochondrial. *Reprinted with permission from BK Siesjo, F Bengtsson. Calcium fluxes, calcium antagonists, and calcium-related pathology in brain ischemia, hypoglycemia, and spreading depression: a unifying hypothesis. J Cereb Blood Flow Metab 1989;9:127.*

free fatty acids act as **membrane detergents and ionophores,** causing vasomotor paralysis and loss of blood-brain barrier integrity.

Lipolysis results in stimulation of the cyclooxygenase and lipoxygenase pathways. During reperfusion, arachidonic acid, which accumulates during ischemia, is oxidized to **leukotrienes** (by the cyclooxygenase pathway) and **prostaglandins and thromboxanes** (by the cyclooxygenase pathway). These eicosanoids act as second messengers, altering synaptic transmission. Leukotrienes constrict blood vessels and increase capillary permeability. Thromboxane A2 is a vessel constrictor and platelet aggregation stimulant, while prostacyclin is a vasodilator and aggregation retardant. **Platelet-activating factor** is proinflammatory, activating platelets and leukocytes and causing leukocyte adherence to endothelial membranes. It may aggravate destructive activity of the arachidonic acid cascade.

Free radicals are produced during reperfusion when there is a sudden increase in tissue oxygen but can also be produced at low oxygen partial pressures. Superoxide (O_2^-) is primarily formed by xanthine oxidase. Hydroxyl radicals (OH^-) and hydrogen peroxides (H_2O_2) also are formed. The damage done

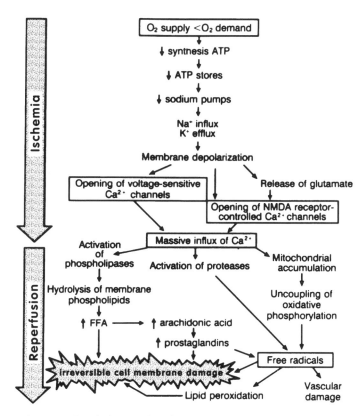

Figure 4.3 The cascade of neuronal ischemia. Irreversible cell injury can result as ischemic injury progresses to reperfusion injury and the multiple ionic and biochemical disruptions inhibit neuronal function. *Reprinted with permission from LN Milde. Anesth Clin North Am 1992;10(3): 595.*

by free radicals also **requires activation of protein-bound iron compounds**. Iron acts as a catalyst for free radical formation (see Table 4.2).

Nitric oxide (endothelial relaxant factor) may be associated with free radical formation preferentially affecting endothelial cells. It produces vasodilatation after activation by calcium and reduced nicotinamide-adenine dinucleotide phosphate, but is inactivated by O_2^-. Nitric oxide and O_2^- may react to form peroxynitrite ions (NO_3^-), which decompose during cellular acidosis; the hydroxyl molecules and NO_2 formed damage endothelial cell membranes.

Excitatory Amino Acids

Aspartate and **glutamate** function as **excitatory neurotransmitters** in brain. Glutamate, the best known of the **excitatory amino acids (EAAs)**, acts on postsynaptic neuronal receptors after release instigated by Ca^{2+} influx **through voltage-sensitive calcium channels**. Increased extracellular glutamate results from

Table 4.2. Mechanisms of Neuronal Injury from Free Radicals

1. Increased intracellular movement of Ca^{2+}
2. Increased release of liposomal enzymes
3. Increased permeability of organelle and cell membranes
4. Mitochondrial disruption
5. Decreased ATP production
6. Amino acid oxidation
7. Protein degradation
8. Increased phospholipase activity

Table 4.3 Postsynaptic Receptors at which Excitatory Amino Acids Exert their Effects

1. N type—the N-methyl-D-aspartate (NMDA) receptor or the voltage-sensitive calcium channel is permeable to both monovalent cations and Ca^{2+}. Aspartate acts only at this receptor.
2. L type—kainate, amino-3-hydroxy-5-methyl-4-isoazole propionic acid receptor, is permeable to Na^+, K^+, and H^+.
3. T type—quisqualate, alpha-amino-3-hydroxy-5-methyl-4-isoxazole (AMPA) receptor.

increased postsynaptic receptors present at membrane cation channels (Table 4.3) Areas sensitive to ischemia have high receptor concentrations.

Release of glutamate and receptor activation cause **Na^+ influx** and **membrane depolarization** with **multichannel Ca^{2+} influx**. Persistent stimulation by EAAs removes Mg^{2+}, which blocks the the N-methyl-D-aspartate (NMDA) channels (the NMDA glutamate receptor) and holds the channels open. Uncontrolled Na^+ and Ca^{2+} influx leads to cell edema and injury. **Inhibitory control of amino acid–induced excitation** is normally maintained by (1) increased K^+ conductance with membrane hyperpolarization, (2) increased Cl^- conductance fixing the membrane potential, (3) transmitters (such as gamma amino butyric acid [GABA]) activating receptors linked to ion channels, and (4) adenosine and noradrenaline (which modify calcium channels) (Figure 4.4).

The Electroencephalogram and Evoked Potential Response to Neuronal Injury

Cortical electroencephalographic activity occurs spontaneously. Evoked potentials record cortical responses to stimulation and monitor subcortical, spinal, and (depending on the stimulation and recording sites) peripheral nerve conduction. Changes in both have wide intersubject variability. However, there is a correlation with both blood flow to cerebral tissues and cellular responses to neuronal injury (Figure 4.5). Decreases of cerebral blood flow to 50–60% of normal change cerebral cortical activity. At 40% of normal (about 20 ml/100 g) or arterial oxygen saturation of 60%, EEG electrical amplitude and evoked cortical responses are depressed. At 25–30% of normal (15 ml/100 g), isoelectricity may occur and evoked cortical responses are absent. There is a rapid loss of

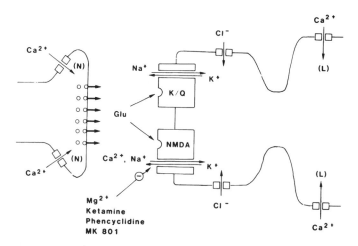

Figure 4.4 Schematic of presynaptic, voltage-sensitive calcium channels and postsynaptic channels gated by glutamate receptors. Presynaptic channels are the N type. The channel activated by kainate/quisqualate (K/Q) opens conductance for monovalent cations. The channel selectively activated by N-methyl-D-aspartate allows calcium influx. *Reprinted with permission from BK Siesjo, F Bengtsson. Calcium fluxes, calcium antagonists, and calcium-related pathology in brain ischemia, hypoglycemia, and spreading depression: a unifying hypothesis. J Cereb Blood Flow Metab 1989;9:127.*

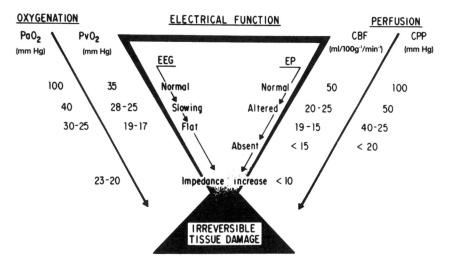

Figure 4.5 Changes in EEG and evoked potential activity occur with decreased cerebral blood flow (CBF), perfusion pressure (CPP), and oxygenation (PaO_2, PvO_2). *Reprinted with permission from H Shapiro. In RD Miller (ed), Anesthesia (2nd ed). New York: Churchill Livingstone, 1986. P 1276.*

EEG activity with neuronal anoxia. Neuroelectric, biochemical, and ionic activity changes occur in unison.

Neurologic damage to the brain and spinal cord results from intracellular events that occur both during ischemia and after restoration of circulation and oxygen delivery to tissues. The end results of this multifactorial cascade of biochemical and ionic disruptions are the functional, physiologic, and pathologic deficits that we sometimes see, but always try to prevent, in our patients.

KEY REFERENCES

Erecinska M, Silver IA. ATP and brain function. J Cereb Blood Flow Metab 1989;9:2. *An excellent review of the overall role of high energy phosphates in cerebral function.*

McBurney RN, Neering IR. Neuronal calcium homeostasis. Trends Neurosci 1987;10:164. *A relatively specific, straightforward view of the role of calcium in neuronal function, injury, and demise.*

Siesjo BK, Bengtsson F. Calcium fluxes, calcium antagonists, and calcium-related pathology in brain ischemia, hypoglycemia, and spreading depression: a unifying hypothesis. J Cereb Blood Flow Metab 1989;9:127.

Siesjo BK. Calcium in the brain under physiological and pathological conditions. Eur Neurol 1990;30(Suppl 2): 3.

Siesjo BK. Pathophysiology and treatment of focal cerebral ischemia. Part I: Pathophysiology. J Neurosurg 1992;77:169.

Siesjo BK. Pathophysiology and treatment of focal cerebral ischemia. Part II: Mechanisms of damage and treatment. J Neurosurg 1992;77:337. *The 1992 papers by Siesjo provide a clear, concise review of the pathophysiology of cerebral injury–related physiologic dysfunction. They are excellent for their thoroughness and clarity.*

RECOMMENDED READING

Bevan S, Wood JN. Arachidonic-acid metabolites as second messengers. Nature 1987;328:20. *The role of arachidonic acid and free fatty acid metabolism in the pathophysiology of neuronal injury is developed. This provides a nice addition to the general information in the pathophysiological reviews.*

Chiappa KH, Ropper AH. Evoked potentials in clinical medicine. Part 1. N Engl J Med 1982;306:1140. *The article, along with Grundy (1983), Leggatt (1991), and Nuwer (1986), provide a broad-based review of neuroelectric activity and the relationship of neuroelectrophysiology and neuronal injury.*

Choi DW. Glutamate neurotoxicity and diseases of the nervous system. Neuron 1988;1:623.

Del Maestro RF. An approach to free radicals in medicine and biology. Acta Physiol Scand 1980:492(Suppl):153. *Oxygen-derived free radicals can do cellular injury. This is part of the neuronal ischemia-induced process.*

Garthwaite J. Glutamate, nitric oxide and cell-cell signalling in the nervous system. Trends Neurosci 1991;14:60.

Grundy BL. Intraoperative monitoring of sensory-evoked potentials. Anesthesiology 1983;58:72.

Hansen AJ. Effect of anoxia on ion distribution in the brain. Physiol Rev 1985;5:101. *Ionic homeostasis is essential for normal neuronal function. A breakdown of the ion pumps and the resulting cellular edema and functional disruption contribute to the continuum of cellular injury.*

Legatt AD. Intraoperative Neurophysiologic Monitoring. In EAM Frost (ed), Clinical Anesthesia in Neurosurgery. Boston: Butterworth-Heinemann, 1991;63–127.

McCord JM. Oxygen-derived free radicals in postischemic tissue. N Engl J Med 1985;312:159.

Murdoch J, Hall R. Brain protection: physiological and pharmacological considerations. Part I: The physiology of brain injury. Can J Anaesth 1990;37:663.

Nicholls D, Attwell D. The release and uptake of excitatory amino acids. Trends Pharmacol Sci 1990;11:462.

Nuwer MR. Basic Electrophysiology: Evoked Potentials and Signal Processing. In MR Nuwer (ed), Evoked Potential Monitoring in the Operating Room. New York: Raven, 1986. Pp 5–48.

Raichle ME. The pathophysiology of brain ischemia. Ann Neurol 1983;13:2.

Rothman SM, Olney JW. Glutamate and the pathophysiology of hypoxic-ischemic brain damage. Ann Neurol 1986;19:105. *Excitatory amino acids form a vital part of the cascade of cellular pathophysiology.*

Siesjo BK. Mechanisms of ischemic brain damage. Crit Care Med 1988;16:954.

Siesjo BK. Calcium, excitotoxins, and brain damage. News Physiol Sci 1990;5:20.

Siesjo BK, Agardh CD, Bengtsson F. Free radicals and brain damage. Cerebrovasc Brain Metab Rev 1989;1:165.

Siesjo BK, Wieloch T. Cerebral mechanisms in ischaemia: neurochemical basis for therapy. Br J Anaesth 1985;57:47.

Wolfe LS. Eicosanoids: prostaglandins, thromboxanes, leukotrienes, and other derivatives of carbon-20 unsaturated fatty acids. J Neurochem 1982;38:1.

5

Technical Standards and Techniques for Basic Electroencephalography

Mary C. Schwentker, B.S.
Debra J. Forney
Robert Gieski
Joyce I. Winters, R.EEG T.

Since the early 1930s, electroencephalographic monitoring has been used in the operating room. This type of monitoring has proven to be a very effective measure of brain activity for both the surgeon and the anesthesiologist. Electroencephalograph recordings are routinely used in surgeries for epilepsy, carotid endarterectomies, and cerebral aneurysms, and procedures where suppression of cortical activity is necessary for cerebral protection, as in barbiturate coma and deep hypothermia.

The electroencephalogram (EEG) itself is a recording of the electrical activity of the brain, specifically the activity of the cortex. In very basic terms, the EEG can be described in two dimensions—amplitude and time. The amplitude or the vertical component of the record is also referred to as the voltage. The voltages associated with the EEG are extremely small, measured in millionths of a volt, called microvolts (μV). The voltage of the EEG is 1,000 times smaller than that of an electrocardiogram (ECG), which is measured in millivolts (mV). This comparison indicates the difficulty involved in recording the EEG.

Time is the horizontal component of the record. The rate of activity is referred to as frequency, measured in cycles per second, or hertz (Hz). EEG frequencies are typically split into four categories, beta (14–30 Hz), alpha (8–13 Hz), theta (4–7 Hz), and delta (0–3 Hz). A recording of the EEG activity will have various ratios of these frequencies depending on the physical state of the patient (i.e., anesthetized, conscious and relaxed, postepileptic seizure, etc.).

The development of a monitoring program for the operating room involves many difficult choices. The pros and cons of each choice must be weighed against available resources. Foremost of the decisions to be made are those surrounding the purchase of the EEG machine and the technical issues of use in the operating room. A machine appropriate for the operating room needs to be easy to use, sturdy, and reliable. The delicate components of the instrument should not be in vulnerable locations. The machine needs to be electronically stable for

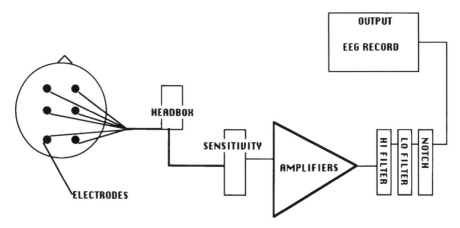

Figure 5.1 Schematic of the components of an EEG monitoring system

long run times; a routine case can run 3–12 hours. The machine should also possess high-quality components such as amplifiers and filters to make the recording and interpretation of the EEG in the operating room possible (Figure 5.1).

THE ELECTRODES

The first step in EEG monitoring begins with the connection to the patient. This is accomplished through the use of **electrodes.** The electrode connection is often the weakest link in the recording system because there is a liquid-to-metal junction at the site of the electrode attachment to the patient's scalp. Great care must be taken in selecting the number, type, and placement of electrodes.

The number of electrodes used is determined in part by the number of recording channels available on the EEG machine and by the surgical procedure and location. As a general rule, the more electrodes applied, the better. If an electrode is lost during the procedure, it is valuable to have another electrode available through a minor montage change, which allows recording from the same general area.

Several different types of electrodes are commercially available. Some of the most common include **subdermal needle electrodes, cup electrodes,** ECG and other **patch electrodes,** an **electrode cap** or **hat,** and **intracranial electrodes** used for recordings directly from brain tissue. Some electrodes are better suited for specific procedures. Stocking several different types of electrodes makes the task of monitoring easier. Proper attachment of the electrodes eliminates potential recording problems.

Needle Electrodes

Needle electrodes are quick and easy to place, although placement is uncomfortable for awake patients. These electrodes have a higher resistance because of their smaller surface areas. This makes artifactual interference more likely. The impedance levels do not usually interfere with the common mode rejection characteristics of the differential amplifier, because they tend to be closely matched (see the section on Amplifiers). When needle electrodes are used, recording the EEG becomes an invasive procedure. This adds a small increased risk for infection to the patient. Small hematomas may also form around the needle portion of the electrode. This may decrease the voltage recorded from that electrode. It is recommended that needle electrodes not be used in patients with transmissible viral illnesses, such as Creutzfeldt-Jakob disease, hepatitis, and acquired immune deficiency syndrome (AIDS).

Application of Needle Electrodes

All needle electrodes used should be sterilized. The skin should be gently abraded with a pumice and the area thoroughly cleaned with alcohol. The skin should be tightly stretched between the fingers and the needle inserted subdermally at an angle nearly stretched parallel to the skin surface. The needle portion of the electrode should not be touched. Once inserted, no metal should show above the skin surface. A small amount of colloid (a commercially available skin glue compound) applied to the electrode helps keep it well anchored. Disposable gloves should be worn when removing the electrodes.

Cup and Disc Electrodes

Cup or **disc electrodes** are noninvasive and comfortable for application on awake patients. These electrodes have lower impedance than needle electrodes because of their larger surface areas. The initial cost is higher than that of needle electrodes, but with proper use the life span is longer. Application of these electrodes is more time-consuming than for needle electrodes, but with practice the difference becomes minimal. This type of electrode is typically used when a technician is available to help with monitoring and set-up. Cup electrodes are commercially available in several metal types. The metal in the electrode used does not make a major difference in the recording as long as all electrodes are the same.

Application of Cup Electrodes

To properly attach cup electrodes, the skin should be gently abraded with a pumice and the area thoroughly cleaned with alcohol. The electrode should be placed on the skin and a small amount of collodion used around both the flange of the electrode and 3 mm of the surrounding scalp. Drying of the collodion can be accelerated with a jet of compressed air from either a wall outlet or a portable air pump. Once the electrode is in place, a blunted needle should be used to fill the electrode through its central hole with a saline electrode contact gel. The use of the contact gel lowers the impedance between the connection of the electrode and the scalp. If the impedance is still high, the blunted needle can be used to gently abrade the skin and lower the skin resistance. To prevent drying of the contact gel for long term monitoring, a small square of gauze soaked with collodion may be placed over the electrode.

Patch Electrodes

Patch electrodes are the same stick-on electrodes used to record ECGs. Other stick-on electrodes are commercially available in many different sizes. There are large rectangular patches that are very effective as grounding electrodes. These electrodes are inexpensive, easy, and very quick to apply. They are limited to use in areas where there is no hair, restricting their use on the head.

The Electrode Hat

The **electrode hat** or **cap** has the electrodes embedded in material that is then stretched over the patient's head. As with patch electrodes, electrode placement is limited, in this case to the fit of the cap. This technique does not work for patients undergoing any type of surgery in which access to the skull is necessary. It also does not allow for normal variation in head size.

Special Electrodes

Other electrodes that may be considered, depending on the procedure and the brain area of interest, are **nasopharyngeal** and **sphenoidal electrodes.** Both types have been specially designed and are commercially available. Nasopharyngeal leads are used to record the activity of the inferior temporal lobe. They are placed through the nostril and threaded along the nasopharynx. Sphenoidal electrodes are used for recording the anterior tip of the temporal lobe. These electrodes are placed through a needle cannula into the temporalis and masseter muscles, with the insertion point between the zygoma and sigmoid notch of the mandible.

Electrodes need to be positioned so that they record data from areas of the brain at risk. A system that has a standardized terminology and electrode location is also needed. This allows similar information to be passed from one monitoring center to another and allows serial studies of the same patient to be run at different times.

THE INTERNATIONAL TEN-TWENTY SYSTEM

A system of electrode placement was developed in 1958 by Herbert Jasper for the International Federation of Societies for EEG and Clinical Neurophysiology. The system is known as the **international ten-twenty system of electrode placement.** This internationally accepted format provides a proven anatomical correlation for each electrode that is consistent from patient to patient, allows for normal variation in head size, and provides uniform spacing of the electrodes.

The system is based on four landmarks of the skull; the nasion, inion, and preauricular points. Electrode placement is based on either 10 or 20% of the distance from one of these landmarks to the other. The first letter of each loca-

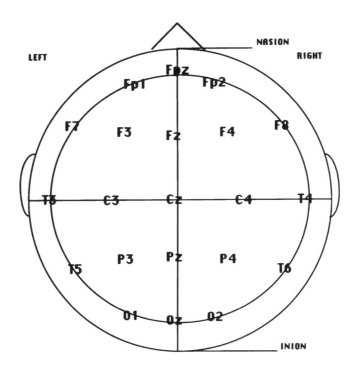

Figure 5.2 Electroencephalograph electrode position based on the international ten-twenty system.

tion corresponds to the anatomical location of the brain over which the electrode is positioned. The subscripted number is used to identify the right or left side of the brain, as well as electrode location. Even numbers represent the right side and odd numbers represent the left side of the head. The subscript "z" refers to the midline of the head (Figure 5.2). Only a tape measure and skin marker are required to use the ten-twenty system (Table 5.1).

One must remain flexible with electrode placement in the operating room. Many variables can force slight modification in electrode placement. These include location of the surgical site, presence of an intracranial pressure monitoring catheter, and skull malformations, among other factors. When modification of electrode placement is necessary, the electrode location must be clearly documented on the record.

THE HEADBOX

The interface that connects the electrodes to the EEG machine is the **headbox** or **jackbox.** The terminal end or the pin end of the electrodes plug is here. Connections are usually marked with the same nomenclature as used in the ten-

Table 5.1 A Method of Placing Electroencephalograph
Electrodes by the International Ten-Twenty System

1. Measure the distance from the nasion to the inion and make a mark at 50% of this distance.
2. Measure the distance from preauricular point to preauricular point and make a mark at 50% of this distance. The intersection of these two marks is Cz.
3. With the tape passing through Cz, measure and mark 10% of the distance from nasion to inion on the forehead for FP, and 10% of the distance from inion to nasion at the back of the head for Oz.
4. With the tape passing through Cz, measure, and mark 10% of the distance from preauricular point to preauricular point. These points are T3 on the left and T4 on the right.
5. Measure the circumference of the head passing through the FP, T3, T4, and Oz.
6. Mark 10% of this distance on either side of FP. These points are FP1 on the left and FP2 on the right. Also mark 10% of this distance on either side of Oz. These points are O1 on the left and O2 on the right.
7. Mark half the distance from T3 to FP1 for F7. Repeat on the right for the location of F8.
8. Mark half the distance from T3 to O1 for T5. Repeat on the right for the location of T6.
9. Mark half the distance from Cz to T3 for C3. Repeat on the right for the location of C4.
10. Mark half the distance from Cz to FP for Fz. Mark half the distance from Cz to Oz for Pz.
11. Mark half the distance from C3 to FP1 for F3. Mark half the distance from C3 to O1 for P3. Repeat for the right side of the head.

twenty system. Some machines also have a **preamplifier** and an **impedance meter** located in the headbox. An impedance meter in the headbox is particularly useful for monitoring in the operating room where the EEG machine and the headbox are often widely separated. The headbox is kept as close to the head of the patient as possible to reduce the amount of artifact recorded. The headbox and the rest of the EEG machine must be designed to handle currents from electrocautery and other electrosurgical units without being damaged or endangering the patient.

The **input cable** connects the headbox to the rest of the EEG machine. This is a long, shielded cable. Solid connections at both the headbox and the EEG machine are necessary for good recordings.

THE IMPEDANCE CHECK

In most EEG machines the next electronic interface is an on-line **impedance meter**. The impedance level of all of the electrodes and their connection to the patient is recorded. The impedance of each electrode should be less than 5 kilo ohms, preferably about 1–2 kilo ohms. It is important to keep the impedance level as low and equally matched as possible to minimize artifact. Matching of electrode impedances allows the highest common mode rejection in the **amplifiers** (see the section on amplifiers). Lower electrode impedance and matched impedances between electrodes make recording less difficult. An EEG machine used in the operating room should give an impedance reading at the main console, not just on the headbox, because during a surgical procedure it is often difficult to get to the headbox once the procedure has started.

SENSITIVITY

The sensitivity selection knob on an EEG machine works as a voltage divider. On most machines it is marked in μV/mm. By selecting the sensitivity, more or less voltage is passed on to the amplifiers. **Sensitivity** is defined as the ratio of the input voltage to the output pen deflection. If 1 μV of input produces a 1-mm deflection at the pen, the sensitivity is 1 μV/mm. This inverse ratio can be confusing, since a lower sensitivity reading refers to a larger pen deflection of the output. A machine used in the operating room should have the same sensitivity range as a machine used in brain death criteria, especially if it is to be used where an isoelectric EEG is desired for cerebral protection.

An **amplifier-blocking mechanism** is another valuable option to have on the EEG mark control panel. Incoming signals can be blocked and the amplifiers returned to baseline quickly. Without amplifier-blocking capabilities it could take several minutes for the amplifiers to return to baseline and valuable data could be lost. This is especially useful when electrosurgical instruments are in use.

AMPLIFIERS

Amplifiers are the heart of an EEG machine. It is here that the electrical activity of the brain is magnified to a point where it can be recorded and analyzed. The amplifier separates unwanted electrical signals from those of the subject's EEG. This is achieved through the use of differential amplifiers with extensive filtering.

There are two amplifier types: **single-ended amplifiers** and **differential amplifiers.** Both have two inputs. In a single-ended amplifier one of the inputs is directly tied to ground, allowing the entire signal of the other input to be amplified. In a differential amplifier the inputs are allowed to "float" or work independently of the ground. The amplifier is grounded internally. This allows the amplifier to only amplify signals that are different or **out of phase** at each input, while canceling the signal that is common or inphase. The ability of the amplifier to cancel the common, or in-phase signal and amplify the out-of-phase signal is known as the **common mode rejection response (CMRR).** A good differential amplifier has a rejection of in-phase signals of at least 10,000 to 1. This value can also be measured in decibels; a good amplifier has a CMRR of 80 dB or more. It is important to select a machine with a very high CMRR. If one of the inputs of the differential amplifier is connected directly to ground, the amplifier becomes a single-ended amplifier, losing CMRR characteristics. The differential amplifier eliminates signals such as 60-Hz interference, which are the same in two electrodes. This also emphasizes the importance of equal electrode impedance.

The **polarity** of the amplifier is determined by convention. For EEG recording the convention is that the pen deflects upward in response to a negative signal at the first input or the first electrode in the montage selection for that channel and downward in response to a positive signal at the first input with respect to the second input. When reviewing an EEG the upward peaks are negative and the downward peaks are positive. Some discrepancies in the direction of polarity may be found with the manufacturers of evoked potential machines. Some of these companies follow the EEG convention while others make positive an upward deflection.

FILTERS

Electronic filters enhance the ability of EEG machines to select only the EEG signal from all signals available. Three basic filters associated with an EEG are (1) the low-end filter, (2) the high-end filter, and (3) the 60-Hz-notch filter. Understanding the filtering mechanisms of the EEG signal is useful to avoid overfiltering the record and losing critical data.

The Low-End Filter

The **low-end filter** has several different names. These include the low-linear-frequency filter, the time-constant filter, and the high-pass filter. The low-end filter works by eliminating in the record contamination by unwanted slow-wave artifact, such as respiration. The low-end filter usually has four settings. The filter is given a numeric value either in hertz (Hz) or time constant (TC). The numeric value stands for the specific amount the filters should attenuate. The filter number, when described in hertz, is the frequency at which the response to a known sine wave input decreases in amplitude to 80% of the initial size. When described as a TC, the filter is the time (in seconds) for a square wave to decay to 37% of its initial amplitude.

The High-End Filter

Like the low-end filter, the **high-end filter** is described in different terms. It is called a high-linear-frequency filter or a low-pass filter. A selection of high-end filter settings is usually available. These filters are also defined in relation to the amount of voltage attenuated. The high-end filter eliminates unwanted fast frequencies, which may contaminate the EEG signal. It depends on the capacitors of the amplifier, which determine the upper limit of the frequencies that will be passed through the amplifier. These filters can be described in two ways. (1) The **rise time** is the time it takes in seconds for a square wave form to attain 63% of the full amplitude. (2) The **frequency** (Hz) at which the response to a sine wave input has decreased to 80% of its initial amplitude is also used. The standard high-end filter for most EEG recordings is 70 Hz.

The 60-Hertz-Notch Filter

The **60-Hz-notch filter** is also known as a **band-stop filter.** It is vital for monitoring in the operating room. This filter is designed to eliminate 60-Hz interference. The operating room environment is electrically hostile. The filter has a very sharp cutoff at the 60-Hz frequency, so it filters out signals at 60 Hz and very little on either side of that frequency. The steep cutoff makes this filter very effective at removing primarily 60-Hz artifacts and not removing useful information at other frequencies.

DATA OUTPUT

The final step in the EEG monitoring system is the **data output.** This output can be recorded electronically to a computer screen or disk or conventionally written to paper. Machines that write to paper may use ink output by mechanical pens, inkjet output (where the ink is sprayed onto the paper), or thermal paper, in which case the writer head is hot and marks special heat-sensitive paper. Because of the large quantity of paper that can be generated, most centers use a reduced paper speed. The normal paper speed used in the diagnostic laboratory is **30 mm/second,** whereas the paper speed routinely used in the operating room is **10 mm/second** or less. Flexibility to increase paper speed should be available. In EEG recording the paper moves from right to left. It is also essential that the pens be easily adjustable to ensure proper alignment.

CALIBRATION

Calibration of the EEG machine ensures that all the amplifiers are intact and functioning properly. A built-in calibration mechanism passes a known DC voltage square wave through the machine components. The rise-time effect of the high-end filter and the TC effect of the low-end filter can be seen and calculated from the calibration signal. The calibration signal should be accurate to 10%, or 0.5 mm, in amplifiers that are correctly calibrated. The calibration signal also gives a known voltage pen deflection to which the amplitude of the EEG record can be compared. It is essential that the machine be calibrated properly, since decisions that will directly affect the patient's care are being made based on the data recorded. Calibration signals should be run before each record at the sensitivity, filter, and paper speed settings routinely used. They should also be run at the end of each record. Calibration signals run are included with each set of parameters in the record.

PATIENT SAFETY

Patient safety is a central concern to operating room neurophysiologic monitoring. The patient in the operating room is more susceptible to injury, because he or she is unconscious with muscles relaxed. One of the major concerns is prevention of burns or electrical shock. Proper grounding of the patient is crucial. **To prevent ground loops, the patient is never grounded more than once.** Ground loops are created when two separate devices are attached to the same patient and have two separate grounding connections. If the voltage between these two connections to ground is not zero, the voltage difference may cause a current to flow through the patient. To avoid grounding loops, use outlets in the same cluster, use only one ground electrode on the patient, and be certain that the patient ground is a **current-limiting device.** There are two types of current-limiting devices: (1) **optical isolation devices** and (2) **isolating diode devices.** Optical isolation devices have photometers and photoreceivers that only allow current beyond a preset value to pass. Isolating diodes have low resistance at low voltages and high resistance at high voltages.

If equipment has a current-limiting device and use of a ground is desired, a large patch electrode (the large surface area creates low resistance), not a cup or needle electrode, is recommended. Some older EEG machines that lack these devices should not be used in the operating room.

In the United States every EEG instrument should be approved as a medical instrument by the Underwriter Laboratories. Equipment so approved will have a "UL" approval code stamped on the back of the main unit.

Most hospital biomedical engineering departments have a strict policy of checking equipment for excessive leakage currents before it is used in the operating room. Leakage currents are caused by stray capacitance and stray inductance. For **stray capacitance** the most common source of leakage current is the instrument's power cord. Stray capacitance is caused by wires, running parallel to each other, acting as capacitors as well as conductors. The amount of stray capacitance often correlates with power cord length. This makes it vital not to use an extension cord when connecting the EEG machine to an outlet. Manufacturers select power cords based on their capacitance per foot of length. Adding an extension cord to the system can increase the leakage current by an unknown and potentially dangerous amount. Other sources of stray capacitance can be found in the internal wiring and electronic components of the instrument.

The other source of leakage current is **stray inductance.** This is a magnetic phenomenon in which each wire carrying current induces a magnetic field that in turn creates currents in other wires. These currents are usually shunted directly to ground but may be conducted through the patient.

Macroshock is a large perceptible current passing from one external surface to another. At most times patients in the operating room are anesthetized, making it difficult to detect a potentially dangerous situation. A leakage current may go undetected.

Microshocks are very low currents; they may be lethal to patients with indwelling electrodes or catheters in the heart, which provide a direct external to internal connection for current. Currents as small as 100 µA, barely perceptible to the arm or hand, may be lethal when applied directly to the heart. The patients at greatest risk of microshock are neonates and patients who have an external source of voltage that connects with indwelling devices such as pacemakers and heart catheters.

There is a potential for sparking during operating room monitoring. Most EEG machines have internal switches that generate sparks as part of their normal use. These machines, as well as machines with thermal recording outputs, should not be used in the presence of flammable gases.

Accidental spillage of liquids, including intravenous fluids and blood, is not uncommon in the operating room. Most monitoring equipment does not have watertight seals. It is important to protect equipment from spills by carefully positioning the equipment or wrapping components in plastic. A spill could result in malfunction of the equipment and an electrical short, placing the patient and the user of the equipment in danger.

There have been reports of patient allergies to the electroconductive gel used with the disk electrodes. Most of these were reactions to calcium, which is not in most gels used today. To minimize the risk of transferring infection from one patient to another all of the equipment should be cleaned with 70–90% ethyl alcohol, isopropyl alcohol, or another noncorrosive disinfectant.

ARTIFACT
Artifact Generation

One of the biggest problems faced during intraoperative neurophysiologic monitoring is identification and elimination of artifact. **Artifact** is defined as any unwanted signal that contaminates the EEG recording. There are four basic sources of artifact. (1) The patient or unshielded electrodes can act as an antenna. (2) Recording electrodes connected to other recording equipment act as conductors. (3) The recording leads or cables connecting the patient with the recording equipment conduct magnetic field artifacts. (4) Interference leaks into the amplifiers from the power lines. Keeping the electrode impedances as low and evenly matched as possible keeps the CMRR ratio high, maximizing elimination of in-phase artifacts. It is better to eliminate the source of artifact than to use a filter to remove it.

There is no practical way to record when the electrocautery is in use. The record must be paused until the surgeon is finished. At the time of purchase, check with the manufacturer that the electrocautery and other electrosurgical devices do not damage the equipment intended for use in the operating room.

Trouble-Shooting Artifacts

Knowing common sources of artifact helps identify and eliminate them. The patient can induce artifacts as well as act as an antenna. Patient artifacts include ECG, which may be eliminated by repositioning the recording electrodes, the ground, or both. Do not cross ECG electrodes with EEG electrodes. Electromyography (EMG), eye blink, and movement are not typically problems for operating room recording. Occasionally EMG is a problem, but this can be eliminated with induced muscle relaxation. Patient movement can be a problem when the surgeon moves the patient or rests a hand on the patient's head or if the surgeon leans on the headbox. Sweating is also a potential problem for electrode contact, especially in cases that use hypothermia and rewarming.

Many electrode-induced artifacts are caused by electrodes that are improperly applied or faulty. If an electrode is suspected of being faulty, the continuity of the electrode should be checked with an ohm meter before application to the patient. The AC line to the room may also cause 60-Hz interference. Sometimes moving to a different electrical outlet resolves the problem.

Airborne artifacts may be picked up by the patient and the EEG electrodes acting as an antenna. The reader may have experienced the antenna effect when trying to tune a radio or television set, when the reception is better as long as one touches the piece of equipment. The main culprits in the operating room include proximity to television or radio stations, electrosurgical devices, devices with mechanical switches, devices with fans, and devices with poorly made power supplies. Other equipment that may give artifacts are respirators, CO_2 analyzers, pacemakers, and fluid pumps. Unfortunately, very little can be done about some of these artifact-generating devices.

Use of the EEG in the operating room can provide important information about the condition of the patient. Understanding the EEG machine is a major part of interpreting the data generated. Proper electrodes, proper electrode attachment, and proper electrode location are essential for a meaningful EEG recording. The impedance level of electrodes must be less than 5 kilo ohms, and impedance levels must be well matched in order to have amplifiers working at their highest CMRR. Calibration of the EEG machine is crucial to ensure that all components are functioning properly. Patient safety should be a central concern. Finding and eliminating sources of artifact is an ongoing challenge in the operating room. Proper attention to all of these issues produces EEG results of the highest possible quality.

KEY REFERENCES

Brittenham DM. Artifacts. In DD Daly DD, TA Pedley (eds). Current Practice of Clinical Electroencephalography. New York: Raven, 1990. Pp 85–106. *This chapter looks in-depth at artifacts that affect all EEG recordings, not just recordings from the operating room. It also provides the reader with EEG records containing identified sources of artifact and describes how these artifacts were eliminated.*

Daube JR, Harper CM, Litchy WJ, Sharbrough FW. Intraoperative Monitoring. In DD Daly, TA Pedley (eds). Current Practice of Clinical Electroencephalography. New York: Raven, 1990. Pp 739–747. *This chapter gives a clear, concise outline of issues to be considered when recording the EEG in the operating room. Included are nice illustrations of actual intraoperative EEG records.*

Litt B, Fisher RS. EEG Engineering Principles. In DD Daly, TA Pedley (eds). Current Practice of Clinical Electroencephalography. New York: Raven, 1990. Pp 11–27. *This chapter provides an easy-to-understand explanation of the engineering principles of each component EEG machine and their interrelationship in EEG instrument development.*

Tyner FS, Knott JR, Mayer WB Jr. Fundamentals of EEG Technology. Vol. 1. New York: Raven, 1983. *This text provides the reader with the foundation for a solid understanding of EEG technology. It is written for the beginning technician with enough depth to be a key source in preparing for the American Board of Registration of Electroencephalographic and Evoked Potential Technologist examinations.*

RECOMMENDED READING

Clark RG. Manter and Gatz's Essentials of Clinical Neuroanatomy and Neurophysiology (5th ed). Philadelphia: FA Davis, 1975

Grass Model 8 Instruction Manual. Part II—Theory and Application. Quincy, MA: Grass Instrument Company, 1973.

Harner PF, Sannit T. A Review of the International Ten-Twenty System of Electrode Placement. Quincy, MA: Grass Instrument Company, 1974.

Prior PF, Maynard DE. Monitoring Cerebral Function: Long-Term Monitoring of EEG and Evoked Potentials. Amsterdam: Elsevier, 1986.

Richey ET, Namon R. EEG Instrumentation and Technology. Springfield, IL: Charles C. Thomas, 1976.

6

Basic Scalp Electroencephalography

Lawrence D. Rodichok, M.D.

Intraoperative monitoring of the electroencephalogram (EEG) is accomplished most commonly by recording scalp activity with a continuous paper printout. EEG may also be recorded digitally on tape or disk and displayed on a monitor, but this technology has not had widespread application in the operating room. The use of computer-processed EEG is discussed in Chapter 7. The EEG recorded in the operating room differs significantly from that recorded in the clinical neurophysiology laboratory, where the study is usually performed with the patient awake and relaxed and with eyes closed, or with the patient in spontaneous sleep. Electrical interference is minimized. It is under these ideal circumstances that the traditional normal waking and sleep patterns may be seen and most types of abnormalities have been described. However, in the operating room the waking portions of the EEG are often recorded with the patient awake and anxious, with the eyes open and considerable electromyographic (EMG) and movement artifact present. The EEG changes abruptly with induction of the state of general anesthesia, which is not at all like spontaneous sleep. Operating room EEG taxes the skill of the EEG technologist to maintain stable electrode contact and to eliminate as much electronic artifact as possible. Similarly, interpretation of operating room EEG requires adequate clinical experience in this state to be familiar with normal patterns expected under general anesthesia and with types of potential abnormalities and their significance to the patient, anesthesiologist, and surgeon. Experience in interpreting "routine" EEGs, although valuable, is not sufficient.

ORIGIN OF SCALP-RECORDED ELECTROENCEPHALOGRAMS

EEG waves, as recorded from the scalp or the surface of the brain, represent the summation of extracellular current fluctuations, due to both **excitatory** and **inhibitory postsynaptic potentials** (**EPSPs** and **IPSPs**, respectively) originating in the most superficial layers of the cortex. These EPSPs and IPSPs are in fact impinging on the apical dendrites of neurons located in the deeper layers. Surface negative waves correlate best with a summation of EPSPs very near the surface, while surface positive waves correlate with a summation of IPSPs. The same synaptic events occurring closer to the soma have the opposite effect on

65

surface EEG. This is a useful oversimplification of the complexity of events contributing to surface electrical activity. Furthermore, EEG recorded from the scalp suffers from the attenuating and filtering effects of the tissues between the brain and recording electrodes, most notably the dura and intervening cerebrospinal fluid. Voltage fluctuations at the scalp probably represent coherent activity from a relatively large area of cortex. Activity in more discrete areas is probably not detected by scalp EEG, although intracranially placed electrodes may be successful in detecting such activity.

TECHNICAL CONSIDERATIONS
Electrode Placement

It is preferable to use the full set of 19 international ten-twenty system electrode locations (the ear electrodes are not always necessary). This allows coverage of each of the major vascular territories, which is especially pertinent during carotid endarterectomy and cerebral aneurysm surgery. It also allows enough overlap within the montage that a failed electrode will not severely limit the adequacy of the study. An adequate number of channels must also be available to simultaneously display activity from a variety of cortical areas as covered by electrode combinations. We prefer 14 or more channels for most studies. We use a combination of "bipolar" longitudinal-linked chains along with **referential derivations**. In some situations, such as for long-term monitoring of barbiturate coma in the intensive care unit, a more limited set of electrodes and channels is appropriate. Neonates may also require fewer than the usual number of adult electrodes. A channel for electrocardiogram (ECG) can also be useful.

Patient Vital Signs

The technologist should record the patient's blood pressure, heart rate, and temperature regularly throughout the record. It is valuable to record the clock time regularly and at every critical surgical point. Always use a clock synchronous with that used for the anesthesiology record. This facilitates later efforts to correlate EEG changes with surgical or anesthetic events.

Recording Parameters

If conditions permit, the **high-frequency filter** setting should be at 70 Hz and **the 60-Hz-notch filter** should be off. It may be critical to be able to recognize attenuation of higher frequency activity at such times as cross-clamping of the carotid artery. However, when necessary, the HFF may be lowered to 30 Hz and the 60-Hz notch filter may be used since most EEG activity during general anesthesia is unaffected, even if both are used. This would not be acceptable for awake patients. For the same reason, **the gain should be sufficient to see the lower-amplitude fast activity**. This allows EEG attenuation on the side of carotid surgery to be recognized immediately.

Most laboratories find a relatively slow paper speed preferable. **Routine EEG is recorded at a paper speed of 30 mm/second, but 10 or even 5 mm/second is preferred in the operating room** because abnormalities are more easily recognized at slower speeds. It is important that at least 5 minutes of artifact-free activity, with the patient as relaxed as possible and the eyes closed, be recorded before induction of anesthesia, to recognize any preoperative abnormalities, especially focal changes. A specific preoperative study is usually not practical or necessary. If the patient has had a previous EEG, the results should be known at the time of monitoring. Intraoperative EEG should be recorded until the patient is removed from the operating table. After carotid endarterectomies, changes due to rethrombosis of the artery may occur.

ELECTROENCEPHALOGRAPHY UNDER ANESTHESIA
The Awake Patient

In the normal awake, relaxed patient with eyes closed, scalp-recorded EEG consists primarily of a prominent posterior frequency between 8.5 and 13 Hz (the **alpha rhythm**) and anterior lower-amplitude activity at 18–25 Hz (beta activity is faster than 13 Hz) admixed with small amounts of 4- to 7-Hz (theta) activity. With the eyes open, the alpha rhythm is blocked or attenuated and the record is then dominated by activity in the beta range with a small amount of random theta activity anteriorly. EMG artifact is often seen in the fronto-temporal leads. The latter pattern is to be expected in the awake anxious patient just prior to induction (Figure 6.1). Unfortunately, it is less likely that any generalized or focal abnormalities will be seen under these circumstances. It is preferable that a short segment of EEG be recorded with the patient's eyes closed and as relaxed as possible to recognize any preoperative focal abnormalities. Patients with an abnormal baseline EEG are more likely to show changes with cross-clamping of the internal carotid artery.

Premedication

Most of the pharmacologic agents used for premedication and for induction and maintenance of anesthesia produce similar EEG changes when given at equivalent doses. At relatively low doses all such agents are associated with the appearance of 18- to 25-Hz beta activity seen predominantly in the more anterior regions. In sedative doses this anterior fast activity is associated with diffuse mixed-frequency slowing, largely in the theta range similar to that seen with simple drowsiness.

Anesthetic Induction and Maintenance

With induction of anesthesia, beta activity often becomes more generalized and paroxysmal high-amplitude anterior rhythmic slowing in the 1- to 3-Hz range is seen (**frontal intermittent rhythmic delta activity**) (Figure 6.2). With

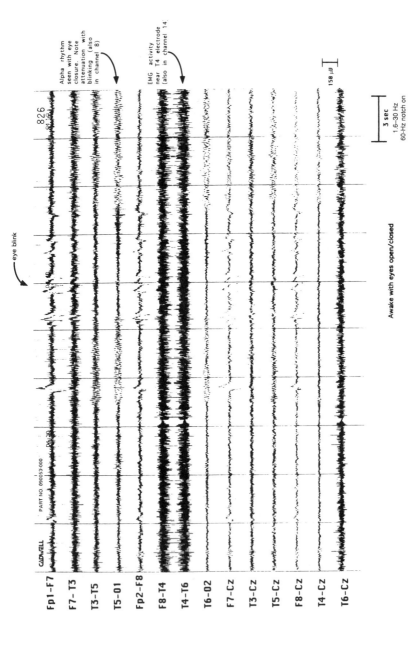

Figure 6.1 Baseline EEG activity in an awake patient prior to induction of general anesthesia. An alpha rhythm is present when the eyes are closed. Blink artifact is seen in the frontopolar leads (Fp1 and Fp2). Electromyographic activity is seen in the channels containing T.

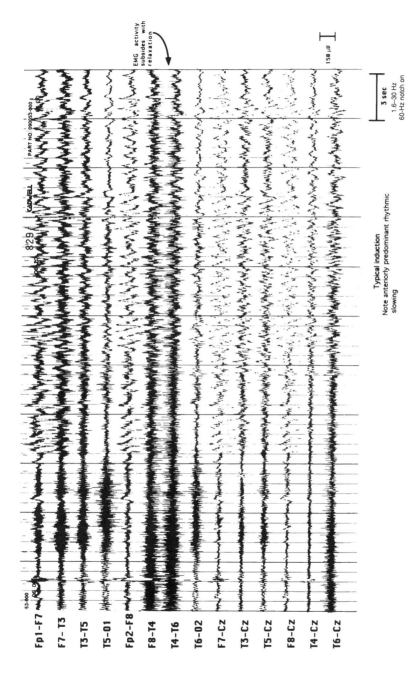

Figure 6.2 Typical EEG changes during anesthetic induction. This is the same patient as in Figure 6.1. Note that the electromyographic activity subsides with muscle relaxation. Note the appearance of high-amplitude rhythmic slowing in the more anterior leads.

very rapid induction there may be a period of 1- to 3-second bursts of diffuse high-amplitude slowing alternating with periods of global attenuation lasting a similar period, a pattern commonly referred to as **burst suppression** (Figure 6.3). This is of variable duration, usually no more than 30–60 seconds. Activity then gradually evolves to a pattern consisting of diffuse rhythmic faster activity, initially in the beta range but gradually slowing to the alpha range. This is mixed with diffuse rhythmic slowing in the theta and delta ranges, initially more prominent anteriorly but becoming generalized as maintenance anesthesia deepens (Figure 6.4). At 1-MAC concentrations of volatile anesthetics, this diffuse and symmetric admixture of theta and delta slowing and the superimposed beta and alpha activity is typical of all agents. Occasional runs of more rhythmic delta activity can also be seen. If this type of activity becomes frequent or prolonged, there should be concern for global cortical dysfunction, as might be seen with significant hypotension. A burst suppression pattern should not be seen after induction unless very deep anesthesia is attained.

Anesthesia-Related Interactions

A variety of exogenous factors may influence the EEG pattern. Lowering the $PaCO_2$ below 40 mm Hg can cause the EEG to be disproportionately slow, suggesting a deeper level of anesthesia. Decreasing blood pressure, hypothermia, hypoxia, or any other systemic metabolic disorder has the same effect. The technologist should first alert the anesthesiologist when such unexpected global changes occur, because they are most often attributable to changes in anesthetic depth, $PaCO_2$, or hypotension. Any focal change, even if it does occur in association with a systemic event, is indicative of focal cortical dysfunction, and the surgeon and anesthesiologist should be informed directly. It is also possible that manipulation of the carotid sinus during surgery in that area can cause EEG changes, even without an effect on blood pressure or pulse.

ELECTROENCEPHALOGRAMS FOR SPECIFIC SURGICAL PROCEDURES
Carotid Endarterectomy

Carotid artery surgery is the most common indication for intraoperative EEG monitoring. There is a good correlation between regional cerebral blood flow (rCBF) and EEG alterations ipsilateral to carotid cross-clamping. EEG changes are seen in nearly all patients with a rCBF below 10 ml/100 g/minute (assuming a normal $PaCO_2$) and in the majority of those with an rCBF below 20 ml/100 g/minute. EEG changes may be more predictive of postoperative deficits than a postocclusion rCBF. The appearance of EEG changes with cross-clamping has been used because (1) it may precipitate efforts to improve perfusion pressure by raising systemic pressure, and (2) the decision to use a surgical shunt may rest on the appearance of EEG changes. Ten to 30% of patients have easily

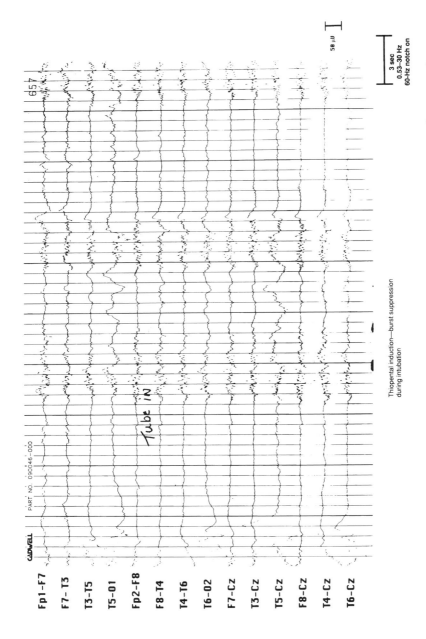

Figure 6.3 Burst suppression pattern during induction of general anesthesia and endotracheal intubation. In this case sodium thiopental was given, but a similar pattern could be seen with most other induction agents in equivalent doses.

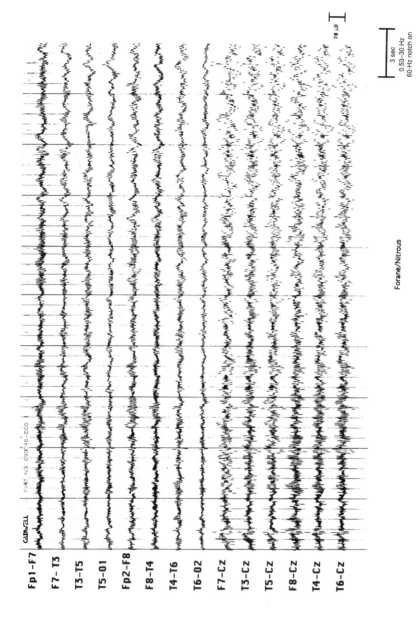

Figure 6-4 Typical EEG background activity during maintenance of general anesthesia with isoflurane and nitrous oxide. Note the diffuse admixture of faster-frequency activity, which is largely in the alpha range, with slower activity in the delta range.

recognizable EEG changes, usually seen within 30 seconds of cross clamping. Patients whose EEG changes are not reversed with shunting are at the greatest risk for awakening with a new neurologic deficit.

The most common type of EEG change is an acute attenuation of the faster-frequency activity ipsilaterally with an increased amount of delta slowing (Figure 6.5). Less commonly, only the former change is seen, and least commonly just the latter. There is no difference in significance for one type of change over the other. Shunting usually reverses these changes (Figure 6.6). Patients with contralateral carotid occlusion or severe (>90%) stenosis are also at especially high risk to show EEG changes and by extension to have intraoperative stroke. However, EEG may be more predictive than the presence of contralateral carotid stenosis or occlusion. Of course the occurrence of focal EEG changes at other points during the procedure may indicate acute ischemia, often due to embolization from the operative site or to thrombosis of the artery. Global slowing may also be seen with cross-clamping (Figure 6.7). Although at other times during surgery systemic causes of global slowing are more likely, during carotid cross-clamping it is probable that perfusion of both cerebral hemispheres depends on one carotid artery. Thus it is important that the EEG be followed for the entire procedure.

Intracranial Aneurysm Clipping

EEG monitoring may be used during surgical treatment of intracranial aneurysms. In some instances this involves **monitoring for the effect of temporary or permanent carotid artery occlusion** as part of the surgical approach to the aneurysm. Similar to what is seen with carotid endarterectomy, there is a good correlation between alterations in EEG activity, reduction in rCBF during test occlusions of the carotid artery, and focal deficit if occlusion is made permanent. There is a small but significant incidence of false-negative EEG after test or permanent occlusions of the carotid artery, in the neck. In the absence of rCBF measurements, EEG is a very useful tool in predicting tolerance to carotid ligation.

In a similar vein, we have found intraoperative EEG useful **during placement of temporary aneurysm clips**. It is usually necessary to place a subdural strip of electrodes in the appropriate vascular territory for this purpose. This should be done as early as possible to establish a baseline pattern since there is no contralateral subdural recording for comparison. Any change from the baseline pattern with placement of the clip suggests that flow through the parent artery has been compromised and repositioning of the clip may be indicated (Figure 6.8).

EEG monitoring for the presence of a **burst suppression pattern** may also be necessary if cerebral protection with deep hypothermia or barbiturate coma is to be used. Continuous EEG monitoring may also be useful in following patients with subarachnoid hemorrhage before and especially after aneurysm clipping. EEG alterations may be an early sign of recurrent bleeding or spasm.

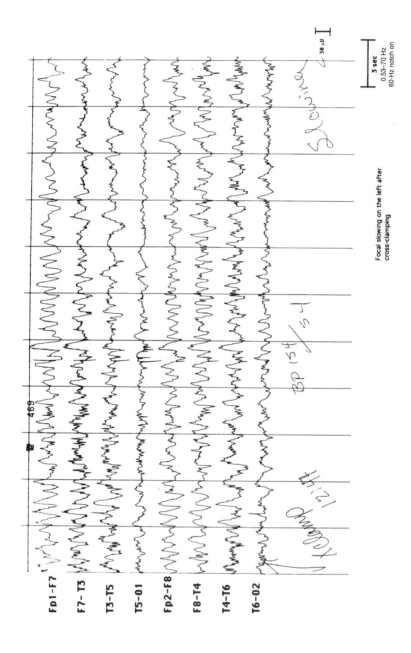

Figure 6.5 Focal EEG slowing over the left cerebral hemisphere (channels 2, 3, and 4) following cross-clamping of the left internal carotid artery. Note the approximately 20-second delay before the appearance of the change. This is the typical time interval before changes occur.

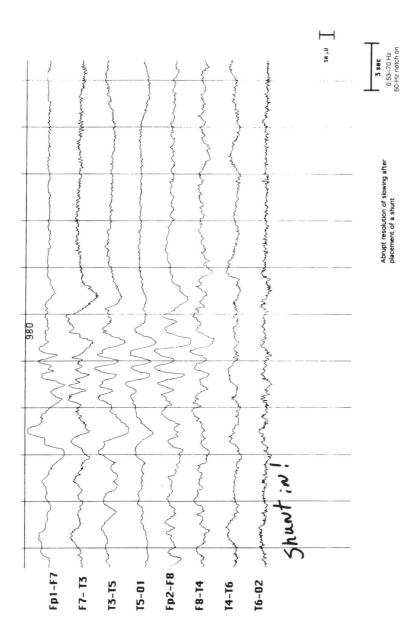

Figure 6.6 Prompt resolution of EEG slowing is seen after opening of a shunt.

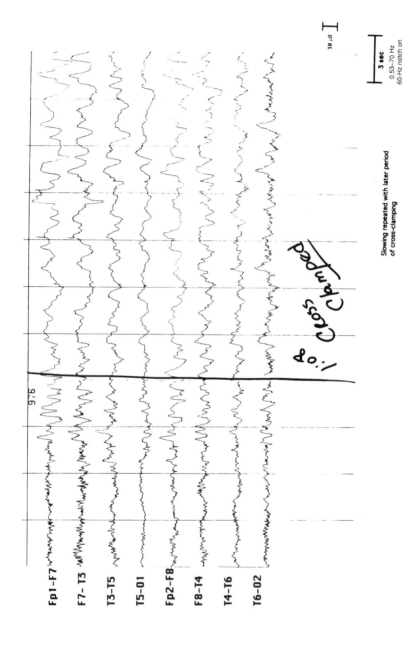

Figure 6.7 Bilateral EEG slowing is seen after carotid cross-clamping. In this case the effect was almost immediate, not delayed as is typical with unilateral changes (see Figure 6.5).

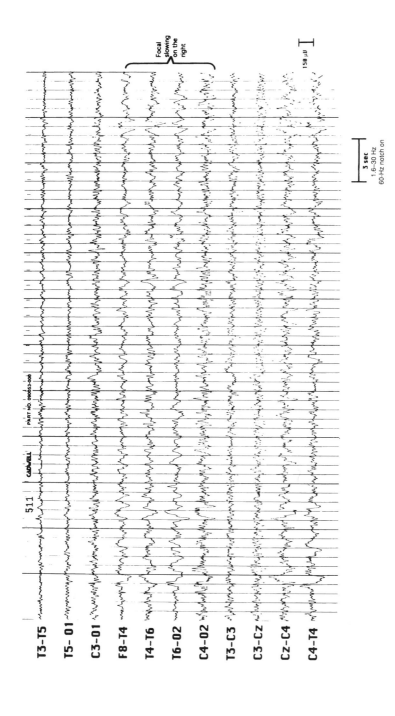

Figure 6.8 Focal EEG slowing seen on the right following placement of a temporary clip on a middle cerebral artery aneurysm. There is limited placement of electrodes due to the craniotomy.

Hypothermic Circulatory Arrest

EEG monitoring is used at some centers during procedures that will include periods of hypothermia with or without reduced or absent cerebral perfusion. This is most commonly the case during correction of congenital heart defects. The EEG shows a characteristic evolution during progressive hypothermia. Most infants have a continuous background of EEG activity at baseline, although some premature infants have brief periods of voltage attenuation. With onset of cardiopulmonary bypass there is often a burst of high-amplitude slowing caused by the cool perfusion fluid reaching the brain. This is followed by a gradual reduction in EEG amplitude and frequency as temperature declines. About 50% of patients show a pattern of **periodic paroxysmal activity (PPA)** at temperatures between 25°C and 20°C (Figure 6.9). In others there is a continuation of the decline in amplitude and frequency. In those with PPA, the interval between bursts of activity gradually lengthens as temperature declines further. There is a gradual decline in amplitude and frequency in those without PPA. Circulatory arrest usually occurs (if indicated) at about 15°C.

In our own experience, approximately 75% of children and adults have persistent EEG activity at this point and require barbiturates, such as thiopental, if suppressing all remaining neuroelectric activity is desired. Once the circulation is completely arrested all EEG activity ceases within 1 minute. EEG activity returns with rewarming in a reversal of the pattern with which it declines—that is, with bursts of activity and gradually shorter "electrically quiet" intervals. PPA is not seen during rewarming. If the circulation had not been arrested, there is almost always a return to a continuous background by the time normal temperature (34°C) is reached. In patients undergoing a period of complete circulatory arrest, nearly half may still have no activity on return to normothermia. The duration of time that EEG activity remains absent is proportional to the length of the arrest. By the end of the procedure, most (88% in our patient series) have a continuous or nearly continuous background EEG rhythm.

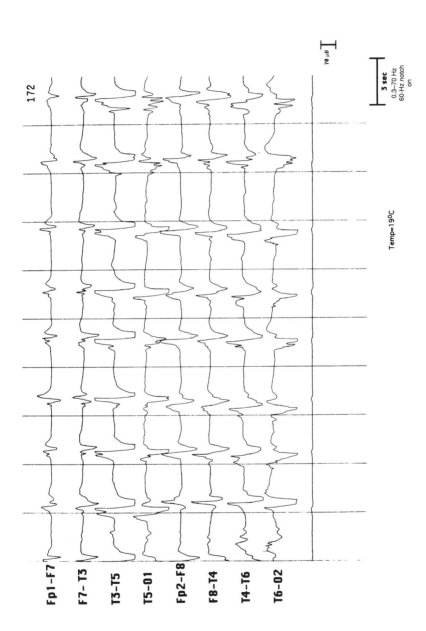

Figure 6.9 Typical EEG seen during progressive hypothermia. This patterned paroxysmal activity may be seen in all age groups.

KEY REFERENCES

Blume W, Ferguson G, McNeill D. Significance of EEG changes at carotid endarterectomy. 1986;Stroke 17:891. *Shunts are not used at the University of Western Ontario so no changes were made in the procedure despite any EEG changes (other than a shorter clamp time probably due to the fact that the attending physician personally performed cases with EEG changes as opposed to supervising the resident). Postoperative deficits only occurred in those with EEG changes.*

Bridgers S, Spencer S, Spencer D, Sasaki C. A cerebral effect of carotid sinus stimulation. Observation during intraoperative electroencephalographic monitoring. Arch Neurol 1985;42:574. *Reports on two cases of diffuse EEG changes with manipulation of the carotid sinus, one during an endarterectomy and one during removal of a schwannoma. No changes in blood pressure or heart rate were seen, but a reproducible relationship to manipulation of the sinus was demonstrated.*

Kalkman C, Boezeman E, Ribberink A, Oosting J, Deen L, Bovill J. Influence of changes in arterial carbon dioxide tension on the electroencephalogram and posterior tibial nerve somatosensory cortical evoked potentials during alfentanil/nitrous oxide anesthesia. Anesthesiology 1991;75:68. *Hypocapnia (PaCO$_2$ <23 mm Hg caused increased power in delta, theta, and beta bands. Hypercapnia caused an increase in alpha and beta.*

Labar D, Fisch B, Pedley T, Fink M, Solomon R. Quantitative EEG monitoring for patients with subarachnoid hemorrhage. Electroencephalogr Clin Neurophysiol 1991;78:325. *EEG changes may precede clinical signs of arterial spasm.*

Miller J, Jawad K, Jennett B. Safety of carotid ligation and its role in the management of intracranial aneurysms. J Neurol Neurosurg Psychiatry 1977;40:64. *Good correlation between rCBF and EEG and between rCBF and safety of carotid ligation. Eighty-six percent of those with a postoperative deficit had EEG changes with the trial occlusion versus 14% of those who did not have EEG changes.*

Redekop G, Ferguson G. Correlation of contralateral stenosis and intraoperative electroencephalogram change with risk of stroke during carotid endarterectomy. Neurosurgery 1992;30:191. *The risk of postoperative deficit was 18% in those with EEG changes and 1.8% in those without EEG changes. EEG was more predictive than the presence of contralateral carotid stenosis or occlusion.*

Rodichok L, Winters J, Myers J, Schwentker M, Marshall W. The evolution of EEG changes during extracorporeal circulation and progressive hypothermia with or without circulatory arrest. Am J EEG Tech 1994;34:66–74. *A technical description of the typical EEG changes during progressive hypothermia with and without circulatory arrest.*

Sundt T, Sharbrough F, Anderson R, Michenfelder J. Cerebral blood flow measurements and electroencephalograms during carotid endarterectomy. J Neurosurg 1974;41:310. *All but one patient with rCBF below 18 ml/100 g/minute had EEG changes.*

Trojaborg W, Boysen G. Relation between EEG, regional cerebral blood flow and internal carotid artery pressure during carotid endarterectomy. Electroencephalogr Clin Neurophysiol 1973;34:61. *Almost all patients with an rCBF below 20 ml/100 g/minute had EEG changes.*

Zampella E, Morawetz R, McDowell H, Zeiger H, Varner P, McKay R, Halsey J. The importance of cerebral ischemia during carotid endarterectomy. Neurosurgery 1991;29: 727. *A more recent study correlating rCBF by xenon injection showed a less frequent incidence of EEG changes with reduction in rCBF than most other studies. There was a high correlation of EEG changes with postoperative deficits, but the correlation with alteration in flow was negative if it appeared at all. The highest incidence of deficits was seen in those with an increase in flow with carotid clamping.*

7

Computerized Electroencephalogram Analysis

Garfield B. Russell, M.D., FRCPC
Lawrence D. Rodichok, M.D.

Traditional interpretation of the electroencephalogram (EEG) relies on visual inspection. While it remains to be proved that mathematical analysis of EEG is superior to traditional methods, there are certainly logical reasons to suspect that this may be the case. Visual inspection relies on the recognition of patterns known to correlate with one or more disease processes. It relies on the more prominent features of the waveforms, which are not necessarily the only important ones. Recognition of lower-amplitude, higher-frequency waves or very-low-frequency waves is not always easy. Automated analysis and display also make it easier for the anesthesiologist to use the EEG as an intraoperative monitor.

The ionic currents reflected in the EEG provide a functional assessment of the central nervous system (CNS). This monitoring capability has extended from standard EEG use for assessment of epilepsy and other CNS pathology to a monitor for anesthetic depth, cerebral ischemia development, and cerebral quiescence during hypothermic cardiopulmonary arrest and barbiturate coma. The EEG has been viewed as a collection of complex and subtle neuroelectric events. In attempts to make these seemingly chaotic waves of cerebral activity interpretable and more functional for day-to-day intraoperative use, mathematical analysis of EEG tracings has been developed to provide correlation between neurophysiologic events and this mathematical representation of the electrical activity.

AUTOMATED ELECTROENCEPHALOGRAM ANALYSIS

A variety of automated methods of EEG analysis have been used. These are divided into **analog** and **digital** techniques. The analog outputs are continuous functions of time. EEG signals are described by both their amplitude and frequency. As the computer analysis proceeds, signal amplitude deviations above and below baseline are squared so that all measurements have a positive value. This is commonly called the **power**, variance, or energy of the signal. In its initial development, this analysis technique was combined with a series of filters tuned to appropriate frequency bands, creating a "wave analyzer," with the output proportional to the power in each of the specific frequency bands. Digital computers have replaced this technique.

The Statistical Basis of Data Interpretation

The analog signal recorded as traditional EEG must be translated (digitized) by computer into a form that can be evaluated and presented in a readily interpretable manner. The EEG waves (amplitude as voltage spread over a time base) are examined at a rapid rate. The sampling rate should be at least twice the highest frequency present; this is called the **Nyquist rule**. A specific digital number is assigned for the voltage of each sampling interval. For example, if the digitizing rate is 100 Hz, 1 hour of sampling would result in 360,000 individual voltage measurements. These sampling intervals, or **epochs**, can often be set for each specific recording and are usually 2–15 seconds, but should be at least as long as the period of the longest frequency present. A mean or variance can be calculated for each epoch. The statistical principle of **stationarity** assumes that the statistics for each epoch do not change with time. Although this is not really true for neurobiological activity, there is relative stability for 15- to 25-second intervals. This makes development of clinically applicable processing algorithms possible.

Condensing and Quantitating the Electroencephalogram

The time-varying signal that forms the analog output of the EEG machine consists primarily of amplitude and rate along with variables that alter their relative effect on direct visual interpretation. The patient's level of anesthesia and physical state of health, the electrode montage and impedances, and individual wave shapes all influence the opinion derived by the electrophysiologist. Most processed EEG data presented to the observer is based on **power spectral analysis**. The amplitude or power of each sine wave component of the EEG waveform is presented as a function of frequency, assuming no interaction between waves. This presents neuroelectric data as epochs of specific, definable information, which may be easier for less experienced personnel to interpret than raw EEG.

ALGORITHMIC APPROACHES TO ELECTROENCEPHALOGRAM ANALYSIS

Computerized analysis uses numerically oriented algorithms to interpret the EEG, although the same variables may influence the computer's analysis as the electrophysiologist's manual interpretation. Specific statistical approaches include **parametric analysis** and **nonparametric analysis**.

Parametric algorithms build statistical models of the EEG but do not reflect the underlying physiology. Future EEG activity is predicted based on statistical analysis. The applications are not for real-time applications but are in digital filters allowing noise input to output as signals with statistical features the same as the EEG signals being monitored.

Nonparametric algorithms do not use modeling based on statistical assumptions about underlying EEG activity. The frequency- and time-domain algorithms commonly used for real-time EEG analysis are nonparametric.

Frequency-Domain Analysis   For **frequency-domain analysis,** the EEG waveforms (voltage over time) for each epoch are processed into spectra (voltage over frequency). **Fast Fourier transform** (FFT) uses specific numbers of raw EEG signals and computes in real time the distribution of electrical energy (or **power**) at each specific frequency interval. If

$$Power = Vp^2/2,$$

where Vp^2 is peak voltage in the EEG signal squared, the EEG data is scaled for a spectral display. For example, a 40 µV peak voltage at 10 Hz would give 0.8 nanowatts on the spectral display.

$$Power = [(40 \times 10^{-6})]^2/2 = 0.8 \times 10^{-9}$$

Time-Domain Analysis   Various **time-domain analysis** techniques have been developed and applied. The square-mean-root or mean of absolute EEG values was used in the quantitation of **average signal amplitude** in early computerized EEG analysis. However, it is inadequate for sophisticated clinical applications because EEG amplitude is not normally distributed. **Zero-crossing frequency** measures time intervals between wave form sequential crossing of the zero voltage axis. Small waves that may "ride" a slow-frequency wave can be ignored because, whatever their frequency, only the slow wave crosses the baseline. Although significant information can be obtained, it often results in large errors in determining **mean frequency.** The **aperiodic algorithm** calculates the peak-to-peak amplitude and duration of each wave with the graphic display showing amplitude as vertical bar height and frequency as the bar position on the x-axis of the display. The **burst suppression ratio** has been used to monitor cortical suppression. The duration of each epoch with EEG amplitude less than 5 µV is the suppression time. The reported value is expressed in seconds as the ratio suppression time/epoch time.

DISPLAYING PROCESSED ELECTROENCEPHALOGRAM DATA

After each epoch of data has been processed, it must be displayed in a way that makes it useful for clinical applications. The purpose of computerized EEG analysis is to produce real-time information, which can be immediately assessed in a "user-friendly" manner and applied to patient care. This processed data can be presented on screen in different formats.

Visual Representations of Electroencephalograms

1. The **analog output of the raw EEG** signal can be presented in real-time on the screen. This is presented in two to eight channels, based on the international ten-twenty system (Figure 7.1).

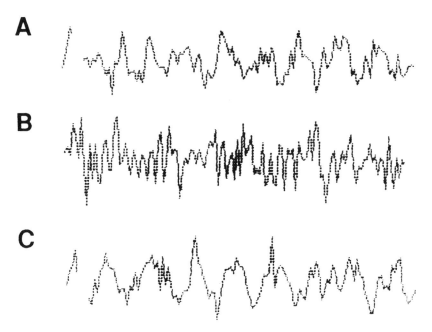

Figure 7.1 Raw analog EEG output. A. Baseline awake fast-wave activity with some background theta activity. B. EEG activation with a sedative dose of midazolam. C. Return of EEG toward baseline after administration of the benzodiazepine antagonist flumazenil.

2. The **compressed spectral array (CSA)** is a pseudo–three-dimensional plot of EEG power (amplitude^2/2) spectral lines (one for each epoch) resulting in a stack of sequential spectra (Figure 7.2). Hundreds of digital steps can be displayed in each graphic presentation.

3. The **density spectral array (DSA)** uses either color distribution or grayscale intensity to represent EEG power at each frequency in each epoch (Figure 7.3). The DSA does not cover as wide a range of power as the CSA since only 8 or 16 levels of color or shade are used in the DSA as compared to many more digital levels in the CSA graph.

4. The **spectral edge frequency (SEF)** is the highest significant frequency present in the recorded EEG spectrum for each epoch (see Figures 7.2 and 7.3). This is usually set to 90–97% of the recorded EEG power. A decline in the SEF suggests that the overall frequency spectrum is shifting to lower frequencies. A unilateral change suggests focal cortical dysfunction. SEF is commonly used during carotid endarterectomies (Figure 7.4).

5. The **spectral histogram** is a bar graph representation of the spectral frequency of the EEG. This can be presented in 0.5- to 1.0-Hz intervals (Figure 7.5).

6. The **median power frequency** is the EEG frequency one-half of the recorded power is below and one-half above.

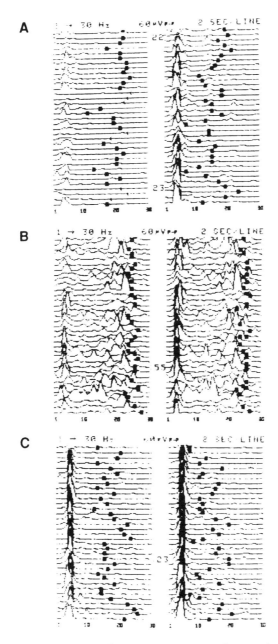

Figure 7.2 The compressed spectral array (CSA). A. Baseline awake fast-wave activity with some background theta activity. Note the marker for spectral edge frequency (SEF) set at 97% power. B. The CSA reflects electrical activation after a sedative dose of midazolam. The SEF moves into higher frequencies and EEG power is increased. C. Return of CSA and SEF toward baseline after administration of the benzodiazepine antagonist flumazenil.

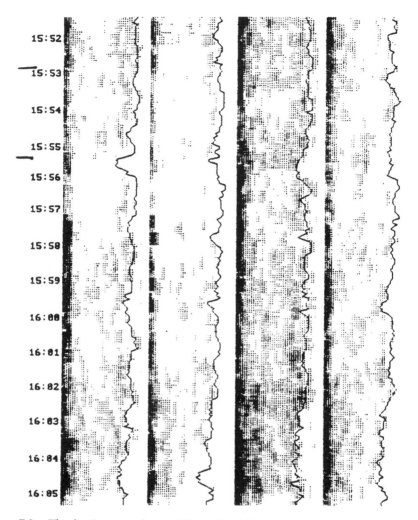

Figure 7.3 The density spectral array. The analyzed data is displayed by varying density of dots in a line. This can also be presented as individual colors or gray-scale shading. The x-axis represents EEG frequency from 0–30 Hz from left to right. Four channels are displayed.

7. The **peak power frequency** is the EEG frequency of each epoch in which the highest power of the current spectrum recorded occurs (see Figure 7.5).
8. **Power bands** are bar graphs of the EEG power in each of the alpha, beta, theta, and delta EEG frequency bands (Figure 7.6).

Derivations from Spectral Histograms

The reliability of the data obtained from computerized EEG analysis depends on the quality of the EEG input. The presence of artifact in a mea-

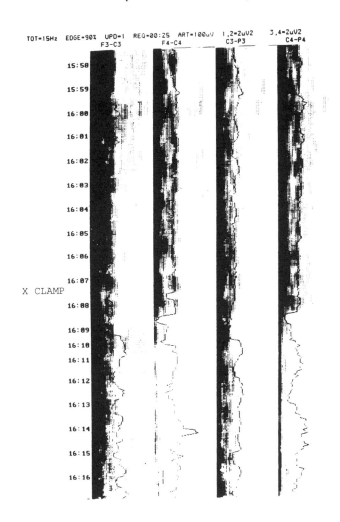

Figure 7.4 The density spectral array and the spectral edge frequency line show bilateral slowing and decreased power with carotid cross-clamp. *Courtesy of the Intraoperative Neurophysiologic Monitoring Service, Milton S. Hershey Medical Center, Penn State University College of Medicine.*

sured frequency band, if not recognized, may confound the analysis. Access is needed to the raw, real-time EEG signals being processed with visual interpretation by the observer. The technique of application and the montage used for electrode placement must be reliable and tailored to the clinical situation. For example, during carotid artery surgery, electrodes generally record from the F7, F8, T3, T4, T5, and T6 regions over the distribution of the middle cerebral arteries. Four channels are preferable, so that two can be analyzed on each side.

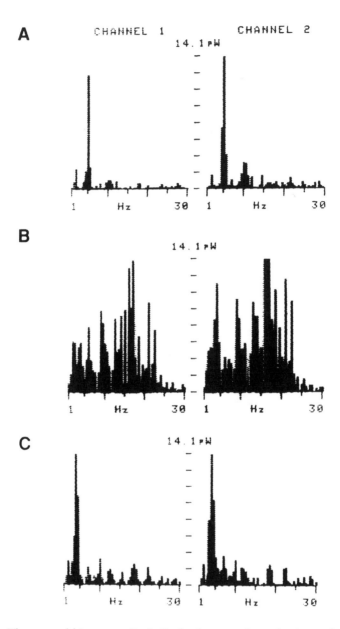

Figure 7.5 The spectral histogram. Each display has two channels. A. Baseline activity across the frequency range. The peak power frequency can be detected as the frequency with the highest EEG power, represented by the column graphs, displayed every 0.5 Hz. B. The spectra reflect electrical activation after a sedative dose of midazolam. The PPF moves into higher frequencies and EEG power is diffusely increased. C. Return of power distribution and PPF toward baseline after administration of the benzodiazepine antagonist flumazenil.

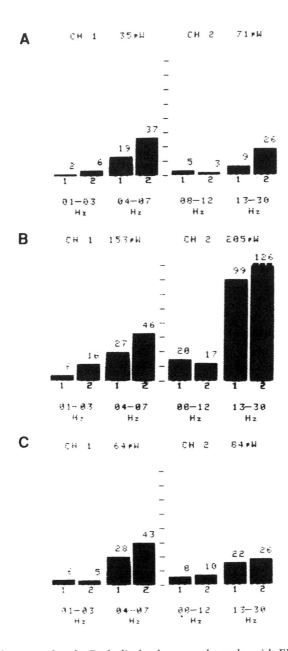

Figure 7.6 The power bands. Each display has two channels, with EEG power (y-axis) displayed in each of the standard beta, alpha, theta, and delta frequencies. A. Baseline with relatively low power spread across frequencies, but maximal in theta and delta bands. B. Electrical activation after a sedative dose of midazolam. Total EEG power increases; changes are not bilaterally symmetrical. C. Return of power bands toward baseline after administration of the benzodiazepine antagonist flumazenil.

In attempts to simplify the data presented as the EEG, numerical representations of computerized analysis have been developed. These include determinations of power in each of the bands and the total EEG power. **Combinations and ratios of these powers have been evaluated** as monitoring parameters. For example, ratios between theta and beta powers and delta and alpha powers have been used, as have left-right **power ratios**. Many of these quantitative techniques have not gained wide clinical application.

CLINICAL APPLICATIONS OF COMPUTERIZED ELECTROENCEPHALOGRAM ANALYSIS

Computerized EEG analysis has been developed in attempts to present large amounts of EEG data in a more easily readable and understandable format for surgeons and anesthesiologists, primarily in the intraoperative situation. Cerebrovascular surgery has probably become the most common application. Monitoring cerebral activity during cardiopulmonary bypass and deliberate hypotension has also been done. Attempts have been made to correlate changes in various analyzed parameters with anesthetic depth.

Most instruments allow selection of sensitivity, frequency range, and epoch length. An epoch that is too short results in erratic results. An epoch of 8–15 seconds can provide more stability. However, this would be inappropriate for monitoring a discontinuous pattern, such as burst suppression. The detectability of EEG changes is influenced by the type of change. During carotid cross-clamping, a commonly seen change is a shift from higher to lower frequencies with minor amplitude changes. This is usually detected with the baseline sensitivity and frequency range settings. Abrupt loss of amplitude across all recorded frequencies is a more severe change, but the overall frequency spectrum and SEF are stable and only total power is decreased. The authors find that abrupt changes are often more easily detected by raw EEG.

Carotid Endarterectomy

Cross-clamping the common carotid artery, with the resulting decrease in cerebral blood flow (generally reported as below 18 ml/100 g/minute), alters EEG activity. Most often there is a marked decrease in fast frequencies or increased delta and theta activity with some fast-wave attenuation. The changes are often unilateral but can be bilateral depending on collateral blood flow and distribution of cerebral vascular disease (Figure 7.7). Although this is considered an excellent monitor for required shunt placement, neurologic deficits can occur during cross-clamp that are not detected by raw or computerized EEG.

Anesthetic Depth

EEG changes vary widely between patients and anesthetic agents making assessment of anesthetic depth based on EEG parameters difficult to document

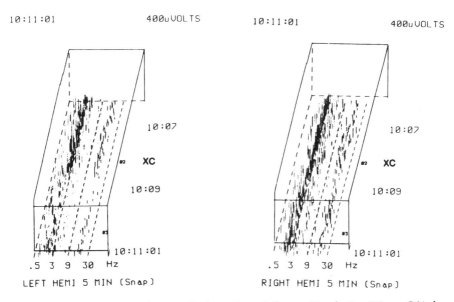

LEFT HEMI 5 MIN (Snap)   RIGHT HEMI 5 MIN (Snap)

Figure 7.7 A periodic time-domain display using a Lifescan (Datek, San Diego, CA) during carotid endarterectomy. Frequency is on the x-axis in a nonlinear scale. Amplitude is the vertical "pole"—the top of the transparent box is 400 µV. The 5-minute data window represented shows attenuation of high-range frequency on the left after carotid occlusion (XC). *Reprinted with permission from TN Spackman, RJ Faust, RF Cucchiara, FW Sharbrough. A comparison of aperiodic analysis of the EEG with standard EEG and cerebral blood flow for detection of ischemia. Anesthesiology 1987;66: 230.*

for clinical use. The spectral edge frequency has been shown to move into lower frequencies with increased anesthetic agents (Figure 7.8). At this point there is no reliable relationship between intraoperative awareness and any of the EEG parameters. New attempts are being made to correlate middle latency auditory evoked potentials rather than EEG with level of anesthesia.

Other Clinical and Physiologic Effects and the Electroencephalogram

Use of computerized EEG monitoring has resulted in application of other clinical findings. Interruption of cerebral circulation with extreme positioning can induce loss of EEG power and the spectral edge frequency (Figure 7.9). Cardiac arrest can result in rapid deterioration in neuroelectric signals (Figure 7.10). Although burst suppression can best be followed on raw EEG, it can also be assessed with computerized EEG analysis (Figure 7.11). These findings have led to use of computerized EEG for monitoring during hypothermic cardiopulmonary arrest, cerebral aneurysm clipping, and barbiturate coma induction for cerebral protection or treatment of refractory intracranial hypertension.

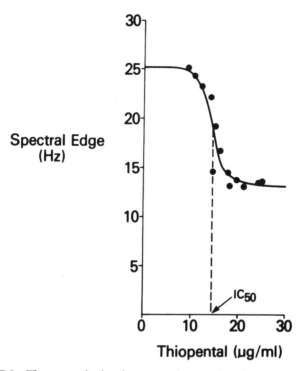

Figure 7.8 The spectral edge frequency decreased with increased thiopental blood levels. *Reprinted with permission from RJ Hudson, DR Stanski, LJ Sandman, E Meathe. A model for studying depth of anesthesia and acute tolerance to thiopental. Anesthesiology 1983; 59:305.*

BISPECTRAL ANALYSIS

Bispectral analysis is an advance in signal processing with high computational requirements applied to quantitation of EEG. Other methods of computerized EEG analysis assume that the EEG is a linear system, a superposition of statistically independent component waves. That is, the idealized neuroelectric sine waves produced by the cerebral cortex are noninteractive. However, the brain, like other natural biology-based systems, is nonlinear. That is, the component waves produced are interactive and produce additional dependent waves. A **quadratic coupling** or **phase-coupling** among various component waves occurs. One of the initial applications of this analysis was for study of the interaction of ocean wave motion. In the EEG, for example, sine waves at 3 Hz and 6 Hz produce a harmonic or an additional sine wave at 9 Hz. Both the harmonic frequency and phase are equal to the sum of the individual wave frequencies and phases, respectively.

Bispectral analysis quantifies cross-coupling, or the interaction between the components. The degree of phase-coupling between possible pairs of frequency waves and the frequency at the sum of the pairs is determined. This measure of

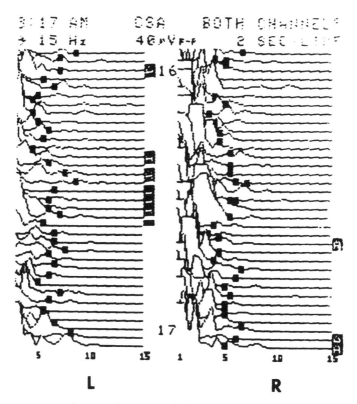

Figure 7.9 Compressed spectral array with the head in extension. Note loss of EEG power and spectral edge frequency in the left hemisphere. *Reprinted with permission from ED Steele, MS Albin, JL Monts, PK Harman. Compressed spectral array EEG monitoring during coronary bypass surgery in a patient with vertebrobasilar artery insufficiency. Anesth Analg 1987; 66: 272.*

phase-coupling at individual frequencies, or **biocoherence**, can be expressed as a percentage variable (0–100%). A noninteractive, or linear, system has a biocoherence of 0%. A nonlinear system, such as EEG, would have biocoherence peaks for the frequency pairs. The amount of neuroelectric activity in a given frequency due to harmonic effects and that due to independent generators can be estimated. Because the biocoherence pattern varies in different cerebral states, the data monitored (frequency, power, and phase of the bispectrum) can be used to generate, by algorithm, the **bispectral index**, a numerical representation of cerebral function. This allows subtle changes in EEG waveforms to be detected for both linear and nonlinear systems. This EEG analysis modality is currently being studied in relation to depth of anesthesia, but full clinical applicability is not yet clear.

Computerized EEG analysis has many clinical applications. It offers easier interpretation to the nonencephalographer, but the information gained can also

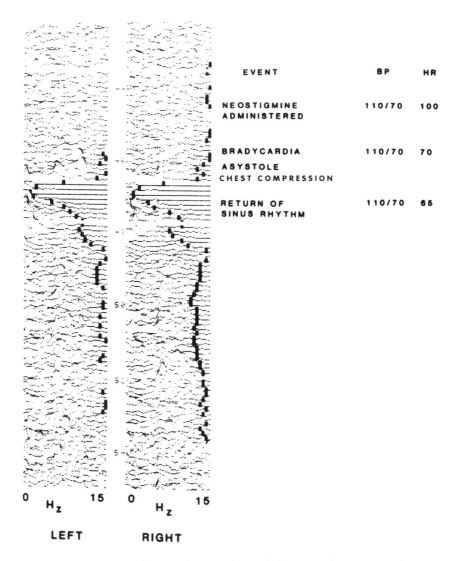

Figure 7.10   Compressed spectral array obtained during cardiac arrest and resuscitation. The numbers between left and right channels are minutes. Dark columns denote spectral edge frequency (SEF). Each line is an 8-second epoch. Cardiac events are noted. *Reprinted with permission from WL Young, E Ornstein. Compressed spectral array EEG monitoring during cardiac arrest and resuscitation. Anesthesiology 1985; 62:537.*

be altered by the parameters requested by the user. Variations in epoch length can influence the data presented. If the user is relying on a derived number or statistical interpretation of fitted data, it is important to realize the potential shortcomings and prevent misinterpretations of the information presented.

BURST-SUPPRESSION

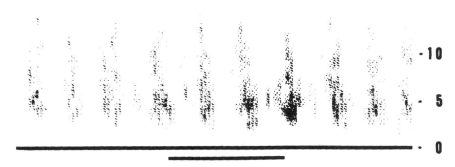

Figure 7.11 The density spectral array demonstrates a burst suppression pattern during cardiopulmonary bypass at a core temperature of 26°C with 1% end-tidal halothane present. Bursts of EEG activity repeat approximately every 20 seconds. *Reprinted with permission from WJ Levy. Quantitative analysis of EEG changes during hypothermia. Anesthesiology 1984; 60:293.*

KEY REFERENCES

Levy WJ, Shapiro HM, Maruchak G, Meathe E. Anesthesiology 1980;53:223. *Although 15 years old, this comparison of available techniques is still relevant in its applicability and basic information.*

McMeniman WJ, Purcell GJ. Neurological monitoring during anesthesia and surgery. Anaesth Intens Care 1988;16:358. *A clear and concise review suitable for an initial introduction.*

Rampil IJ. What every neuroanesthesiologist should know about electroencephalograms and computerized monitors. Anesthesiol Clin North Am 1992;10:683. *An excellent and thorough review. A good introduction to the background of EEG, computerized EEG data presentation, and clinical applicability.*

RECOMMENDED READING

Archibald JE, Drazkowski JF. Clinical applications of compressed spectral analysis (CSA) in OR/ICU settings. Am J EEG Techn 1985;25:13. *A useful collection of clinical applications and recordings of the CSA.*

Barnett TP, Johnson LC, Naitoh P, Hicks N, Nute C. Bispectrum analysis of electroencephalogram signals during waking and sleeping. Science 1971;172:401.

Fleming RA, Smith NT. Density modulation—a technique for the display of three-variable data in patient monitoring. Anesthesiology 1979;50:543.

Long CW, Shah NK, Loughlin C et al. A comparison of EEG determinants of near-awakening from isoflurane and fentanyl anesthesia. Spectral edge, median power frequency, and delta ratio. Anesth Analg 1989;69:169.

Rampil IJ, Holzer JA, Quest DO, Rosenbaum SH, Correll J. Prognostic value of computerized EEG analysis during carotid endarterectomy. Anesth Analg 1983;62:186.

Steele ER, Albin MS, Monts JL, Harman PK. Compressed spectral array EEG monitoring during coronary bypass surgery in a patient with vertebrobasilar artery insufficiency. Anesth Analg 1987;66: 271.

Vernon J, Bowles S, Sebel PS, Chaumon N. EEG bispectrum predicts movement at incision during isoflurane or propofol anesthesia. Anesthesiology 1992;77: A502.

8

Intraoperative Electrocorticography

David P. Archer, M.D., M.Sc., FRCPC
Francis E. LeBlanc, M.D., Ph.D., FRCSC

Intraoperative diagnostic testing to localize resectable epileptogenic lesions includes tests of epileptic excitability (electrocorticography and intraoperative depth electrode recording) and tests of focal functional deficit (intraoperative psychometrics and interictal functional brain mapping). Functional brain mapping alone may guide the limits of a safe resection of a nonepileptogenic lesion that encroaches on a brain region vital for normal function.

WHO? THE PATIENT AND PREOPERATIVE EPILEPTOGENIC LESION LOCALIZATION

The patient referred for resective surgery will have undergone a thorough evaluation to identify the type of seizures and the brain tissue in which they are most likely to originate. Diagnostic tests to localize epileptogenic lesions include diagnostic imaging (computed tomography, magnetic resonance imaging, positron emission tomography) and tests of epileptic excitability—videotaped ictal behavior, ictal and interictal electroencephalography (EEG), and chronic intracranial monitoring. To lateralize the location of essential structures, the evaluation also includes tests of focal functional deficit such as psychometric testing, and the intracarotid injection of amobarbital (Amytal)—the Wada test—to evaluate and localize speech and memory functions. Although the reliability of each of these testing modalities is controversial, a thorough diagnostic evaluation will identify patients with a resectable epileptogenic focus and will locate the lesion according to side and the intracerebral anatomic system.

WHY? GOALS OF ELECTROCORTICOGRAPHY
Electrocorticography

Electrocorticography (ECOG) refers to the intraoperative recording of potentials directly from the cortical surface. Jasper and Penfield developed this technique to guide cortical resection during surgery for intractable epilepsy. In current practice ECOG may help to (1) identify the epileptogenic zone, (2) delineate the extent of the resection, and (3) guide for additional resection when residual ECOG abnormalities persist after the initial removal. Brain stimulation can (1) identify landmarks on the cortical surface (e.g., the sensorimotor cortex), (2) evoke the initial aura characteristic of the patient's habitual seizure, (3) reproduce the interictal EEG, (4) locate brain regions (e.g., speech) that must be preserved, and (5) characterize the epileptogenic region by determining the distribution of thresholds for afterdischarge. The value of ECOG and stimulation in each of these roles varies with the type of epilepsy being treated, the brain region or regions involved, and the specific ECOG abnormalities present. The specific use of ECOG and brain mapping in determining the extent of excisions varies among different epilepsy surgery centers.

Brain Mapping with Cortical Stimulation
Temporal Lobectomy

During anterior temporal lobectomy, ECOG and hand-guided depth electrode recording refine the preoperative localization of the epileptogenic focus. In some circumstances, information obtained from cortical stimulation may allow the surgeon to extend resection limits defined by anatomical landmarks and measurements. Interference with naming and counting caused by cortical stimulation identifies speech areas in the posterior temporal lobe.

Frontal Excisions

Frontal resections can be quite extensive. The team may have difficulty localizing epileptogenic zones in the frontal lobe for two reasons: (1) Only a small portion of the cortex is accessible to ECOG, and (2) frontal lobe seizures tend to spread rapidly. It is common to observe simultaneous spiking in several frontal gyri; this does not preclude a successful resection. The resection must avoid the speech areas (Broca's area) usually located in the third frontal gyrus, immediately above the sylvian fissure (Figure 8.1). The specific cerebral location is highly variable. Since failure to interrupt speech by stimulation is no guarantee that the stimulated cortex is not functionally significant, some surgeons choose to limit their resection anatomically rather than pursue a prolonged search for a positive response to stimulation.

Sensorimotor Seizures

In patients with sensorimotor seizures without associated hemiparesis, localization of the epileptogenic lesion by ECOG and the demonstration of the potential postoperative functional deficits provide the basis for the limits of resections. Under the appropriate circumstances, the patient can experience what his or her postoperative condition might resemble and play a decisive role in the limits of the resection.

HOW? TECHNOLOGICAL ASPECTS OF ELECTROCORTICOGRAPHY AND STIMULATION
Recording the Electrocorticograph

The ECOG is recorded with sterile, flexible electrodes placed directly on the brain surface and connected to standard electroencephalographic amplifiers and

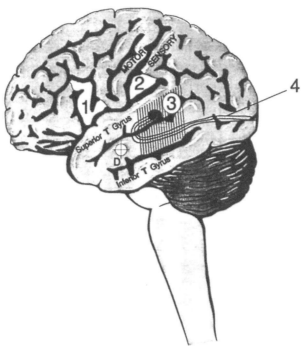

Figure 8.1 Lateral view of the brain surface showing regions of importance during cortical resection. 1. Broca's speech area in third frontal gyrus. 2. The region of the sensory cortex that commonly serves the tongue. 3. Wernicke's speech area (dominant hemisphere). 4. The visual pathways for the superior quadrant, radiating from the lateral geniculate nucleus to the visual cortex. This pathway limits the posterior resection margins for nondominant temporal lobectomy. D identifies the surface location on the middle temporal gyrus for insertion of a depth electrode, 4 cm from the temporal pole.

recording devices. A frame attached to a skull pin provides a stable platform for the array of 16 electrodes. A ball-joint attachment allows independent manipulation of each electrode. Electrodes are made from 10-cm lengths of insulated silver wire tipped with a smooth ball of carbon or silver-silver chloride. To record from the depths of the brain, the surgeon inserts a 3-cm insulated blunt needle equipped with ring-shaped contacts 1 cm apart. Depth recordings of paroxysmal activity from the medial aspects of the temporal lobe are particularly useful as a guide to the need for resection of the amygdala or the hippocampus or both.

To facilitate localization of foci, the surgeon arranges the electrodes on the cortical surface in four equally spaced parallel rows. The equidistant array of electrodes facilitates the production of horizontal or vertical sets of recordings when in bipolar mode.

Characteristics of Interictal Epileptiform Activity

During an interictal recording of the ECOG, the presence of random spikes may help to locate an epileptogenic area. Jasper first identified the random **spike discharge** as the principal interictal cortical electrographic manifestation pathognomonic of a locally discharging focus. He described a surface negative wave of 10- to 20-msec duration and an amplitude of 500–2,000 µV recorded at the brain surface (Figure 8.2A). Recorded from the scalp, random spikes are of 20- to 40-msec duration and 50–500 µV amplitude. When conducted across a distance, the spikes become temporally dispersed with a rapid rising phase and a more prolonged declining phase. These waves are called **sharp waves**. The site of the cortex in which they originate does not affect the electrocorticographic characteristics of spikes and sharp waves. The absence of normal background cortical rhythms, a visible lesion, and poststimulation afterdischarges all strengthen the diagnosis of an epileptogenic zone in a brain region with cortical spiking. Sharp waves, superimposed on a normal cortical background activity, may suggest conducted discharges.

Accurate evaluation of the significance of interictal activity on the ECOG requires considerable experience in EEG and ECOG interpretation to separate epileptiform activity from nonspecific spikes and sharp waves.

Effects of Anesthetics on Electrocorticography

Anesthetics may markedly alter both background and epileptiform activity. Our epilepsy service commonly suspends anticonvulsant administration preoperatively to increase the frequency of interictal discharges intraoperatively. Accordingly, the anesthesiologist should avoid the use of benzodiazepines. The influence of general anesthesia on the ECOG is more controversial. While some centers prefer to avoid general anesthesia, others have found that "light anesthesia" with nitrous oxide and isoflurane provides conditions suitable for ECOG. In early studies, Jasper noted that "light" general anesthesia with thiopental caused fast activity (17–24 Hz) whereas cyclopropane–nitrous oxide anesthesia produced slow waves. At low doses, thiopental, methohexital, and propofol (Figure 8.2B) increase the background fast activity and the spike and wave generation. For this reason, thiopental and methohexital are commonly used to "activate" the ECOG after the principal recordings have been obtained. Propofol may obscure epileptiform discharges on the ECOG. Drummond et al. have reported a case in which the fast activity from a propofol infusion outlasted the sedative effects of the drug and interfered significantly with the ECOG interpretation.

Techniques of Cortical Stimulation and Brain Mapping

Cortical stimulation may provoke a focal or generalized seizure. Consequently, cortical stimulation begins with nonepileptogenic regions with low thresholds for response (e.g., postcentral gyrus) and progresses to regions requiring stimuli of greater intensity. From subthreshold levels, the neurosurgeon slowly increases stimulus intensity until the patient feels a tingling sensation in the tongue, face, or hand. This procedure establishes the threshold for

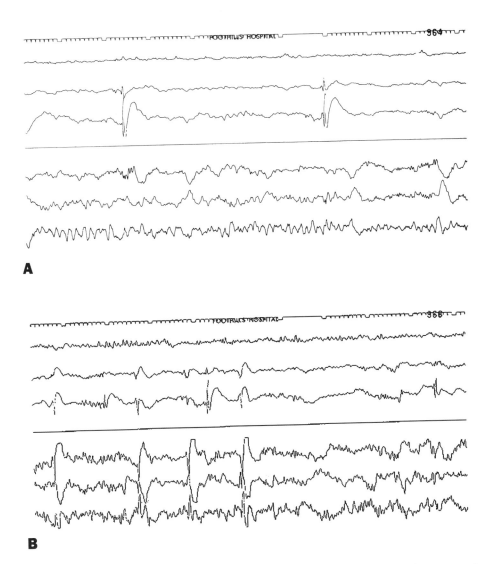

Figure 8.2 ECOG tracings from six electrodes on the surface of the anterior temporal lobe in a patient with partial complex seizures. A. Two of the three upper recordings demonstrate cortical spikes followed by waves, typical of interictal epileptogenic activity. B. ECOG recordings from the same electrodes following the administration of propofol, 30 mg. The spiking frequency in the upper tracings is increased and there is spread to previously unaffected sites.

stimulation in sensory cortex, which usually has a slightly lower threshold than motor cortex. The subsequent pattern of stimulation depends on the goals of brain mapping.

For patients with focal motor seizures, the surgeon may stimulate a series of cortical sites along the precentral gyrus to outline the somatotopic representation of the motor cortex. Finally the surgeon stimulates the region with the highest frequency of interictal epileptiform discharges on the ECOG. The goal is to identify a region that, when stimulated, reproduces the initial symptoms or aura of a patient's seizure with an accompanying electrographic after-discharge, although this is not always possible.

In patients with seizures of temporal lobe origin, stimulation frequently focuses on identifying the location of sensation for the tongue (see Figure 8.1). This landmark helps define the posterior extent of the temporal resection. In the dominant hemisphere, stimulation of the posterior aspects of the temporal lobe can locate the region essential for speech (Wernicke's area). In this role, cortical stimulation has both stimulatory and inhibitory effects. Stimulation in the association cortex outside the primary motor and sensory areas for speech disrupts an ongoing language task. It is generally accepted that a lesion in such an area within the temporal lobe will result in aphasia. Most aphasias are characterized by naming deficits; consequently, naming tasks are used to screen cortical sites for language function.

Stimulation parameters vary among different centers. Commonly, bipolar electrodes deliver 4- to 8-second trains of 1.0- to 2.5-msec duration biphasic waves at 50–60 Hz. Current levels range from 0.5–10.0 mA. The stimulus intensity required to evoke a response varies inversely with the stimulus frequency—60-Hz stimuli require a lesser stimulus intensity than 20-Hz stimuli. The stimulus intensity can also vary with the anesthetic level.

ECOG recording continues during cortical stimulation, to identify targets for stimulation, to observe the emergence of foci activated by the stimuli, and to detect the onset and spread of afterdischarges that may herald the beginning of a seizure.

HOW? ANESTHETIC CONSIDERATIONS FOR PROCEDURES REQUIRING INTRAOPERATIVE ELECTROCORTICOGRAPHY AND BRAIN MAPPING
Awake Craniotomy

Neurosurgeons recommend craniotomy in the awake state to patients whose intraoperative cooperation is necessary to map and preserve eloquent areas of cerebral cortex. While craniotomy under local anesthesia is most often performed for the resection of epileptogenic cerebral tissue, the surgical excision of brain tumors or vascular malformations that border on or invade eloquent brain areas can more safely be performed with the cooperation of the awake patient. Whatever the reason, the key to successful craniotomy in the awake patient lies in the communication skills of the surgeon, the anesthesiologist, and the nursing staff. These patients require constant explanation of the proceedings and reassurance both before and during the surgical procedure to maintain their motivation and their cooperation.

The Preoperative Visit

During the preoperative visit, the anesthesiologist must assess the specific issues concerning the patient, the lesion, and the surgical plan that determine the choice of anesthetic conditions.

A sequential description of the planned procedure as it will unfold helps establish a relationship between the anesthesiologist and the patient. This discussion should not be rushed. The anesthesiologist should encourage the patient to ask questions and make comments concerning such issues as the length of the procedure, pain, nausea and vomiting, and the plan for control of a seizure. The anesthesiologist should review the reasons for planning an awake procedure and the principal anesthetic risks (intraoperative pain and pulmonary aspiration during sedation or during a seizure).

Phase I: Positioning, Conscious Sedation, Scalp Infiltration, and the Opening

The combination of a scalp block with neuroleptanalgesia is popular for craniotomy in awake patients. Preoperative sedation is commonly avoided. The patient is transferred from the bed or stretcher to a comfortably padded table and placed in the lateral recumbent position. Monitoring devices for electrocardiogram, blood pressure (noninvasive), pulse oximetry, and respiration are applied. The anesthesiologist then administers light sedation with droperidol (5–15 mg) and an opioid, either by intermittent bolus or by continuous infusion. The goal is to provide analgesia and sedation while preserving the patient's ability to maintain the airway and to respond to verbal command. This state has been called "conscious sedation." In this setting equivalent infusion strategies of opioids appear to be (1) fentanyl—bolus 0.75 µg/kg, infusion 0.01 µg/kg/minute; (2) sufentanil—bolus 0.075 µg/kg, infusion 0.0015 µg/kg/minute; (3) alfentanil—bolus 7.5 µg/kg, infusion 0.5 µg/kg/minute. With these strategies, the total dose of opioid administered is similar to the total amount given by intermittent injection. If a sedating antinauseant (e.g., dimenhydrinate, 0.25 mg/kg) is given, the dose of droperidol should be reduced to 0.014 mg/kg.

The neurosurgeon infiltrates the scalp with a dilute solution of long-acting local anesthetic beginning with the auriculotemporal, supraorbital, and supratrochlear nerves. Infiltration continues along the planned incision line in the subcutaneous plane and down to the galea. In our center, 60–80 ml of 0.25% bupivacaine with epinephrine, 5 µg/ml, is injected, giving a total dose of 2–3 mg/kg. Arterial bupivacaine concentrations peak during the 5–10 minutes after the infiltration is complete. Signs and symptoms of local anesthetic toxicity following infiltration are uncommon.

Following the surgical preparation, the team applies the surgical drapes so that the patient has a clear view of the anesthesiologist. Oxygen is supplied, either through nasal prongs or simply under the drapes around the patient's face. The anesthesiologist should position the draping supports to facilitate access to the patient's head should assisted ventilation or tracheal intubation become necessary. The neurosurgeon may suture the drapes to the scalp to preserve the sterile field if there is an intraoperative seizure. This is an opportunity to supplement any deficiencies in the scalp block.

It is essential that the anesthesiologist and neurosurgeon maintain communication with the patient during this initial phase of the operation. To ease the patient into the procedure, each step is introduced slowly; explanations, support, and additional analgesia or infiltration are provided when required. To avoid a startle response, the team warns the patient that the drill and craniotome produce noise and vibrations during the turning of the bone flap. The elevation of the bone flap may be painful and the neurosurgeon should be ready to provide additional local anesthesia around the middle meningeal artery and the dural nerves as required. Additional sedation and analgesia may be provided until this infiltration is complete.

Phase II: The Electrocorticography Recording, Stimulation, and the Resection

The full cooperation of the theater team is essential during recording and stimulation. The anesthesiologist must have planned the management so that there is minimal interference between anesthetic agents and the ECOG. In patients managed with conscious-sedation analgesia, the patient must be sufficiently comfortable to be cooperative yet alert enough to respond to stimulation, to provide useful answers to questions, and to alert the anesthesiologist to the onset of an aura. During stimulation, communication among the team members is essential. The ECOG team must monitor carefully for the onset and spread of after-discharges. The electroencephalographer or the neurosurgeon must alert the anesthesiologist when stimulation is likely to provoke convulsions. This occurs particularly when epileptogenic areas are being stimulated or when stimuli of high intensity are being delivered. During these periods, the anesthesiology, neurosurgery, and theater support teams must be thoroughly prepared for emergency management of a seizure.

After completion of electrocorticography and mapping, the neurosurgeon performs the resection. At this time the patient may be heavily sedated as a result of thiopental or methohexital administered as an activating agent.

Phase III: The Closure

Following a postresection ECOG recording, the craniotomy is closed. For patient comfort the anesthesiologist may administer small intravenous doses of benzodiazepines or additional opioid, either as boluses or as an infusion as outlined above. Droperidol or other long-acting drugs given early in the procedure may exaggerate the effects of any of these intravenous drugs, so the anesthesiologist must carefully titrate small doses against the patient's level of sedation. With propofol infusions, we have found that a small induction dose (20- to 30-mg bolus), followed by a low-dose infusion such as 1.75–2.50 mg/kg/hour (25–40 µg/kg/minute) can produce adequate sedation in many patients. We aim for a minimally depressed level of consciousness, hoping to preserve the patient's capacity to maintain and protect the airway. It is often very tempting to sedate the patient heavily (i.e., to the point that the patient will not respond purposefully to verbal command). However, it is likely that once consciousness is lost, the patient is at greater risk for airway complications such as obstruction and aspiration. Occasionally, the patient requires deeper levels of sedation. In such situations the anesthesiologist and the neurosurgeon must decide whether to secure the airway or to continue without tracheal intubation. The team usually bases the decision on the patient's behavior, including any nausea or vomiting. The anesthesiologist will also have observed the ease with which the patency of the patient's airway could be maintained during the case. It is the anesthesiologist's role to balance the difficulty and risks of continuing without tracheal intubation against the problems of securing the airway. Although the closure may be a trying period for the patient, in our institution it is very uncommon that we convert to general anesthesia with tracheal intubation at this time. Encouragement and support from the anesthesiologist and the neurosurgeon usually enable the patient to complete the procedure under conscious sedation.

General Anesthetic Conditions Suitable for Electrocorticography

If the team plans to perform the resection under general anesthesia, the anesthesiologist should explain that the patient may be aware during periods when the depth of anesthesia is reduced to optimize ECOG recording. To provide pain relief during these periods, the neurosurgeon may infiltrate the scalp with local anesthetic as for awake craniotomy. Positioning and preparation are the same as for awake craniotomy. Since the patient may move during periods when the depth of anesthesia and neuromuscular blockade are reduced, we avoid, when possible, the use of rigid skull fixation.

There is little agreement concerning the effects of light levels of general anesthesia on interictal epileptiform activity. Low concentrations of GABA-ergic agents such as propofol, methohexital, and thiopental accentuate beta activity in the ECOG, which may obscure spikes. As in awake craniotomy, we avoid benzodiazepines. We usually select either an opioid-relaxant technique with nitrous oxide or a balanced technique in which we also add low concentrations of isoflurane. Before ECOG recording and cortical stimulation, we administer additional opioid and then eliminate any volatile anesthetic used during the opening. We monitor neuromuscular blockade and adjust the depth to enable visualization of three of four twitches on the train-of-four. This usually permits hand, arm, or face movement when the neurosurgeon stimulates the corresponding motor cortex.

WHAT DO I DO NOW? COMMON PROBLEMS AND SOLUTIONS

The most serious anesthetic challenges are dysphoric or panic reactions and generalized tonic-clonic convulsions. Either of these problems may provoke the team to initiate general anesthesia. Although an intravenous bolus of barbiturate (thiopental, 25–50 mg, or methohexital, 30–40 mg) may quickly abort a seizure, the patient is often confused and combative in the postictal period. The team should anticipate the possibility that if the anesthesiologist cannot regain verbal control of the patient, general anesthesia will have to be induced. Generalized seizures may generate a severe metabolic acidosis, for which the patient usually compensates with marked hyperventilation. Consequently, the anesthesiologist should, if possible, avoid rendering the patient apneic until it is certain that the airway can be rapidly secured and mechanical hyperventilation begun. There is no "method of choice" for tracheal intubation in these trying circumstances. The best method is the most rapid and reliable technique for the anesthesiologist in charge.

Nausea and vomiting are common despite the administration of relatively large doses of droperidol. Some centers routinely add dimenhydrinate while others administer antinauseants as required. Unfortunately nausea and vomiting are not simply a discomfort for the patient. Unexpected movement during delicate dissections can be extremely dangerous, and if the patient vomits while deeply sedated, aspiration is a possibility. In our hands, the best solution is to maintain close communication with the patient, who will warn the team if nausea becomes a problem. At that point, delicate surgery is suspended while antinauseants are administered. If the neurosurgeon suspects that traction on unanesthetized mesial dural structures is provoking the nausea, then additional local anesthetic infiltration may be indicated.

Brain swelling is an uncommon problem and occurs most frequently following a generalized seizure. However, the conditions present during awake craniotomy differ from those provided by general anesthesia with hyperventilation. During the opening, the brain often fills the dura and may start to herniate through the initial dural incision. At this time, we request that the patient hyperventilate briefly, relaxing the brain until the dura opening is large enough to avoid laceration of cortical vessels. After the opening, drainage of CSF usually reduces brain volume significantly, providing for excellent conditions for closure even in a heavily sedated patient with spontaneous respiration.

SO WHAT? OUTCOME OF AWAKE CRANIOTOMY WITH ELECTROCORTICOGRAPHY AND BRAIN MAPPING
Intraoperative Anesthetic Morbidity and Mortality

Anesthetic techniques may influence the outcome of resections performed with ECOG and brain mapping in two different ways. First, the anesthetic technique may affect operative conditions and may affect the usual measures of perioperative morbidity and mortality. Second, the anesthetic technique may influence the reduction of seizures by the surgical resection.

Intraoperatively, the main morbid events are (1) seizures (16% of cases), (2) nausea and vomiting (8%), (3) excessive sedation (3%), (4) "tight" brain (1.4%), and (5) possible local anesthetic toxicity (2%). In approximately 2% of patients, the team intraoperatively elected to convert the anesthetic to general anesthesia. We are not aware of any study that has systematically examined intraoperative patient comfort. Craniotomy for temporal lobe resection using conscious-sedation analgesia appears to be safe. In a study of over 2,000 awake procedures, Rasmussen did not report any intraoperative pulmonary aspiration or death.

Influence of the Anesthetic Technique on Surgical Success

It is difficult to evaluate the influence of awake techniques on the effectiveness of cortical resection. Clinicians measure the outcome of epilepsy surgery by the reduction in the seizure frequency. Epilepsy centers commonly classify postoperative outcome into four categories: (1) seizure-free, (2) reduction of seizure frequency by 75% or more, (3) reduction by 50%, and (4) slight improvement or no change. Although this measure appears quite reasonable, two experienced investigators classifying results from the same group of patients differed by more than 20%.

If anesthetic techniques affect the outcome of procedures with relatively standardized resections (e.g., anterior temporal lobectomy), they probably do so by altering the sensitivity or specificity (or both) of ECOG. However, the role of ECOG in guiding resection limits is controversial, with some centers relying more heavily on anatomic landmarks. Thus, it is likely that current outcome measures are not sufficiently sensitive to detect the effects of anesthetic techniques.

RECOMMENDED READING

Archer DP, McKenna JMA, Morin L, Ravussin P. Conscious-sedation analgesia during craniotomy for intractable epilepsy: a review of 354 consecutive cases. Can J Anaesth 1988;35:338. *This is a retrospective review of anesthetic results and complications during awake craniotomy for epilepsy surgery.*

Bernier GP, Saint-Hilaire J-M, Giard N, Bouvier G, Mercier M. Commentary: intracranial stimulation. In J Engel Jr (ed), Surgical Treatment of the Epilepsies. New York: Raven, 1987. P 324. *This is an excellent summary of the methods and interpretation of stimulation techniques used worldwide.*

Drummond JC, Iraqui-Madoz V, Alksne JF, Kalkman CJ. Masking of epileptiform activity by propofol during seizure surgery. Anesthesiology 1992;766:652.

Gignac E, Manninen PH, Gelb AW. Comparison of fentanyl, sufentanil and alfentanil during awake craniotomy for epilepsy. Can J Anaesth 1993;40:421.

Gloor P. Contributions of electroencephalography and electrocorticography to the neurosurgical treatment of the epilepsies. In DP Purpura, JK Penry (eds), Advances in Neurology. Vol 8. New York: Raven, 1975. P 66. *This paper provides an excellent overview of the role of ECOG in epilepsy surgery.*

Jasper HH. Electrical signs of epileptic discharge. EEG Clin Neurophysiol 1949;1:11–18. *This paper provides the original description of the interictal ECOG findings in focal epilepsy.*

Manninen P, Contreras J. Anesthetic considerations for craniotomy in awake patients. Int Anesthesiol Clin 1986;24:157.

McBride MC, Binnie CD, Janota I, Polkey CE. Predictive value of intraoperative electro-corticograms in resective epilepsy surgery. Ann Neurol 1991;30:526. *This is one of the few prospective evaluations of ECOG.*

McCarthy FM, Soloman AL, Jastak J et al. Conscious sedation: benefits and risks. J Am Dent Assoc 1984;109:46

Ojemann, GA. Brain organization for language from the perspective of electrical stimulation mapping. Behav Brain Sci 1983;6:189. *This paper provides a detailed description of the localization of speech function during epilepsy surgery.*

Olivier A. Commentary: Cortical resection. In J Engel Jr (ed), Surgical Treatment of the Epilepsies. New York: Raven, 1987. Pp 404–416. *This is a summary of many of the current controversies in epilepsy surgery.*

Penfield W, Jasper H. Epilepsy and the Functional Anatomy of the Human Brain. Boston: Little, Brown, 1954. *This is the original comprehensive textbook describing the techniques for epilepsy treatment developed by the Montreal School.*

Rasmussen, TB. Surgical treatment of complex-partial seizures: results, lessons, and problems. Epilepsia 1983;24:S65. *This study reports results from the largest series of cortical excisions for epilepsy.*

Trop D. Conscious-sedation analgesia during the neurosurgical treatment of the epilepsies—practice at the Montreal Neurological Institute. Int Anesthesiol Clin 1986;24:175. *This and the article by Manninen and Contreras provide a comprehensive description of the anesthetic techniques used in two different centers doing cortical resection under local anesthesia.*

Wilder BJ, Musella L, Van Horn G, Schmidt RP. Activation of spike and wave discharge in patients with generalized seizures. Neurology 1971;21:517. *One of the first descriptions of "activation procedures" for identification of epileptogenic tissue.*

9

The Epilepsy Monitoring Unit As an Extension of the Operating Room

Lawrence D. Rodichok, M.D.

Although intraoperative electroencephalography (EEG) is used in some epilepsy centers as a guide during surgical resection, it may be impractical and inadequate in localizing the epileptic focus itself. In those patients in whom scalp EEG monitoring has failed to localize the focus sufficiently or other diagnostic studies have failed to provide concordant localizing information, it may be necessary to record ictal onsets from intracranial electrodes. Although intraoperative electrocorticography can provide information concerning areas of irritability, in most cases this alone is not sufficient to permit resection.

SEIZURE IDENTIFICATION

It is necessary to record both electrically and on videotape a series of the patient's habitual seizures in an epilepsy monitoring unit (EMU) to properly identify an area of brain for therapeutic resection. It is unlikely that a sustained ictal discharge will occur in a short operative period. It is certainly unlikely that a clinical seizure will occur such that it can be identified clinically as the patient's habitual seizure type. It would also be impossible to record a series of seizures to confirm a stereotyped clinical pattern in the operating room.

INTRACRANIAL ELECTRODES

It has become the standard in most epilepsy centers that intracranial electrodes are placed stereotactically in locations appropriate to the patient's seizure pattern and the patient is then placed in an intensive video and EEG monitoring unit to record as many ictal onsets as necessary (Figure 9.1). In some instances a large area of the brain may be covered with grids of subdural electrodes to detect the source of seizures that had been previously localized to that general region (Figure 9.2). The use of this type of intracranial electrode allows for extensive coverage so that areas that might be the source of the patient's seizures can be recorded. With modern digital telemetry equipment as many as 128 or more contacts can be recorded simultaneously and continuously and later reformatted in any desired montage (Figure 9.3).

109

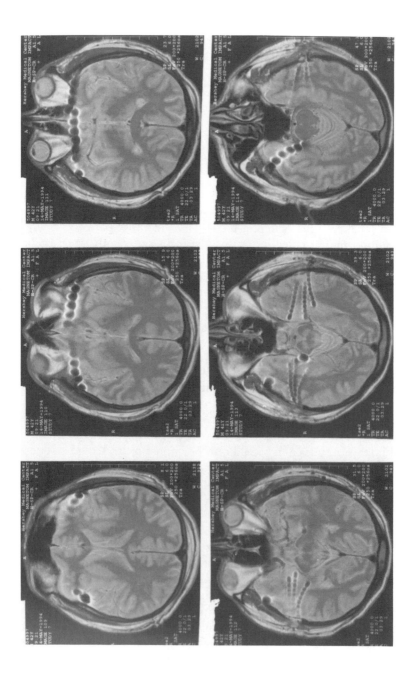

Figure 9.1 Magnetic resonance imaging scans showing placement of both intracerebral "depth" electrodes and subdural strip electrodes in a patient being evaluated for epilepsy surgery.

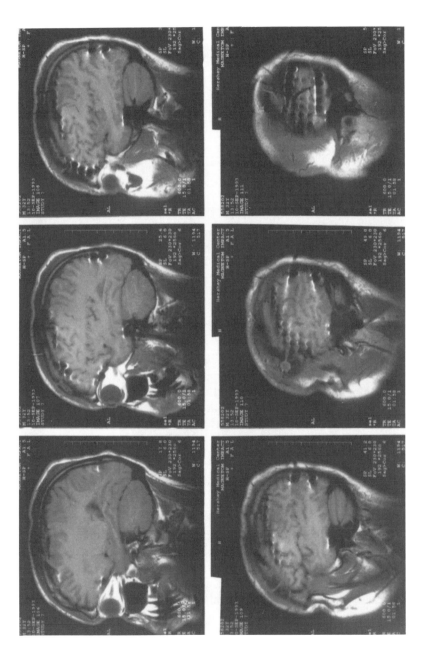

Figure 9.2 A series of sagittal magnetic resonance imaging scans shows the presence of a large (8 contact by 8 contact) grid of electrodes over the left hemisphere. This grid (along with other subdural strips) was used both for recording ictal onsets and for later stimulation studies for functional cortical mapping.

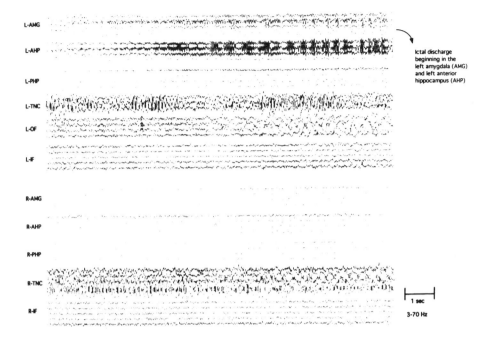

Figure 9.3 Example of a recording of an ictal onset using modern digital equipment and an array of intracerebral and subdural electrodes. Onset is seen in channels 1–8 as a high-frequency discharge beginning in second number 2.

Subdural strips and depth electrodes are placed through burr holes. They are removed after monitoring is complete and the patient is then discharged to return for surgery, if indicated, at a later date. Placement of subdural grids requires a craniotomy; therefore, the patient will have surgery, if indicated, immediately after monitoring is completed.

Monitoring in the Epilepsy Monitoring Unit

While the recording of seizures in an EMU has largely replaced intraoperative monitoring for interictal spikes, the EMU has also become an alternate site for functional cortical mapping. In the operating room this is accomplished with direct cortical surface stimulation, often while the patient is awake, especially if language and other areas of higher cortical function are to be localized. This approach is limited by all the constraints of an awake craniotomy, including time limitations. In many instances it is preferable to implant subdural grids that will be used both for recording seizures and for stimulation studies to be performed in the EMU. With this approach more time is available for functional mapping and the patient is much more comfortable and therefore capable of the concentration required for some of the tasks involved. Often this type of functional mapping takes place over a day or two. This allows detailed testing of language and other types of higher cortical function, in a setting comfortable and quiet for the patient and staff. Results can be corroborated by repetition if necessary, without the concern for the time limitations of the intraoperative setting. This type of mapping has the disadvantage that stimulation is limited by the location of the electrodes on the grids and strips and also by the current density allowed by their size and proximity to the cortex. Intraoperative stimulation is usually applied with a handheld stimulator that can be moved at will to any desired location that is exposed. At the present time many centers use both procedures when necessary to fully localize areas of critical function to be avoided during resection.

KEY REFERENCES

Engel J Jr (ed). Surgical Treatment of the Epilepsies (2nd ed). New York: Raven, 1993.
Luders HO. Epilepsy Surgery. New York: Raven, 1992. *Multiple chapters in each of these sources deal with the techniques involved in recording seizures and the performance of functional mapping in the epilepsy monitoring unit.*

10

Intraoperative Evoked Potentials: Technical Standards and Instrumentation

Lawrence D. Rodichok, M.D.

In nearly all instances, "evoked potentials" represent electrophysiologic responses to stimulation of an afferent pathway. Most often it is possible to record a sequence of such potentials along the pathway of interest and to measure the latency between potentials. Through comparison with established norms it is then possible to detect the presence and approximate location of areas of pathology affecting the pathway being tested. This comparison has become especially useful in detecting areas of demyelination, which are often asymptomatic, in patients with multiple sclerosis. In a few instances, such as with motor evoked potentials, an efferent pathway is stimulated and responses are recorded peripherally.

NEUROPHYSIOLOGIC BASIS OF EVOKED POTENTIALS

Most evoked potentials appear to represent one of two general types of electrical phenomena: (1) a wave of depolarization as it travels along an axonal bundle (such as a peripheral nerve) or central pathway (such as the posterior columns), or (2) the synchronized depolarization of a nucleus in such an afferent pathway (like the posterior column nuclei or the cochlear nucleus). The first is sometimes called a "traveling wave" and is usually detected by an electrode placed near the pathway. Its latency depends on the location of the electrode; that is, it will be earlier if placed distally and later if placed more rostrally. These potentials are also examples of "near-field potentials"; their detection depends on placing an electrode close to the generator, and their amplitude falls off as distance from the source lengthens. An example of a near-field potential is that recorded over a peripheral nerve after distal stimulation. Some near-field potentials are from neuronal sources (the cortical component of the somatosensory evoked potential [SSEP]) or from depolarization of the afferent endings themselves, as with wave I on the auditory evoked response. In the latter cases the amplitude does fall off with distance, but the latency is not affected by electrode location. Far-field potentials occur at the same latency no matter where the recording electrode is placed. These are most often generated at a nucleus by the temporal summation of excitatory postsynaptic potentials. An example of a far-field potential is the N13 of the SSEP by median nerve stimulation. Waves II–V of the auditory response are also far-field potentials.

INSTRUMENTATION

Most of the clinically useful evoked potentials are in the microvolt and often submicrovolt range. Thus, they are considerably smaller than the non–event-related, spontaneous biologic activity such as that measured by electromyography, electrocardiography, and even electroencephalography (EEG). In addition there are invariably numerous sources of electronic interference, such as from 60-Hz power sources and from other instruments. The operating room (OR) is an especially "hostile" environment in this regard.

Signal Averaging

Sophisticated computer averagers are required to recognize and analyze these small event-related potentials. The stimulus generator triggers acquisition of a series of samples for a prescribed interval after the stimulus. This is repeated until background activity, having a random relationship to the stimulus, is "averaged out" and the stimulus-related potential can be identified. The contribution of the random activity is reduced by a factor equal to the square root of the number of events in the average—i.e., $\sqrt{N}$. The signal-to-noise ratio is improved by a factor of 10 when 100 events are averaged. This rule applies to wide-band background noise. Many EEG events are single transients that are unlikely to occur in the same location again. The contribution of these is reduced by a factor of $1/N$. Of course, the more averages acquired the better the signal-to-noise ratio, although the proportional improvement diminishes with continued averaging.

Sampling Frequency

The response to the stimulus must be sampled often enough to identify the series of relatively high-frequency waves that follow. When the samples are taken more frequently, the instrument recognizes the presence of a triggered potential more easily. By the Nyquist theorem, the minimum sampling rate is twice the rate of the highest frequency of interest. For example, the frequencies of the early components of an auditory evoked potential are in the range of 1,000 Hz (about one wave every millisecond). Thus, the sampling rate of the A-to-D converter must be at least 2,000 Hz (2,000 samples per second) to resolve the response. This is sometimes referred to as "horizontal resolution." Most modern instruments are capable of much higher sampling rates—up to 1 MHz. For an instrument with a sampling rate of 250 KHz, each sample would represent a 4-μs epoch. This is sometimes called the "dwell time" or the "intersample interval."

Vertical Resolution

The ability of the instrument to resolve vertically is determined in part by the analog-to-digital (A/D) converter since this determines the number of possible increments in amplitude that can be detected. Most current instruments have at least a "12-bit" A/D converter allowing 2^{12} (4,096) possible vertical steps. The value of a powerful A/D converter is lost if the amplification of the signal is not adequate. This is, in turn, determined by the differential amplifier system. Gains of 100,000–250,000 are necessary for auditory and somatosensory studies. Sensitivity is often in the range of 1–10 μV full scale. As with horizontal resolution, the number of responses in the average does affect vertical resolution. The actual vertical resolution may be calculated by dividing the full-scale sensitivity by the number of possible vertical steps and then by the number of responses in the average. Thus, at 10 μV full scale, using a 12-bit A/D converter, after 100 responses are averaged, the vertical sensitivity would be 10/4,096/100 or 2.44×10^{-3} μV.

Filtering

The differential amplifier plays a critical role in the initial acquisition and amplification of the biological signals of interest. It also provides the initial rejection of interfering electrical activity. This is accomplished through the use of common-mode rejection and filtering. Differential amplifiers have two inputs (often called "grid 1" and "grid 2," or the negative and positive). The output of this type of amplifier is the algebraic difference between the two inputs (input 2 is inverted and then added to input 1). Thus, signals that are common to the two inputs, such as 60-Hz interference, cancel each other, while those unique to one or the other inputs, such as an underlying biological event, are amplified. The common-mode rejection ratio, an expression of the ability of the amplifier to reject activity common to the two inputs in comparison to noncommon signals such as the biological event of interest, is in the range of 20,000 to 1 for modern systems. The use of digital or analog filters may further refine the signal before it is passed on to the A/D converter. These filters must be used so as not to distort the biological signal. The high-frequency filter may be used to eliminate interference, but excessively low settings may also distort or even eliminate the evoked response. The high-frequency filter may also cause a phase shift in the frequencies of interest such that latencies are erroneously delayed. For this reason, in the OR it is undesirable to change this filter during a procedure. Excessive low-frequency filtering can also distort or even eliminate the biological signal as well as cause a phase shift in the direction of earlier latency. The use of a 60-Hz notch filter is also discouraged because of its effect on frequencies of interest and because of "ringing"—i.e., the production of a frequency of about 60 Hz that can be mistaken for a biological response. Standards set by the American EEG Society for routine evoked potentials should serve as guidelines, although they may require slight modification in the OR. Usually slightly narrower bandpasses are permissible.

Electrodes

The final technical elements are the recording electrodes. These are usually metal cup electrodes made of gold or of silver and silver chloride. Some centers prefer to use subdermal needles. Electrodes must be placed in the proper locations, which vary depending on the type of study. Usually the head should be measured according to the standard ten-twenty system of electrode placement (see Chapter 5). Attention to proper skin preparation is essential for surface electrodes. Impedance below 5,000 Ω but above 500 Ω is essential. It is of equal importance that impedance be balanced between electrode pairs or the common-mode rejection capabilities of the differential amplifier will be partially defeated. Cup electrodes must be secured with collodion.

The Recorder

The characteristics of the recording instrument itself are also important. It must usually be specifically modified for OR use. Multiple recording channels are imperative, as it is for routine testing. This permits use of multiple recording sites along the pathway of interest as well as some redundancy of electrode derivations. For example, SSEPs may be recorded over the peripheral nerve stimulated, often at a spinal level and at the scalp level, sometimes using more than one derivation. At least four channels are needed for adequate intraoperative SSEPs. Automatic artifact rejection is essential. Most instruments reject any signal that is above a preset percentage of the maximum amplitude setting, usually 90%. Decreasing the sensitivity setting also lessens artifact rejection. Efforts to increase sensitivity result in increased automatic rejection. Some instruments permit operator specification of the artifact rejection level. Rejection should be set such that responses containing large-amplitude components that are probably artifact are eliminated from the average. OR instruments must provide the ability to compare the current average to one acquired at baseline, and preferably they should reveal the trend in responses over an extended time so that gradual deviations from the baseline can be recognized. For an increasing number of OR applications, it is very useful that the instrument be capable of displaying more than one type of signal, such as both evoked potentials and free-running electromyographic (EMG) activity.

Of course, all instruments used in the OR must meet intraoperative safety standards. Instruments used in the routine neurophysiology laboratory do not necessarily meet those standards. All intraoperative instruments must meet the most stringent standards for regular safety inspections. These should be well documented in a log book.

TECHNICAL STANDARDS

In general, it is best to start with the standards established by the American EEG Society for routine diagnostic evoked potentials. Some of these standards must be modified for the OR.

Personnel

The technical personnel involved in intraoperative evoked potential monitoring must be specifically trained both in recording evoked potentials and in applying them to the OR setting. Most such individuals have been previously trained in routine EEG and possibly intraoperative EEG. However, evoked potential recording is generally more difficult than EEG, and it cannot be assumed that an individual with experience in the diagnostic lab only or with only EEG training can master these skills. Furthermore, the level of responsibility involved in the OR is considerably higher than in a routine lab, and not all individuals are suitable for this responsibility.

Somatosensory Evoked Potentials

Upper Limb Stimulation

In the diagnostic laboratory the minimum electrode derivations used for recording with upper-extremity stimulation are as follows:

Epi-Epc (Epi: Ipsilateral Erb's point referred to contralateral Erb's point or other noncephalic reference)

C5s-Epc (C5 spinous process referred to contralateral Erb's point or other noncephalic reference)

CPi-Epc (Ipsilateral sensory cortex referred to contralateral Erb's point or other noncephalic reference)

CPc-CPi (Contralateral sensory cortex referred to ipsilateral sensory cortex)

These should yield a series of recorded potentials (Figure 10.1). The potential at Erb's point (EP) is a near-field potential that serves as a useful reference point for calculating conduction times and also demonstrates that stimulation is adequate. The use of a peripheral nerve recording site to confirm effective stimulation is very important in the OR. The potential derived from the C5 spinous process is a far-field or stationary potential felt to originate from postsynaptic activity in the dorsal gray matter of the cervical spinal cord. This is an example of a subcortical potential that is largely unaffected by anesthetic agents and therefore very useful intraoperatively. The CPi-Epc derivation yields two more subcortical potentials. The P14 potential is felt to originate in the caudal portion of the medial lemniscus, while the N18 appears to originate from multiple subcortical generators in the upper brain stem and thalamus. N20 is the near-field potential from the contralateral sensory cortex. It may be difficult to resolve each of these components intraoperatively.

Lower Limb Stimulation

The posterior tibial nerve is the usual lower-extremity stimulation site (Figure 10.2). The following electrode derivations are recommended:

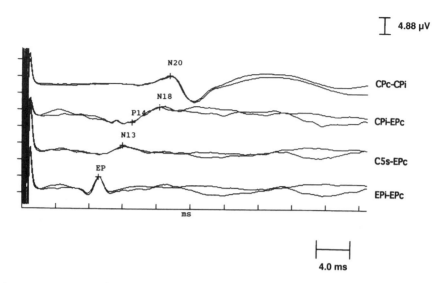

Figure 10.1 Normal somatosensory evoked potential with median nerve stimulation. (Epi = ipsilateral Erb's point; Epc = contralateral Erb's point; C5 = spinous process of C5; CPi = ipsilateral sensory cortex; CPc = contralateral sensory cortex.)

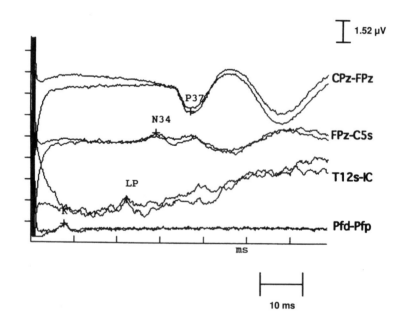

Figure 10.2 Normal somatosensory evoked potential with posterior tibial nerve stimulation. (Pfd = distal popliteal fossa; Pfp = proximal popliteal fossa; T12 = spinous process of twelfth thoracic vertebra; IC = iliac crest; CPz = midline sensory cortex; FPz = as in the international ten-twenty system.)

Pfd-Pfp (Two electrodes are placed 3–4 cm apart along the course of the sciatic nerve in the popliteal fossa)

T12s-IC (An electrode at T12 or so referred to an inactive reference such as the iliac crest)

Fpz-C5s (An electrode at Fpz referred to the C5 spinous process, which in this case serves as an inactive reference)

CPz-Fpz

Cpi-Fpz (Two derivations are used to record near-field cortical potentials. The electrode designation "CP" refers to a point midway between Cx and Px in the ten-twenty system. For example, CP3 is midway between C3 and P3. This is a change from the previous guideline that recommended using a point 2 cm posterior to C3 or C4 to record SSEPs.)

The two electrodes over the sciatic nerve in the popliteal fossa are used to record the afferent volley and serve the same purpose as those at EP with median or ulnar stimulation. The electrode over the lower thoracic spine may record a small potential that is the equivalent of the N13 with median nerve stimulation. This potential is small and difficult to obtain even in the diagnostic lab. It is not commonly used intraoperatively. Fpz-C5s may detect an N34, which is the equivalent of the N18 with median nerve stimulation. It may be preceded by a small P31, probably the equivalent of the P14 with median stimulation. Both Cpi-Fpz and CPz-Fpz are intended to record the P37 potential, which is the equivalent of the N20 from the upper extremity. Because of the medial position of the leg representation on the sensory homunculus, the potential is paradoxically recorded best ipsilateral to the side of stimulation. In some individuals, however, the potential is seen better with the CPz-Fpz derivation. In the OR it is often preferable to use less selective electrode derivations that yield larger, more reproducible responses that often represent the summation of several subcortical and cortical components.

The recording sweep is usually 40 ms for the upper extremity and 60 ms for the lower extremity, although either may be made longer, especially in the OR. A bandpass of 30–3,000 Hz is recommended. A narrower bandpass (30–1500 Hz, for example) may be used in the OR. Since the patient serves as his or her own control in the OR, this narrower band should not have a significant effect as long as it is not altered during the procedure.

Brain Stem Evoked Potentials

The stimulus for brain stem evoked potentials is usually a click delivered by earphones. The opposite ear is masked by "white noise" 30 dB below that of the stimulated ear to prevent any contribution from that ear. The clicks are either "rarefaction" or "condensation" clicks depending on whether the initial deflection of the diaphragm is away from or toward the tympanic membrane,

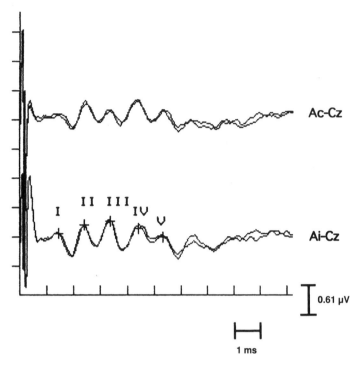

Figure 10.3 Normal brain stem auditory evoked response. (Ai = ipsilateral ear; Ac = contralateral ear; Cz = vertex as defined in the international ten-twenty system.)

respectively. These produce slightly different latencies so that, in the diagnostic laboratory, normative data must be established for each click polarity. Alternating click polarities may also be used. This method can be helpful in canceling the early cochlear microphonics and thus making it easier to identify wave I. In the OR, earphones are impractical. Ear inserts that fit into the auditory canal are used with the actual sound generator at the end of a short length of tubing. This introduces a slight delay and therefore longer absolute latencies. The stimulus rate is usually about 11/second, although faster rates such as 31/second may be used for some purposes at the expense of some definition of the component waves. The faster rates may be advantageous in the OR.

The recording electrode pair is the ipsilateral ear (Ai) referred to the vertex (Cz). In the diagnostic laboratory an electrode on the earlobe or mastoid is used. In the OR the recording electrode is usually in the auditory canal and is in fact gold foil-wrapped around the outside of the insert used for stimulation. Occasionally a needle electrode in the external canal is used. In the diagnostic lab and in the OR a second derivation is used, namely the contralateral ear (Ac) referred to the vertex. The ipsilateral derivation results in a series of waves at about 1-ms intervals beginning with wave I at about 2-ms latency (Figure 10.3). A small wave II may be identified, followed by wave III at about 4 ms. This is followed by the IV-V complex. The upper limit of normal for wave V latency using earphones is about 6.5 ms. As with SSEPs, each laboratory must establish its own normative data so these are only approximate values. The derivation to the opposite ear may help identify some of the waves. In this derivation, wave I may not be seen, II becomes larger, III smaller, IV a little earlier, and V a little later so that the IV-V complex splits apart slightly. In the OR it is usually only possible to identify waves I, III, and V and sometimes only wave V.

KEY REFERENCES

American EEG Society. Guidelines in electroencephalography, evoked potentials, and polysomnography. J Clin Neurophysiol 1994;11(1):1.

Emerson RG. Anatomic and physiologic bases of posterior tibial nerve somatosensory evoked potentials. Neuroligica Clin 1988;6(4):735.

Yamada T. The anatomic and physiologic bases of median nerve somatosensory evoked potentials. Neurol Clin 1988;6(4):705.

11

Somatosensory Evoked Potentials

John C. Keifer, M.D.

This chapter demonstrates the strategy for placing stimulating and recording electrodes to obtain reliable somatosensory evoked potentials (SSEPs). It also briefly describes the variety of intraoperative scenarios where SSEP monitoring has proved beneficial for monitoring the integrity of the sensory system.

ANATOMIC PLACEMENT OF RECORDING ELECTRODES
Cortical Electrodes

The currently used surface landmark method for placing cortical recording electrodes was initially presented in 1958 by the Committee on Methods of Clinical Examination in Electroencephalography. These guidelines have become known as the international ten-twenty system (see Chapter 5) because each half of a cerebral hemisphere is divided into quadrants measuring 10%, 20%, and 20% of the hemispheric length to locate the position of the electrodes (Figure 11.1).

Sagittal Landmarks

To determine electrode position, a tape measure is placed over the midline of the cranium extending from the nasion (bridge of the nose) to the inion (occipital protuberance). The tape overlies a line called the "central line" (the subscript z, applied to electrodes located on this line, means zero). The length of the central line is noted. The first electrode, Fpz (frontal pole), is located 10% of the central line length back from the nasion. The second electrode, Fz (frontal), is placed by measuring back 20% of the central line length from the first electrode. The third electrode, Cz (central), is located 20% of the central line length back from the second electrode. (We have now reached a distance halfway between the nasion and the inion (10% + 20% + 20% = 50%). The fourth electrode, Pz (parietal), is located 20% of the central line length from the central electrode. The fifth electrode, Oz (occipital), is located 20% back from the fourth electrode.

Coronal Landmarks

Lateral measurements are based on the central coronal plane. The tape is passed from the left to the right preauricular points (felt as depressions at the root of each zygoma just anterior to the tragus). The tape passes over the vertex

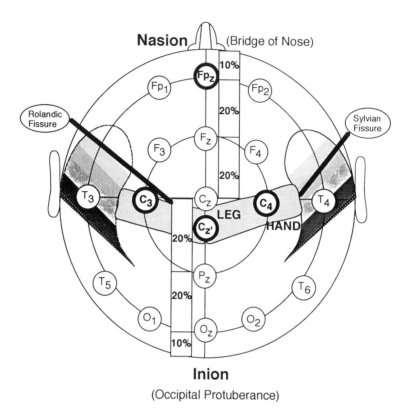

Figure 11.1 A schematic of the international ten-twenty system of electrode placement. Placement is demonstrated in relation to the sensory strip.

through the previously determined central point, Cz, to measure a coronal length. Ten percent of this distance above the preauricular points determines the T (temporal) points. T3 is left and T4 is right. Twenty percent above the temporal points are the lateral central points. C3 is left and C4 is right.

Horizontal Landmarks

To place the electrodes over the temporal lobes, horizontal coordinates are required. The horizontal line length is determined by a tape placed at Fpz and extended around the side of the head to reach Oz. Ten percent of this horizontal length is measured lateral from the Fpz to reach Fp1 on the left and Fp2 on the right. Twenty percent farther back on the horizontal line determines F7 on the left and F8 on the right.

If one then measures from the occipital point along the horizontal line, 10% of the horizontal length determines O1 on the left and O2 on the right. An additional 20% of the distance determines T5 on the left and T6 on the right.

Parasagittal Placement

The remaining cortical electrodes (F3, F4, P3, and P4) are placed along the frontal and parietal coronal lines equidistant between the midline and horizontal line of electrodes. The two auricular electrodes are placed on either ear.

Modified Electrode Placement

Since the sensory cortex is the site of neuronal activation from sensory stimulation, some configurations have moved the central electrode posteriorly to better cover the entire sensory strip. This modified site has been called Cz'. Selecting the electrode pair to monitor a particular SSEP may also be dictated by the area of the postcentral sensory strip is most likely to be affected by the stimulation (Figure 11.2). A central electrode located closer to the midline (e.g., Cz') will detect sensory strip activity following lower-extremity stimulation. More laterally placed electrodes (e.g., C3 and C4) will detect sensory strip activation following upper-extremity stimulation.

Extracortical Recording Electrodes
Upper Extremity

Erb's Point To follow electrical activity from the peripheral nerve (usually the median nerve), an electrode is placed at Erb's point, which is located in the supraclavicular fossa just lateral to the clavicular insertion of the sternocleidomastoid muscle. This electrode is well situated to detect the electrical potential, Erb's point peak, that is thought to arise from trunks and divisions of the brachial plexus.

Cervical Spine Electrodes can be placed on the skin overlying the cervical vertebral spines to distinguish three peaks, which probably arise from (1) the dorsal root entry zone, (2) the posterior column–nucleus cuneatus interface, and (3) the medial lemniscus.

Lower Extremity

The course of electrical activation can be monitored in the peripheral nerves following tibial nerve stimulation at the ankle. Popliteal fossa electrodes are placed at the inferior and superior borders of the fossa. Recording electrodes can be placed on the skin overlying the spinal column or can be placed within the ligamentum flavum, spinous process, or epidural space to record electrical activity within the spinal cord.

SENSORY TRACTS

Cell bodies of the large-fiber dorsal column sensory system lie in the dorsal root ganglia; their central processes travel rostrally in ipsilateral posterior columns of the spinal cord and synapse in the dorsal column nuclei at the cervicomedullary junction. Second-order fibers cross to the other side shortly after

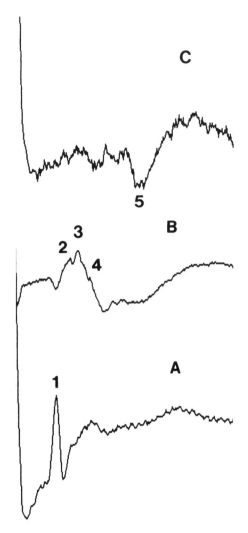

Figure 11.2 Somatosensory evoked potential recorded from Erb's point (A), cervical spinous process (B), and contralateral scalp following ulnar nerve stimulation at the elbow (C). (1 = Erb's point peak; 2 = cervical peak A; 3 = cervical peak B; 4 = cervical peak C; 5 = N18/20 peak.) (See Table 11.1 for approximate latencies.)

origination and travel to the primary receiving nucleus of the thalamus through the medial lemniscus. Third-order fibers continue from the thalamus to the frontoparietal sensorimotor cortex. Whether any of the activity-generating SSEPs in humans travel in ascending paths other than the posterior columns is not known. Therefore, until further evidence is forthcoming, short-latency SSEPs can reasonably be considered to be generated by volleys traversing the posterior columns and medial lemnisci.

PLACEMENT OF STIMULATING ELECTRODES
Upper Extremity
The Median Nerve
For median nerve stimulation, the electrodes are placed at the distal wrist skin crease at a point between the palmaris longus tendon and the flexor carpi radialis tendon. Stimulation of this nerve should result in flexion of the wrist; opposition of middle finger, forefinger, and thumb; and flexion of the lateral three forefingers. The median nerve is especially suited for upper-extremity SSEPs because of the relatively large area occupied on the sensory strip by thumb sensation.

The Ulnar Nerve
The ulnar nerve lies on the medial side of the ulnar artery on the volar aspect of the wrist. Stimulation of this nerve should result in flexion of the wrist, adduction of all fingers (clenched together), and flexion and opposition of the lateral two fingers and thumb.

Lower Extremity
The Tibial Nerve
The tibial nerve is commonly monitored posterior to the medial malleolus. The tibial nerve also lies within the popliteal fossa. The fossa has the appearance of an inverted kite. The nerve is stimulated or recorded by placing the electrode in the midline of the kite at a point above the skin crease at the back of the knee. Stimulation of this nerve results in plantar flexion of the foot.

Common Peroneal Nerve
The common peroneal nerve is stimulated by placing electrodes at the lateral side of the fibular head. Stimulation of this nerve should result in dorsiflexion and eversion of the foot.

WHAT ARE EVOKED POTENTIALS?

The electrical potentials detected from stimulation differ based on (1) which nerve is stimulated, and (2) the location of the recording electrodes. A variety of recording electrodes can be useful in identifying a typical pattern of electrical potentials, especially when the latency of a given potential is altered by normal physiologic variability (such as length of the nerve or limb temperature) and the disease process present. Even though the latency of the impulse is recorded from the time of stimulation, it is possible to measure the latency from the particular reference potential for that nerve. This reference potential is usually selected as one that develops from the ascending volley arriving at the cord from the peripheral nerve. This technique minimizes variability in nerve conduction time along the peripheral nerve. Latency is measured in milliseconds. Peaks are identified by the direction of the deflection (P for positive and N for negative). A subscript number refers to the latency in milliseconds (N11 refers to a peak with a negative deflection and a latency of

Table 11.1 Somatosensory Evoked Potentials Detected After Median Nerve Stimulation

Name	Recording Electrode	Latency	Proposed Generator	Comments
Erb's point	Erb's point	9 ms	Trunks or divisions of plexus	Largest amplitude point
Cervical A	Cervical	11 ms	Dorsal root entry zone of cervical spinal cord	
Cervical B	Cervical	12–13 ms	Posterior column/ nucleus cuneatus	
Cervical C	Cervical	14 ms	Brain stem	May appear as a shoulder on the previous 13-ms peak
N18	Contralateral scalp	18 ms	Subcortical	
N20	Contralateral scalp	20 ms	Somatosensory cortex	May be seen along with N18 as one negative complex in the scalp recording electrode

11 ms). Alternatively, and to remove ambiguity due to interpatient variability, some authors refer to peaks with a numerical subscript that refers to the order in which the peak is seen (e.g., N_2 refers to the second negative peak in a series).

Upper-Extremity Potentials

The normal potentials detected following median nerve stimulation can best be appreciated if one looks for these potentials in three recording sites: (1) Erb's point, (2) the cervical spine, and (3) the contralateral scalp (Table 11.1).

Lower-Extremity Potentials

As with the upper extremity, it is possible to measure electrical activity from the periphery following tibial nerve stimulation. This is accomplished by placing recording electrodes within the popliteal fossa. More proximal activity can be measured over the spinal cord at lumbosacral or thoracolumbar levels prior to recording cortical potentials (Table 11.2).

CLINICAL INDICATIONS FOR MONITORING SOMATOSENSORY EVOKED POTENTIALS
Scoliosis with Posterior Spinal Fusion

The incidence of postoperative paraplegia following scoliosis surgery is 1.7%. There is an increased risk of paraplegia with preexisting conditions such

Table 11.2 Somatosensory Evoked Potentials Detected after Tibial Nerve Stimulation

Name	Recording Electrode	Latency	Proposed Generator	Comments
N20	Lumbar spine	20 ms	Spinal roots/spinal cord	Usually followed by a broad positive peak
P27	Cervical spine	27 ms	Nucleus gracilus at the cervicomedullary junction	May correspond to the 13-ms potential from median nerve stimulation
N35/P40	Scalp	35/40 ms	Somatosensory cortex	40-ms peak is analogous to the 22-ms peak following median nerve stimulation

as kyphosis, congenital scoliosis, and preoperative traction. Impairment of spinal cord function may be due to stretch, compression, mechanical trauma during placement of instruments, or compromised perfusion.

Spinal Cord Mass Lesions

SSEP monitoring may be useful for determining the number of feeding vessels that can be sacrificed before a tumor or arteriovenous malformation (AVM) is excised without significantly impairing spinal cord perfusion. Anecdotal case reports document either improvement in the SSEPs after decompression of the cord following spinal tumor removal, or abrupt loss of the SSEPs from unrecognized compression of the cord by disk material during decompressive surgery.

Aortic Cross-Clamping

A variety of studies confirm that spinal cord ischemia during aortic cross-clamping can be detected by changes in SSEPs generated by tibial nerve stimulation. The mechanism of this spinal cord ischemia may be a distal aortic pressure insufficient for cord perfusion. Alternatively, cord ischemia may result from a sacrifice of the critical radicular arteries. Laschinger (1983) reported that SSEP changes did not occur in experimental dogs if the distal aortic pressure was kept above 70 mm Hg pressure. SSEPs were stable in 25 human patients undergoing aortic cross-clamp for aneurysm repair if the distal aortic pressure remained above 60 mm Hg. Controversies over the use of SSEPs for aortic cross-clamping include an unacceptably high rate of false-positive and false-negative studies and technical and anesthetic problems that may render the SSEP unreliable. However, important points emerge:

1. SSEPs are lost on patients at increased risk for neurologic complications following aortic cross-clamp.

2. Immediate loss of SSEPs (within minutes of cross-clamp) is a poor prognostic sign requiring therapeutic intervention.
3. Gradual loss of SSEPs is commonly encountered without neurologic sequelae.
4. Prolonged absence of SSEPs is associated with increased morbidity even if the loss is gradual.

Pelvic and Acetabular Surgery

Vrahas et al. reported the results of SSEP monitoring in a combined retrospective and prospective study of 82 patients undergoing repair of pelvic and acetabular fractures. This study identified two features associated with intraoperative SSEP changes and risk for iatrogenic neurologic complication: the presence of a preoperative sciatic nerve injury and the presence of an unstable pelvic fracture. Operative events associated with SSEP changes that improved with a change in surgical technique were (1) reduction of a fracture that involved superior and posterior migration and sagittal rotation of the hemipelvis, and (2) insertion of a guide wire, noncannulated screw, or drill into the lateral sacrum for fractures of the lateral sacrum or sacroiliac joint. The incidence of iatrogenic nerve injury in the first 40 patients studied retrospectively was 7.5%. The rate of iatrogenic nerve injury fell to 0 of 42 in the prospective group following institution of more stringent criteria for diagnosing an SSEP abnormality and establishment of surgical protocol for quicker response to SSEP changes.

Carotid Surgery

Median nerve SSEPs show alterations when the cerebral blood flow falls to 18 ml/100 g/minute. The SSEPs become systematically smaller and then disappear when cerebral blood flow falls to 15 ml/100 g/minute. Carotid endarterectomy patients whose cortical amplitudes decrease by more than 50% perform worse on postoperative neuropsychologic testing than patients who experienced a lesser degree of SSEP attenuation. In carotid endarterectomy patients (eight of whom had decreased carotid stump pressure following cross-clamping) in whom a shunt was not placed because there were no SSEP changes documented, no significant postoperative neurologic complications were found. Similar data are documented for carotid aneurysm repair and for AVM surgery.

The merits of SSEP monitoring during carotid artery surgery have been assessed. In a review of 994 carotid surgery patients, SSEPs detected cerebral ischemia in 7 of 8 patients who developed neurologic deficits, for a sensitivity rating of 87.5%. Kearse et al. concluded that SSEPs were not sufficiently sensitive to detect cerebral ischemia during carotid cross-clamp. However, they did not use an independent measure of ischemia and simply compared the rate of abnormalities registered with SSEP to the rate of abnormalities registered with raw EEG. Twenty-three of 53 cases showed signs of ischemia by EEG criteria.

It is apparent that SSEP monitoring will change during cerebral ischemia induced by carotid artery cross-clamping. However, whether SSEPs possess sufficient sensitivity or specificity to augment or supplant raw cortical EEG monitoring during carotid surgery remains controversial.

KEY REFERENCES

Haupt WF, Horsch S. Evoked potential monitoring in carotid surgery: A review of 994 cases. Neurology 1992;142(4):835.

Jasper HH. Report of the Committee on Methods of Clinical Examination in Electroencephalography. EEG Clin Neurophysiol 1958;10:370.

Kearse LA Jr, Brown EN, McDeck K. Somatosensory evoked potentials sensitivity relative to electroencephalography for cerebral ischemia during carotid endarterectomy. Stroke 1992;23(4):498.

Laschinger JC, Cunningham JN, Catinella FC, Nathan IM, Knoop EA, Spencer FC. Detection and prevention of intraoperative spinal cord ischemia after cross-clamping of the thoracic aorta: use of somatosensory evoked potentials. Spine 1982;92:1109–1117.

Vrahas M, Gordon RG, Mears DC, Krieger D, Sclabassi RJ. Intraoperative somatosensory evoked potential monitoring of pelvic and acetabular fractures. J Orthop Trauma 1992;6:50.

RECOMMENDED READING

Chiappa KH. Evoked Potentials in Clinical Medicine. New York: Raven, 1990;307–507.

Nuwer MR. Evoked Potential Monitoring in the Operating Room. New York: Raven, 1986.

Salzman SK. Neural Monitoring: The Prevention of Intraoperative Injury. Clifton, NJ: Humana Press, 1990.

12

The Use of Brain Stem Auditory Evoked Potentials in Intraoperative Monitoring

C. William Erwin, M.D.
Andrea C. Erwin, B.A., R. EP T.

The term *brain stem auditory evoked potentials* (BAEPs) was suggested by the American Electroencephalographic Society in its guidelines covering both diagnostic and intraoperative applications of these electrophysiologic signals. Others have called them *brain stem auditory evoked responses*, which, though more phonetic, is redundant in that all responses are, by definition, evoked. *Auditory evoked potentials* (AEPs) are used by some to describe these responses. AEPs include middle- and late-latency responses in addition to the earlier components. However, it is only the events of brain stem origin, recorded over the first 10–15 ms, that are known to be sufficiently state-independent to be used in assessing neural integrity. This state-independence is of particular importance during anesthesia and surgery.

HISTORY

The intraoperative use of BAEPs was first reported in 1978. The recording of end-organ (cochlear) potentials occurred much earlier. Primarily due to their much higher amplitude, end-organ potentials could be recorded without the use of averaging techniques. In current use, posterior fossa surgery uses BAEP monitoring, often combined with other forms of neural monitoring such as somatosensory studies of central responses to median nerve stimulation and monitoring of cranial motor nerves. Other than the acoustic division of VIII, cranial nerves VII and V are most commonly monitored, but depending on the structures at risk, the motor components of III, IV, VI, IX, X, XI, and XII have all been monitored.

A 1991 review of experience with 150 microvascular decompression cases revealed that as the surgeon gained experience, all complications associated with the procedure decreased with the exception of retrocochlear hearing loss. This implies that in posterior fossa surgery via a retromastoid approach there are inadequate visual clues as to the occurrence or severity of auditory compromise. Types of

135

posterior fossa neoplasms suitable for BAEP monitoring include vestibular neurile-momas, other extraaxial tumors, and, rarely, intrinsic pontomedullary tumors. Vascular and compressive disorders in which BAEP monitoring is useful include hemifacial spasms, tic douloureux, aneurysms, arteriovenous malformations, and posterior fossa decompressions. The general and specific monitoring techniques are essentially the same for these different disorders and will not be discussed separately.

GOALS

The goal of intraoperative monitoring of BAEPs is to provide early warn-ing of impending neurologic deficits that may occur as a result of surgery. Hearing function should be preserved to the degree possible, and, more impor-tant, brain stem function should be maintained.

Auditory function is at risk whenever surgery in the posterior fossa is under-taken. The literature suggests that the potential for impending auditory damage is greatest in dealing with tumors involving the acoustic nerve either directly or by close approximation. The majority of eighth-nerve tumors arise from the vestibu-lar division of the eighth nerve. Tumors of other cell types, including menin-giomas, are not uncommon. Audition may be lost or seriously compromised before surgery begins due to the pathologic consequences of the tumor itself. There is usually a good correlation between tumor size, the degree of presurgical hearing compromise, and prognosis for a good acoustic surgical outcome.

Retromastoid microvascular decompressive surgery for hemifacial spasm and tic douloureux produces a significant incidence of hearing impairment (10%), which can be reduced to essentially zero by the appropriate application of BAEP monitoring techniques. Although preservation of hearing is an important goal of BAEP monitoring, clearly justifying its application, it is in preservation of brain stem function that such monitoring is most critical for preservation of patient function.

METHODS
Electrode Types

Electrode types include either subdermal (needle) or disc-shaped surface electrodes. Although electrode polarization is not usually a problem, gold-plated disc electrodes reduce this problem and are highly stable. Depending on the size of the operating room and required placement of neurophysiologic monitoring equipment, long-lead electrodes may be of great value. Many suppliers will pro-vide leads of any length requested. Seventy-two–inch leads are long enough for most applications. In theory, very long leads could contribute to artifact by act-ing as antennae. In practice, this does not appear to be a problem.

Electrode Placement and Designation

Electrode placements are the same for diagnostic studies and intraoperative moni-toring. All waves of the BAEP can be recorded at the vertex of the head and in the region of the ears. The majority of BAEP components, waves II through VII, are much higher in amplitude at the vertex, while wave I and the preceding cochlear microphonic are recorded with the highest amplitude at the ear ipsilateral to stimulation. After years of confusion, today clinical neurophysiologists use an electrode location terminology developed by an international terminology committee. The location strategy, called the international ten-twenty system, is based on percentage measurements from skull bone landmarks. In this system the vertex location is called Cz and is located in the midline 50% of the distance from the nasion to the inion. The ear locations are called A1 and A2. "A" stands for auricular, and in the ten-twenty system odd numbers are for locations left of the midline and even numbers for right of the midline. Thus, A1 is the left ear and A2 is the right ear. Ai and Ac are abbreviations for the ipsilateral and contralateral ears (in reference to the ear receiving sound stimulation). M1 and M2 are abbreviations for left and right mastoid locations, respectively. The maximal amplitude of wave I is recorded from an electrode on the mesial side of the lower part of the ear lobe.

Methods of Application

Recording electrodes must have good electrical contact (low impedance) and firm mechanical attachment. These factors are critically important in intraoperative monitoring, where it is usually impossible to improve faulty electrodes due to surgical drapes and sterile technique. Electrodes must remain useful for extended periods of time, and drying of conductive electrode gels must be avoided.

Excellent mechanical stability of a surface electrode is attained by taping or gluing the electrode to the skin. The most common technique is to use collodion as a glue. It is very fast-drying, given its 70% ether base, and it is easily removed with acetone. Subdermal electrodes are used in some centers. They are faster to apply than collodion applications. Subdermal electrodes lack good mechanical stability and have an inherently higher impedance.

Evaluation of Contact Integrity

Measuring impedance with an impedance meter is the only certain method of assuring adequate electrode contact. The oily outer epidermal layers must be breached if low impedance to electron flow and good-quality recording are to be attained. Skin preparation agents, acetone to remove skin fat, abrasive skin paste, and punctation with sterile needles are the most common techniques to reduce electrode-skin impedance. The impedance meter measures the quality of skin preparation and electrode contact. Measurements should be made immediately after electrode application (before the first recordings) and periodically throughout the surgical case.

Recording Instrumentation

A basic evoked potential system includes three conceptually different components, which are usually housed in the same cabinet: a stimulator, an amplifier-filter system, and an averager. Additional components include a display module, electronic data storage, and provisions for remote monitoring. The potential (difference between two recording electrodes) is amplified, filtered, and then processed by the averager. The stimulator is time-locked to the averager. Following amplification and filtering, the analog signal enters the averager, where analog-to-digital conversion, display, and storage functions take place and averaging and other mathematical computations are accomplished.

The averager must have a constant relationship (time-locked) to the stimulus, such that when a stimulus is delivered, the averager is triggered to analyze the biological activity. Almost any sensory stimulus, particularly if it has an abrupt onset, will elicit physiologic responses with electrical manifestations.

Signal-to-Noise Ratio

The majority of short-latency evoked potentials are in the microvolt and submicrovolt range and are invisible in the usual analog recording. This is because the potential (signal) is smaller than that of the ongoing, non–event-related activity (noise). This may be described as an adverse signal-to-noise ratio. Indeed, components of a BAEP may be more than 100 times smaller than the spontaneous cortical rhythms, muscle activity (measured with electromyography [EMG]), cardiac activity (measured with electrocardiography [ECG]), eye movements (measured with electrooculography [EOG]), 60-Hz artifact, slow skin potentials, respiratory artifact, and so on, that comprise the mix of non–event-related activity.

Evoked potentials may be subdivided by their neural origin, being referred to as near-field or far-field potentials. Although there are exceptions to the rule, near-field potentials are generally of greater amplitude, later latency, and slower frequency, with greater topographic specificity. Conversely, far-field potentials are of lower amplitude, earlier latency, faster frequency, and diffuse distribution. Near-field potentials are often of cortical origin, but there are many exceptions. An example of an evoked potential of cortical origin is the visual pattern-reversal response, which is generated in the visual cortex of the occipital lobe. BAEPs are far-field potentials (with the exception of wave I) because they are generated in the brain stem and transmitted through the electrically conductive fluids and tissues of the hemispheres and generate broadly distributed electrical fields recorded at the scalp. Wave I is a near-field potential, although it is early and not of cortical origin. No neural pathways are involved in BAEP transfer from the generator to the surface (skin).

To be visualized, the evoked potential must be extracted from a sea of noise from EEG, EOG, EMG, skin potentials, 60-Hz interference, and other sources. Analog processing by the amplifier provides not only an increase in gain but also common-mode rejection (CMR) and selective filtering. Although the principal technique to selectively attenuate noise components is averaging, an understanding of common-mode rejection and analog filtering is necessary to achieve technically adequate, interpretable data.

Principles of Averaging

Averaging of individual potentials to a sequence of sensory stimuli is done to improve the signal-to-noise ratio. This is the ratio of the amplitude of the time-locked activity (signal) to the random activity (noise). Increasing the number of averaged potentials increases the likelihood that noise components will be attenuated. The total number (N) of responses is summed (Σx) and divided by N ($Avg = \Sigma x/N = \bar{x}$). Time-locked or stimulus-related (signal) activity is preserved by the averaging process, while random noise components unrelated to the stimulus are attenuated. Thus, signal averaging enhances the signal by reducing noise.

Intraoperative Setup Procedures

During the preoperative study, gold-plated disc electrodes with braided 72-inch leads are applied at Cz, Fz, and the mesial sides of the left (A1) and right (A2) ear lobes using collodion technique. Duplicate electrodes are placed at each recording site in case of electrode malfunction. Often the ear lobe is not large enough to accommodate two electrodes, in which case only one electrode is applied. Then gauze squares soaked in collodion are placed over each electrode to provide additional mechanical bonding. Braiding the electrode leads reduces tangling and various forms of common-mode artifact.

The morning of surgery, scalp electrodes are regelled, impedances are checked, and Grass subdermal electrodes are inserted at the vertex (Cz) and in each tragus. These electrodes serve as redundant recording electrodes should the disc electrodes malfunction. If the ear lobe disc electrode becomes defective, the subdermal electrode in the tragus may be used but it should be referred to a subdermal electrode. A derivation with one disc and one needle electrode is likely to have a severe impedance imbalance, causing a degradation of the CMR response and increased artifact. Insert transducers are placed in auditory canals, and the ears are carefully taped to anchor the transducer in place. Standard headphones cannot be used because of their size; they are so large that they invade the operative field. A popular ear insert consists of transducers connected by plastic tubing with a compressive sponge collar at the patient end. This is inserted into the ear canal. The collar provides some acoustic shielding. The length of tubing produces a delay of almost 1 ms. This device is available from audiometric supply houses and all equipment manufacturers. We prefer less expensive transducers (Radio Shack—Micro Stereo Earphones, item no. 33-980). After placement of the tube or transducer the entire ear is covered with a waterproof tape (Steri-Drape) to prevent liquids from entering the auditory canal.

While the operative field is being scrubbed, the transducers are connected to the recording instrument via a 10- to 15-foot extender cable, and the electrode headboard is placed in a location convenient for access during the procedure. An IV pole is commonly used; it is important to protect the headboard from fluids by elevating it and covering it with waterproof material. Fluids could short the electrically isolated ground to true earth ground and produce an electrical hazard to the patient. The technologist turns on the auditory stimulator to confirm proper functioning of the transducers.

Recording Parameters
Montage

The standard montage for BAEP recording is two channels. These consist of Cz-Ai and Cz-Ac. This not only provides some redundancy but reveals the distribution of components critical to accurate component identification. Some have recommended the use of a transverse montage (Ac-Ai) to enhance the recording of wave I. Wave I is a near-field response, negative in polarity, recorded primarily by the ipsilateral electrode. It does project as a dipole with the positive "end" oriented toward the opposite ear. Therefore electrodes on opposite ears are on opposite ends of the dipole and maximize the recording of wave I. This is true but unfortunately not the whole story. The positive dipole projection is seen with equal amplitude at Cz. As a result, the standard, vertical derivation of Cz-Ai already takes advantage of the dipole recording principles.

Analog Filters

Common settings for high- and low-frequency filters are 3,000 and 150 Hz, respectively. The appropriate use of analog filters in the amplifier allows for selective amplitude attenuation of frequencies not of clinical interest. For example, the BAEP has relatively little activity of reported clinical value below 100 Hz or above 3,000 Hz. Suppressing frequencies below 100 Hz greatly diminishes background EEG, EMG, and 60-Hz, while suppressing frequencies above 3,000 Hz reduces inherent amplifier noise, radio frequencies, and other high-frequency components.

While the EEG technologist is encouraged to change filter settings to maximize the display of pertinent features in the EEG, evoked potential technologists have no such freedom. In addition to attenuating the amplitude of clinically nongermane frequencies, analog filters have the unfortunate effect of causing a phase shift. This results in an apparent shift in the latency of peaks in an evoked potential as well as potential morphologic distortion. With excessive filtering of low-frequency activity, there is an apparent shortening of the apparent absolute latency. This is called "phase lead." Excessive high-frequency filtering has a clinically more serious effect of producing an apparent lengthening of the absolute latency that is called "phase lag." Although the potential looks "cleaner" following more harsh filtering, it may be significantly distorted in biological terms to the degree that a false-positive interpretation could be rendered. In clinical diagnostic studies, filters selected must be demonstrated to not alter the latency of the potential as compared to less harsh filters.

In the operating room, more freedom with filtering is allowed and filter changes may be necessary if unexpected noise develops. High-frequency oscillators sometimes found in other monitoring equipment, microscopes, video, and several tumor-debulking devices can be so severe as to prevent further monitoring if not dealt with by filtering. In general, high-frequency filtering should not exceed 1,000 Hz. At the point that filters are changed, a phase shift can be expected (waves appear later) and therefore new baselines must be obtained. Some investigators have used restrictive filters in somatosensory studies in an attempt to reveal low-amplitude, high-frequency components otherwise obscured by high-amplitude slow components. Such applications have generally not been used in clinical BAEP studies.

Stimulating Parameters

Currently most clinical BAEP studies are performed with earphones (transducers). These devices transform one form of energy to another form (i.e., electricity to sound). Separate left- and right-ear transducers allow each ear to be stimulated separately and allow the nonstimulated ear to be acoustically masked.

The acoustic output of the click stimulus usually has its major energy in the 3,000- to 4,000-Hz range, but some energy can be detected from several hundred to more than 6,000 Hz. For this reason, the click is called a "broad band click," referring to the broad band of frequencies generated. Transducers made by different manufacturers and even different models made by the same manufacturer generate different acoustic waveforms and consequently generate different BAEPs from the same individual. The BAEP differences are most marked in morphology, relative amplitudes of different components, and absolute latencies of peaks occurring within the first 10 ms. The most important features for clinical neurologic diagnosis, the interpeak latencies (IPLs), are relatively little affected by these transducer considerations. These considerations have little importance to intraoperative monitoring where the subject serves as his or her own control. It is change from a baseline rather than comparison to a multisubject normative data base that has clinical significance.

Click Polarity

When the initial movement of the transducer diaphragm is away from the tympanic membrane, the click is defined as a rarefaction click. When the initial movement of the diaphragm is toward the tympanic membrane the click is defined as a condensation click. These are frequently abbreviated as "R" and "C" clicks. Alternating R and C clicks are appropriately called alternating "A" clicks. Responses to R and C click stimulation differ, particularly in those with sensory-neural hearing impairments. Clicks of A polarity may produce cancellation of out-of-phase BAEP components present in such patients.

A stimulus artifact is produced by the magnetic fields of the transducer coil cutting across the wire of the electrode. The electrode becomes the secondary coil of a transformer. The higher the intensity in dB, the greater the current flow, the greater the magnetic field, and the greater the potential induced in the electrode wire. Alternating the pulse polarity and averaging greatly reduces the stimulus artifact. Stimulus artifact is not a significant problem in the diagnostic BAEP lab, where intensities are higher. In the operating room, where noise contamination is a greater problem, higher-intensity stimulation is the rule and significant data corruption by stimulus artifact is a problem. As a result, A clicks are commonly used. They are less a necessity when insert transducers with tubes are used that physically remove the transducer from proximity with the electrode lead.

Click Intensity

The reference for 0 dB is defined by several different techniques: a single individual's subjective response threshold (sensation level [dBSL]), the mean threshold of a group of individuals (normal hearing level [dBHL]), or by reference to a physical measure taken from test apparatus (peak equivalent sound pressure level [dBpeSPL]). Most measures of dB in intraoperative monitoring are based on dBHL.

Click Rate

When monitoring surgical cases it is important that one be able to obtain sequential responses rapidly. Two or more averaged responses may be needed to have convincing evidence that meaningful change has occurred. The time required to obtain such an averaged response can be reduced by increasing the rate of stimulation.

The click rate or rate of stimulation is usually defined by the term *per second*. Thus, one frequently encounters such terminology as "clicks were delivered at a rate of 11.1 per second." To avoid locking into some component of 60-Hz line frequency, it is necessary to avoid any stimulation rate that is an exact multiple of 60. The term "Hertz" (Hz) is also commonly used, although some prefer to reserve it for pure sine wave activity. Based on initial publications, rates of approximately 10 per second were historically the norm for most laboratories. Using a 15-ms (0.015 second) analysis time, which is common in BAEP operative monitoring studies, the theoretical fastest stimulation rate would be 66.67 per second (1/0.015) unless more than one stimulus per sweep is desired.

Using a faster rate of stimulation has no effect on the magnitude of noise components. Unfortunately, for BAEP components, faster rates reduce the amplitude as well as having minor effects on morphology (broadening of peaks). Since this produces an adverse impact on the initial signal-to-noise ratio (S/N), more responses are required to achieve the same improvement in S/N as compared to slower rates. Efficiency calculations have been published for BAEP data indicating that rates of approximately 30 per second can be used to advantage. Thus, high-quality data can be obtained in one-third the time required at a more "standard" 10 per second.

Faster rates of stimulation produce longer absolute and interpeak latencies of BAEP components. In the diagnostic lab it is necessary to have normative data at each of the different rates of stimulation to be used. Fortunately, in intraoperative monitoring each subject serves as his or her own control.

Obligate Components

Seven major peaks are usually present in the first 10 ms in the BAEP of normal adult humans. Severely abnormal adult responses and responses from very young infants may have components falling outside the 10-ms window. Thus, when studying neonates and in operative monitoring, a 15-ms analysis time is commonly used.

Appropriate clinical interpretation mandates that major components be accurately and consistently identified. A number of recording and stimulation parameters affect the morphology and latency of the BAEP components. In some instances, manipulation of these variables facilitates component identification.

Methods of Peak Identification

It is not possible to correctly and consistently identify BAEP components by their latency or peak order. The latency of a component may be delayed due to changes in stimulus parameters or due to pathology of the end organ or central auditory pathways. It is true that wave III usually occurs between 3 and 4 ms, but a late wave I or II can also fall in that time window.

Counting waveforms to identify the peak order and thus the identity of a component in question is particularly hazardous. Waves I, III, and V are considered obligatory, meaning they are present in all normal subjects and therefore pathology can be assumed if these waves are absent. Waves II, IV, VI, and VII may be and often are absent in asymptomatic neurologically and audiologically intact individuals.

Given the above problems it is clear that a less ambiguous method (than latency or peak order) of peak identification is needed. Fortunately each component has a different field distribution on the scalp. The field distribution may be demonstrated by the use of two or more recording channels. Of the major BAEP components, wave V is of greatest importance in intraoperative monitoring. The reason is simple: It is the one wave most likely to be present despite hearing deficits and manipulation of stimulation and recording parameters. Identification of all components is occasionally required; Table 12.l presents the guides on field distribution.

Effects of Anesthetic Agents on Brain Stem Auditory Evoked Potentials

Only minimal direct effects of any anesthetic agent on BAEP components are recognized. There is a shift of 0.1–0.2 ms in the latency of all components with anesthetic induction similar to the changes occurring with unsedated sleep. This is presumably due to changes in muscles of the ossicular chain (middle ear). The result is an apparent attenuation of sound activation of the cochlear apparatus and thus the delay of absolute latencies. Correlated with duration and depth of anesthesia are prolongations of interpeak latencies, but the mechanism for these IPL changes is brain temperature and not the agent itself. Various authors have reported a prolongation of wave-V latency of approximately 0.2 ms per degree Centigrade.

Table 12.1 Brain Stem Auditory Evoked Potentials Field Distributions

	Cz-Ai	Cz-Ac
Wave I	Upgoing, later than 1.3 ms	Virtually absent
Wave II	Usually present but absent in some normal individuals (not an obligate wave)	If present, similar amplitude to Cz-Ai ~0.1 ms later
Wave III	Present in normals	Lower amplitude (sometimes virtually absent, ~0.01 ms earlier than Ai
Wave IV	Not obligate	If present, ~0.01 ms later than Ai
Wave V	Obligate, largest of waves, followed by major down-going negativity	Larger, more separated from IV than in Ai, usually ~0.01 ms later than Ai

Surgical Factors

Retractor Placement

Latency changes of wave V to as much as 4.0 ms can be seen in some surgical cases. The most frequent surgical event preceding such changes is retractor placement during retromastoid approaches to brain stem structures. Cerebellar retraction for visualization of brain stem structures may induce compression, traction, ischemia, or a combination of factors affecting acoustic nerve function. The changes may be slow and progressive or develop rapidly over a 30- to 60-second period. There may be considerable change in wave-V latency during the time required for a single average. At a stimulation rate of approximately 30 per second, 1,000 responses are averaged in 30 seconds. A camera might reveal a blurred image, but current instrumentation can only reveal a single average. One might suspect temporal dispersion by a broadening of the time base of components. It is better to start a new average than to increase the number of responses; taking the latter course still yields an average, whereas starting a new average is more revealing of the current severity of change.

Operating Room Acoustic Noise

Environmental sound masks target sounds. A subject may detect stimuli at 0 dB (at some specific frequency) when in a sound-attenuated acoustic chamber but fail to detect the same level of sound out of the chamber. Outside the chamber the acoustic mechanism is activated not only by the specific stimulus but also by environmental building noises. The loss (approximately 10 dB) is usually more pronounced in the lower frequencies that characterize most building noises.

Operating rooms are usually noisier than other hospital environments. The most intense noise is generated by drills used to remove bone. The translabyrinthine approach is often used to improve the chances of preservation of facial nerve function at the sacrifice of acoustic nerve function. It requires

Table 12.2 Increase in Amount of Artifact

Problem/Cause	Detection	Action
High-impedance electrode	Check electrode impedance	Switch to duplicate electrodes
Increased EMG	View input signal, check anesthetic level	Patient may be "light"; request increased anesthesia or use NM block; increase number of stimuli
Electrocautery	High-amplitude noise causing amplifier block (saturation)	Wait, resume when cautery stops and amplifiers recover
Other equipment	Rhythmic, high-amplitude noise. View input to determine frequency	Turn off one source of noise at a time while looking at input

EMG = electromyography; NM = neuromuscular.

extensive drilling, which causes acoustic masking not only on the operated side but also by bone transmission to the contralateral ear.

Intraoperative Troubleshooting

Before alerting the surgeon that significant changes or loss of BAEP components have occurred, there should be vigorous attempts to rule out technical problems. The technologist-interpreter should be well prepared for such events and have a checklist of causes, methods of confirmation, and actions to be taken (Tables 12.2 and 12.3). Troubleshooting should be accomplished in less than 5 minutes.

False-Positives and False-Negatives

A false-negative occurs when there is no report of significant change in monitored parameters but the patient awakens with a neurologic or audiologic deficit. There are several reasons for this: (1) The lesion occurs in a structure not involved in the pathway being monitored (i.e., normal BAEPs are to be expected in a medullary or midbrain lesion). (2) The quality of the data is so poor (for either physiologic or technical reasons) that change is not appreciated. To avoid these problems the surgeon should be aware of (a) the anatomy, physiology, and inherent limitations of the pathway being monitored, and (b) low-quality data encountered for whatever reason.

False-positives occur when the surgeon is told there are significant changes and the patient awakens with no deficit. This may be a misnomer because the monitored parameter may have correctly indicated significant physiologic change that fortunately was reversible. Furthermore, some pathologic states appear to make the patient susceptible to evoked potential alterations not corre-

Table 12.3   Shift of Latency or Loss of Response

Problem/Cause	Detection	Action
Transducer defect	Suspect during surgery, confirm later by testing transducer	Increase stimulus intensity, later discard transducer
Transducer dislodged	Suspect during surgery, confirm by inspecting placement	Increase stimulus intensity, improve placement and securing techniques next time
Conductive loss (fluid in ear canal)	Suspect during surgery, confirm by inspecting placement	Increase stimulus intensity, improve sealing of ear canal (Steri-Drape, etc.)
Cable	Change cable	Replace cable
Stimulator fault	Attach new transducer to stimulator and confirm proper function	Note latency shift or response loss, repair or replace as soon as possible
Excessive high-frequency filtering	Check filter settings	Return filter to baseline settings
Noise masking, drilling, etc.	Noise apparent in input and average	Increase stimulus intensity, pause averager during drilling

lating with clinical change. Specifically, we have encountered three patients with tic douloureux associated with multiple sclerosis. All had firm clinical diagnoses and presurgical abnormal BAEP IPLs. Wave V was lost during surgery despite prompt retractor removal when significant change was reported. Wave V remained absent at closing of skin and the end of monitoring. Postoperative audiometric assessment revealed normal audiograms unchanged from the presurgical studies.

Intraoperative Feedback to the Surgeon

The guidelines of the American EEG Society on intraoperative monitoring state that "the monitoring team should be under the direct supervision of a trained clinical neurophysiologist (M.D., Ph.D., or D.O.) experienced in EPs." This person should have specialized training in problems related to intraoperative monitoring. The interpreter should be available to communicate to the surgeon about the stability of responses throughout surgery. The interpreter should be familiar with the indications for surgery, the possible neurologic complications of the planned surgery, and the results of any presurgical studies that would relate to the monitoring. In the case of BAEP monitoring, the audiologic status of the patient as revealed by preoperative BAEP and audiogram would constitute a minimum of data. The surgeon should be advised of any preoperative abnormalities before surgery begins. The general quality and reliability of the data should be revealed to the surgeon as this will affect the credence to be given to changes. In the case of lesions affecting the auditory nerve, data quality may be very marginal. The interpreter should have criterion values, beyond which the surgeon will be notified of impending problems. Usually these are in the form of latency and amplitude. It is rare to encounter postoperative deficits unless BAEP responses are entirely lost. However, when changes begin, it is impossible to predict how severely altered responses will become.

A shift in latency of any component of 1.0 ms or more or an amplitude attenuation of 50% should be reported to the surgeon. Rapid latency changes are of greater concern because responses can be lost quickly. Amplitude changes are problematic. A change from 0.50 μV to 0.25 μV is a 50% change but a robust amplitude remains, whereas a change from 0.10 to 0.06 is only a 40% change but the response is virtually lost and may be entirely lost on the next average.

The surgeon should understand the physiology and significance of BAEP monitoring. The interpreter should report the nature of the change and reliability of the data. He or she should be ready to correlate the changes with prospective mechanisms and offer a likely prognostic outcome.

Brain Stem Generators of Brain Stem Auditory Evoked Potential Components

Both the interpreter and surgeon should understand the neural structures involved in the generation of BAEP components. The topic is complex and beyond the scope of this chapter. The components present in all normal subjects (obligate waves) are limited to waves I, III, and V. Waves II, IV, VI, and VII are commonly absent in audiologically and neurologically normal individuals.

Wave I is the action potential of the distal portion of the acoustic division of the eighth cranial nerve. As such it is not a brain stem potential but a peripheral nerve action potential. Wave III is attributed to brain stem, lower pontine generation. Wave V presents some controversy, but the majority attribute its generation to lower midbrain regions. The potentials are probably not a direct result of synaptic activity. Work continues in this elusive area.

Intraoperative Record Keeping

It is imperative to maintain and archive accurate records throughout a surgical case. The interpreter will occasionally need to refer to earlier events in the surgery to appreciate the significance of current electrophysiologic data. When there are adverse outcomes, well-maintained records may shed light on the events associated with a functional loss. It is appropriate to treat each surgical case as having a high potential for an adversarial action. Thus, a log of important events should be maintained by the individual responsible for acquiring and maintaining records. All electrophysiologic data should be stored electronically and archived. This means recording to disk all responses for a given case and downloading the disk to some semipermanent media on a regular basis. This may be floppy disks, removable disks, optical disks, or digital tape. All have a definable life expectancy, and paper records are the only permanent storage. There are no national and usually no state regulations governing appropriate media or duration of storage. It is important to have a written storage policy for the institution.

In our view the important events to log include:

1. All recording and stimulation parameters if not separately and automatically stored by the recording instrumentation.
2. Important milestones in surgery (i.e., time of beginning, opening of dura, use of microscope, placement of retractors, biopsy, tumor debulking, vascular clamps, and so on).
3. Important physiologic parameters (as the anesthesiologist would), especially blood pressure, core temperature, blood loss, electrolyte values, and so on.
4. Anesthetic agents and their concentration that have little or no effect on BAEP components. It is common that the same team recording BAEP responses will record other physiologic activity such as upper-extremity somatosensory responses or cranial nerve motor activity (both spontaneous and evoked). Both can be affected by various anesthetic agents.
5. The time and essence of reports made to the surgeon by the technologist and data interpreter.
6. Any changes in the surgical approach or anesthetic regime made in response to a change of monitoring parameters.

The Postoperative Report

The postoperative report is of little value to the patients. If they benefit, it is from communications in the operating room between the interpreter and surgeon. However, it is mandatory that a permanent record of the monitoring activities be included in the patient's chart. The report should include the following:

1. A brief history
2. A description and interpretation of the preoperative electrophysiologic studies
3. A description of the monitoring, including significant changes and their duration and eventual resolution
4. An interpretation in clinical terms of the findings

CASE STUDIES

The following cases illustrate some of the problems commonly encountered during intraoperative monitoring. Also described are the general technique and the quality of data one might expect. The data was photographed exactly as collected without improvements from postacquisition filtering or medical illustration (other than labeling).

85 dBHL C Clicks

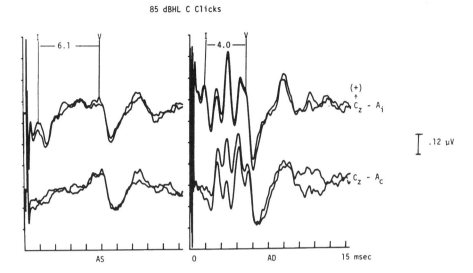

Figure 12.1A Preoperative BAEPs recorded from a 46-year-old patient (Case 1) with an acoustic neuroma. The recording parameters for this and following BAEP illustrations are identical except where noted. Analysis time = 15 ms; filters: LF = 150 Hz; HF = 3,000 Hz; rate = 31.1 per second; number of stimuli = 2,000/trial. Positivity at the vertex will produce an upward deflection.

Case 1

Figure 12.1A shows a preoperative BAEP study on a 46-year-old patient who was to undergo posterior fossa surgery for removal of a presumed eighth nerve tumor. It is a two-channel recording with responses to left ear (AS) stimulation on the left of the figure and right ear (AD) stimulation on the right. Channel 1 is recorded from the vertex (Cz) to the ear ipsilateral to stimulation (Ai) and channel 2, Cz to the ear contralateral to stimulation (Ac). Two trials are superimposed to demonstrate reproducibility. Responses to AD stimulation are entirely normal with a I-V IPL of 4.0 ms. Responses to left-ear stimulation are abnormal with absence of wave III and a severely prolonged I-V IPL of 6.1 ms.

Figure 12.1B demonstrates intraoperative responses on the patient in Case 1 with the eighth nerve tumor. Displayed are responses from stimulation of the ear ipsilateral to surgery as recorded from Cz-Ai. A stimulus rate of 31.1 per second allows rapid assessment, as the acquisition time for a completed average is approximately 1 minute (1,800 stimuli in 1 minute). An unchanged wave V is often visible in less than 5 seconds (150 stimuli). In this instance, the stimuli are 85-dBHL condensation clicks delivered to the Ai while Ac received 55-dBHL white noise masking. The most commonly used intraoperative click polarity is alternating rarefaction and condensation (R/C), the advantage being cancellation of the stimulus artifact. Responses were recorded from 11:08 AM to 12:31 PM. Wave V is the major component of interest because it is the most stable

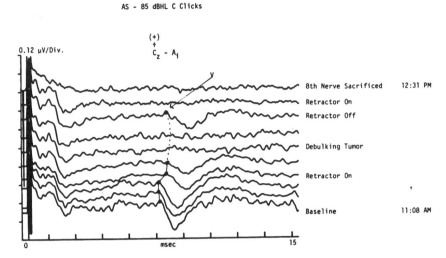

Figure 12.1B Same patient. Intraoperative BAEPs to left-ear stimulation.

BAEP component. At baseline wave V is reproducible although the BAEP is abnormal due to an absence of wave III and prolongation of wave V. When a retractor is placed on the cerebellum, the wave-V latency increases from trial to trial and the V component is not detectable as the tumor is being debulked. The retractor is released and wave V is seen within seconds after an average is initiated. The retractor is replaced and wave V is again lost. The top tracing was recorded after the auditory nerve was sacrificed as required for tumor removal.

Figure 12.1C is from the patient in Case 1 and contrasts left- and right-ear responses. This figure illustrates that while the ear on the side of surgery may (depending on whether the nerve will be sacrificed) be monitored continuously to evaluate auditory nerve and brain stem function, the opposite ear should be monitored at regular intervals to evaluate brain stem function. Likewise, median nerve responses should be recorded regularly, particularly the median nerve contralateral to the side of surgery so that electrophysiologic function caudal to the cerebellopontine angle and rostral to the caudal midbrain can be assessed. In this case, there is no evidence of physiologic change. The cochlear and vestibular nerves were sacrificed primarily due to significant preoperative auditory compromise and size of the tumor.

Case 2

Case 2 is a patient undergoing posterior fossa exploration for tic douloureux.

Figure 12.2A shows intraoperative BAEP responses. Vascular compression of the fifth nerve is a common finding in this condition. Displayed are responses from stimulation of the ear ipsilateral to surgery. The stimuli are 85dBHL rar-

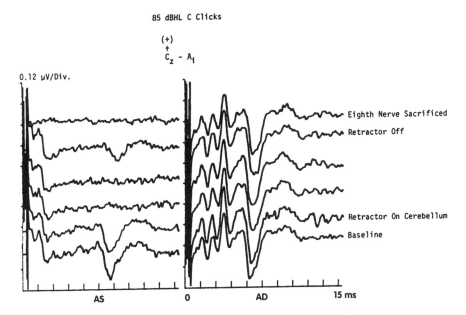

Figure 12.1C Same patient. Comparison of intraoperative BAEPs to left- and right-ear stimulation.

efaction clicks with the opposite ear receiving 55dBHL white noise masking. Responses on the bottom were recorded at baseline at 12:15 PM. Wave V has an absolute latency of 5.88 ms. A retractor was placed on the cerebellum at 12:42 PM. Fifteen minutes later wave V has shifted nearly 1 ms to 6.87 ms and further prolongation occurs. The surgeon is advised that a shift greater than 1 ms has occurred. The retractor is repositioned at 1:24 PM. Wave V has now shifted to 7.71 ms, nearly 2 ms later than baseline. Finally, retraction is released at 1:27 PM. The absolute latency of wave V is 8.01 ms. In the following 9 minutes, wave-V latency moves back to 7.35 ms, and at closing, 30 minutes after retraction is released, the absolute latency of wave V has returned to 6.81 ms—that is, within 1 ms of baseline values.

Figures 12.2B and 12.2C are intraoperative left and right median nerve responses at baseline and at the conclusion of surgery of the Case 2 patient. There is no change from baseline, further demonstrating the electrophysiologic integrity of the somatosensory system traversing brain stem structures. Figure 12.2D illustrates normal intraoperative BAEPs recorded from the ear contralateral to surgery at baseline and at the conclusion of surgery.

Case 3

Case 3 is a 43-year-old patient undergoing a left retromastoid craniotomy for hemifacial spasm. Figure 12.3 shows intraoperative BAEPs. At baseline, the

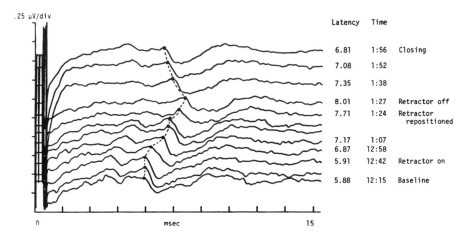

Figure 12.2A Intraoperative BAEPs of a 58-year-old patient (Case 2) with tic douloureux.

Intraoperative
Left Median Nerve

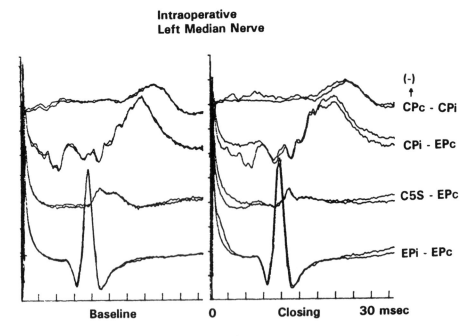

Figure 12.2B Intraoperative left median nerve responses at baseline and at the conclusion of surgery in Case 2.

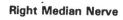

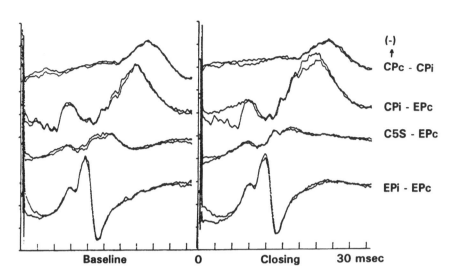

Figure 12.2C Intraoperative right median nerve responses at baseline and at the conclusion of surgery in Case 2.

absolute latency of wave V is 6.48 ms. The retractor is positioned on the cerebellum and wave-V latency increases to a maximum latency of 8.43 ms before retraction is released. Morphology is preserved throughout. By the end of surgery, wave-V latency has shortened to 7.74 ms, 1.3 ms later than baseline values. As is our procedure, the surgeon was notified as the prolongation of wave-V latency approached 1 ms.

Case 4

Case 4 is of a patient with tic douloureux involving the third division of the trigeminal nerve. Eight years previously the patient suffered tic douloureux in the second division of the trigeminal nerve and following drug failure was successfully treated by surgery. Symptoms developed 7 years later in the third division, and, after a brief success with anticonvulsants she again become refractory. Figure 12.4A shows the intraoperative BAEP changes. At this time (1981) we were not yet monitoring median nerves intraoperatively. The patient had an entirely normal preoperative BAEP study. Responses from the ear ipsilateral to surgery are displayed. The wave-V component is stable until a retractor is placed, following which wave-V latency increases. Arterial bleeding was encountered, requiring further retraction to visualize and stop the source of bleeding. Concomitantly there is progressive attenuation of wave V and finally it is absent. As soon as bleeding was controlled the retraction was released and wave

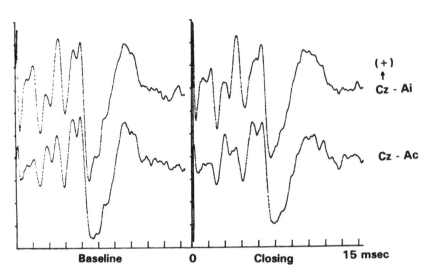

Figure 12.2D Normal intraoperative BAEPs from the ear contralateral to surgery recorded at baseline and at the conclusion of surgery in Case 2.

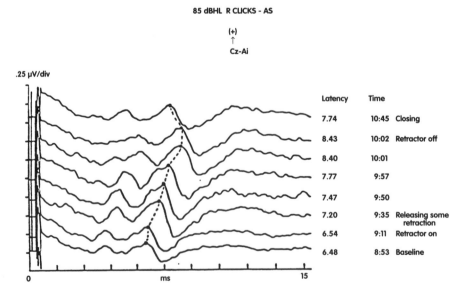

Figure 12.3 Intraoperative BAEPs in a 43-year-old patient (Case 3) with retromastoid craniotomy for hemifacial spasm.

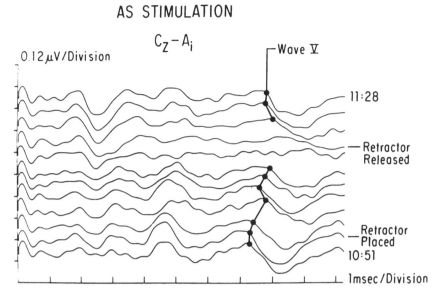

Figure 12.4A Intraoperative BAEPs on a patient (Case 4) with tic douloureux.

V returned within seconds. The absolute latency was initially prolonged but by the end of surgery it had returned to baseline values. In the recovery room, it became apparent that the patient had suffered a dense right hemiparesis, and subsequent clinical examination and imaging studies confirmed a rostral brain stem infarction, which went undetected by BAEP monitoring. Her BAEPs 4 days postoperatively were entirely normal (Figure 12.4B). Postoperative median nerve responses (Figure 12.4C) were demonstrated to be bilaterally normal to the level of P14 generation (caudal pons), but with severe attenuation and asymmetry of the responses from more rostral generators. Her tibial nerve studies demonstrated essentially the same findings (Figure 12.4D). This case, although a false-negative at the time, illustrates that a rostral brain stem lesion is not expected to alter BAEP responses. Had median nerve responses been monitored in addition to the BAEP responses, the lesion would not have gone undetected.

Our current protocol is to monitor BAEPs and median nerves in an alternating fashion. The critical time in these cases appears to be when the retractor is positioned on the cerebellum.

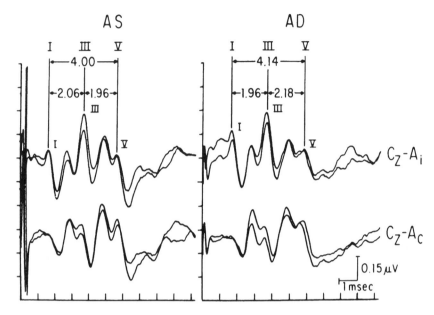

Figure 12.4B Normal BAEPs 4 days postoperatively in the Case 4 patient.

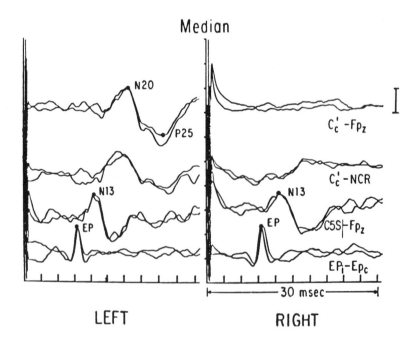

Figure 12.4C Abnormal median nerve responses 4 days postoperatively.

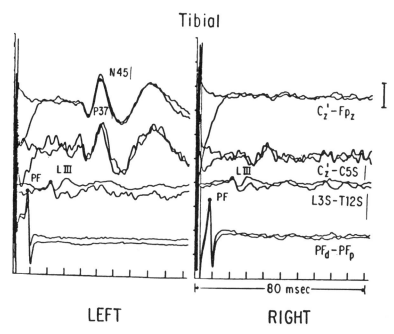

Figure 12.4D Abnormal tibial nerve responses 4 days postoperatively.

KEY REFERENCES

American Electroencephalographic Society guidelines on evoked potentials. J Clin Neurophysiol 1994;11:40.

Drake ME, Erwin CW. Brainstem auditory evoked responses: Validity of adding responses to opposite click polarities to synthesize alternating click responses. EEG Clin Neurophysiol 1982;53:92.

Erwin CW, Cahill WT, Griffiths MF. A mathematical model to explain derivation-specific latency shifts in BAEP studies. Neurology 1986;36:30.

Erwin CW, Gulevich SJ. The evaluation of transducers for obtaining intra-operative short-latency auditory evoked potentials. EEG Clin Neurophysiol 1985;61:194.

Erwin CW. Brainstem auditory evoked potentials: Investigation of latency-amplitude differences from ipsilateral and contralateral ear derivations. EEG Clin Neurophysiol 1981;52:S133.

Janssen R et al. Differential impact of hypothermia and pentobarbital on brain stem auditory evoked responses. EEG Clin Neurophysiol 1991;80(5):412.

Jasper H. The ten-twenty electrode system of the international federation. EEG Clin Neurophysiol 1958;10:367.

Jiang ZD, Wu YY, Zhang L. Amplitude change with click rate in human brainstem auditory-evoked responses. J Audiol 1991;30(3):173.

Kakizawa T, Shimizu T, Fukushima T. Monitoring of auditory brainstem response (ABR) during microvascular decompression (MVD): Results in 400 cases. Brain Nerve 1990;42(10):991.

Legatt AD, Arezzo JC, Vaughan HG Jr. The anatomic and physiologic bases of brainstem auditory evoked potentials. Neurol Clin 1988;6:681.

Levine RA et al. Evoked potential detection of hearing loss during acoustic neuroma surgery. Neurology 1978;28:339.

Lloyd-Thomas AR, Cole PV, Prior PF. Quantitative EEG and brainstem auditory evoked potentials: Comparison of isoflurane with halothane using the cerebral function analyzing monitor. Br J Anaesth 1990;65(3):306.

Lueders H et al. Origin of far-field subcortical evoked potentials to posterior tibial and median nerve stimulation. A comparative study. Arch Neurol 1983;40:93.

Markand ON et al. Effects of hypothermia on brainstem auditory evoked potentials in humans. Ann Neurol 1987;22:507.

Moller AR. Evoked Potentials in Intraoperative Monitoring. Baltimore: Williams & Wilkins, 1988.

Piatt JH, Radtke R, Erwin CW. Limitations of brainstem auditory evoked potentials for intra-operative monitoring of posterior fossa surgery. Case report and technical note. Neurosurgery 1985;16:818.

Piatt JH, Wilkins RH. Treatment of tic douloureux and hemifacial spasm by posterior fossa exploration: Therapeutic implications of various neurovascular relations. Neurosurgery 1984;14:462.

Sebel PS, Erwin CW, Neville WK. Effects of halothane and enflurane on far- and near-field somatosensory evoked potentials. Br J Anaesth 1987;59:1492.

Sindou M et al. Intraoperative brainstem auditory evoked potential in the microvascular decompression of the 5th and 7th cranial nerves. Rev Laryngol Otol Rhinol 1990;111(5):427.

Slavit DH et al. Auditory monitoring during acoustic neuroma removal. Arch Otolaryngol Head Neck Surg 1991;117(10):1153.

Stockard JJ, Stockard JE, Sharbrough FW. Nonpathologic factors influencing brainstem auditory evoked potentials. Am J EEG Technol 1978;18:177.

Wilkins RH, Radtke RA, Erwin CW. The value of intraoperative brainstem auditory evoked potential monitoring in reducing the auditory morbidity associated with microvascular decompression of cranial nerves. Skull Base Surgery 1991;2:106.

13

Motor Evoked Potentials

Garfield B. Russell, M.D., FRCPC

Development of motor evoked potential (MEP) monitoring has allowed improved care of the anesthetized patient at risk for intraoperative spinal cord injury. Somatosensory evoked potentials (SSEPs) have allowed intraoperative assessment of the dorsal and lateral sensory tracts of the spinal cord (see Chapter 11) and have been thought to provide some reflection of changes in integrity of the anterior motor tracts. (See Chapter 2 for description of spinal cord tracts.) However, motor deficits during spinal surgery have occurred without changes in SSEPs. The capability of monitoring both the sensory and now the motor tracts has improved the perceived completeness of spinal cord monitoring and has maximized the likelihood of preserving the electrical and functional integrity of the spinal cord.

MOTOR EVOKED POTENTIALS
Eliciting and Recording Motor Potentials

MEPs can be elicited by either electrical or magnetic stimulation. Stimulating impulses can be applied either transcortically to the brain or to the spinal cord. Although transcortical stimulation for spinal cord monitoring involves transcranial application of either electricity or a magnetic field, during neurosurgical procedures direct electrical stimulation may be applied to the motor cortex (see a description of the motor homunculus in Chapter 2) to elicit a physical or electrical motor response and help define functional motor cortex borders. The electrical responses are recorded distal to the site of stimulation. These responses can be neurogenic potentials from the spinal cord itself or peripheral nerves, or myogenic potentials elicited from muscle fibers after activation of the motor-end plates.

Contrasting Neurogenic and Myogenic Motor Potentials

Both neurogenic and myogenic responses can be elicited by electrical and magnetic stimulation. Neurogenic recordings from the spinal cord can be made with surface or needle electrodes, but less technical interference is obtained from a catheter/electrode in the epidural or subdural space. For intraspinal recordings, two catheter/electrodes are placed so that one is rostral and one caudal to the spinal segments at risk, allowing localization of changed potentials and comparison with the proximal "control" recording. During spinal surgery, these recording electrodes can be placed through a laminectomy site, between lamina if a laminectomy is not done, or percutaneously through a Tuohy needle if the spine is not exposed at the insertion site.

Neurogenic recordings from peripheral nerves are usually made from needle electrodes inserted percutaneously over the nerves being monitored after stimulation of the cortex or electrical stimulation of the spinal cord. Muscle artifact can distort these low-amplitude responses, and administration of muscle relaxants improves quality.

Myogenic potential recordings are made from needle electrodes inserted into peripheral muscles. Careful titration or avoidance of muscle relaxants is needed since neuromuscular blockade can eliminate the recordable compound muscle action potential. Because the stimulation is usually transcranial, these motor potentials can be easily suppressed by anesthetic agents (see Chapter 18).

TRANSCRANIAL ELECTRICAL STIMULATION FOR MOTOR EVOKED POTENTIALS

Monitoring the functional integrity of the spinal cord expanded with recording of responses to noninvasive transcranial electrical stimulation of the motor cortex (TceMEPs) and spinal cord in 1980. A high-voltage, short-duration stimulus overcomes the high impedance of scalp and cranium to induce a current in brain tissue and stimulate motor cortex with depolarization of pyramidal neurons or their axons and activation of corticospinal tract neurons.

Technical Aspects

One of the electrical stimulators used is the Digitimer D180A (Digitimer Ltd., Welwyn Garden City, UK). Stimulus intensity is adjustable as a percentage of maximum output up to 1,200 volts with a time constant of 50 or 100 ms to 0.4 Hz. The higher intensity stimulus is usually used for stimulation over the vertebral column, whereas up to 750 V is used for transcranial applications (Figure 13.1). Stimulation rates can vary from 5–17 Hz, although higher repetition rates are less frequently used. Typically 30–250 repetitions are used intraoperatively.

Bipolar and unipolar stimulation methods have been used. For bipolar stimulation, either Ag/AgCl$_2$ cup electrodes (9-mm diameter) or spiral electrodes are applied to the scalp. Anodal stimulation is thought to be superior, with better quality recordable responses. For upper-extremity stimulation, the anode is 1 cm in front of C3/C4 and the cathode at Cz. (For a description of the international ten-twenty system, see Chapter 5.) For lower-limb stimulation, the anode is positioned at Cz and the cathode 6 or 7 cm in front of Cz or 1 cm in front of C3/C4.

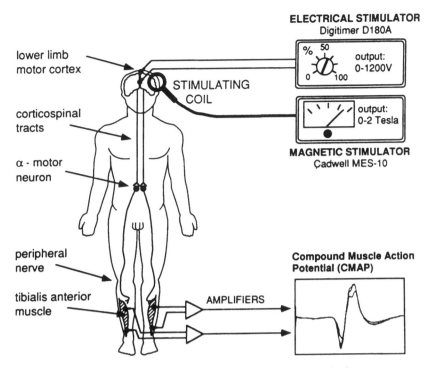

Figure 13.1 Both magnetic and electrical stimulation of the cerebral motor cortex can be used to produce compound muscle action potentials. Neurogenic responses can be recorded but are not usually used at this time. *Reprinted with permission from CJ Kalkman et al. Effects of propofol, etomidate, midazolam and fentanyl on motor evoked responses to transcranial electrical or magnetic stimulation in humans. Anesthesiology 1992;76:503.*

For unipolar stimulation the anode is placed over the appropriate area of the motor cortex, and the cathode consists of eight electrodes placed in a circle above the nasion-inion line.

Myogenic responses are usually recorded, although neurogenic potentials can also be monitored. Compound action potentials (CMAPs) are recorded from gold-disk electrodes placed on the bellies of peripheral muscle or needle electrodes inserted into the muscle. Signal amplification is used as appropriate for the size of the signal, which can vary. Single sweeps of 100–ms duration can be used with filtering usually between 10 and 3,000 Hz.

Disadvantages and Reservations

The disadvantages of TceMEPs include (1) susceptibility to anesthetic depression (see Chapter 18), (2) inability to separately stimulate upper and lower extremities, and (3) discomfort on stimulation, although this is not a problem in anesthetized patients.

Electrical current may result in significant neuronal injuries. Damage depends on the charge density to tissue and the charge with each stimulation. Attenuation of the electrical stimulus by the high resistance of the skull diminishes this intensity. The electrical current induced is much less than that with electroconvulsive therapy.

Many contraindications are relative; risk-benefit ratios must be considered for many patients.

1. A history of seizures or an EEG indicative of a seizure disorder must be considered. Kindling, or the production of a self-sustaining seizure focus secondary to repeated stimulation with subthreshold electrical stimulation, may be a risk. This concern is more relevant to awake patients.
2. Skull fractures or other defects in the calvarium may result in current shunting with excessively high local current densities resulting.
3. Implanted metallic devices may focus current density.

TRANSCRANIAL MAGNETIC STIMULATION FOR MOTOR EVOKED POTENTIALS

A strong pulsed magnetic field applied over the scalp activates cortical and probably subcortical motor neurons generating motor tract potentials (TcmMEPs), which can be recorded as neurogenic potentials from the spinal cord or peripheral nerves, or myogenic potentials, which can be recorded as standard electromyography (see Figure 13.1). A high-voltage capacitor bank discharges a high current (approximately 4,000 A) into a coil producing a magnetic field (usually 1.5–2.0 tesla). The center of the stimulating coil, which is in contact with the scalp, is the reference point. Stimulation is painless, but the TcmMEP responses are very easily suppressed by anesthetic agents (see Chapter 18).

Technical Aspects

Magnetic stimulation of the brain with recording of muscle action potentials was initially introduced in 1985. Although clinical use is still experimental, available magnetic stimulators include the Digitimer D190 (Digitimer Ltd., Welwyn Garden City, U.K.), the Magstim 200 (Novametrix, Wallingford, CT), and the Cadwell MES-10 (Cadwell Laboratories, Kennewick, WA). With the Cadwell MES-10, a transient 2-tesla magnetic field can be induced through a 9-cm–diameter isolated coil firmly held against the scalp. A rotary dial is calibrated in terms of percentage of maximum output. The 20-mV to 100-V CMAPs are not averaged and gain settings are individually determined. A 3- to 3,000-Hz bandpass filter is used. The average latencies for proximal upper limbs (14–18 ms), distal upper limbs (19–25 ms), and lower limbs (40 ms) make 50- to 100-ms sweep times reasonable.

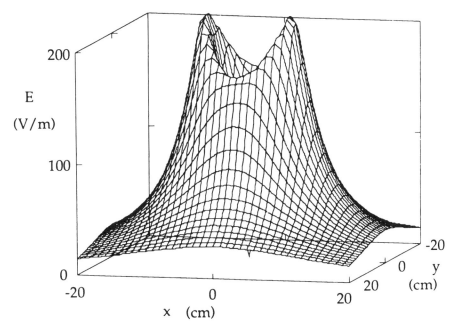

Figure 13.2 The contour plot of a magnetic field generated by a cap coil. A symmetrical field is shown with the drop in the field between peaks representing the center of the band of coil windings over the cranium. *Reprinted with permission from WJ Levy et al. Transcranial Magnetic Evoked Potential Monitoring. In CM Loftus, VC Traynelis (eds), Intraoperative Monitoring Techniques in Neurosurgery. New York: McGraw-Hill, 1994.*

Magnetoelectric Stimulation

In 1831, Faraday discovered that a changing magnetic field induced an electric current in a conductor under it (Faraday's law). This stimulatory effect was found to extend to excitable tissue in 1896, neural tissue in 1968 and 1972, and finally to CMAP response recordings in 1985.

The flow of electricity through a magnetic coil generates a magnetic field with invisible lines of magnetic flux. The magnetic field and so the electric current induced is proportional to the total teslas of this flux density, which depends on coil area and number of turns in the coil.

The intensity of magnetic fields induced by coils is maximal under the edge of the coil and minimal in the center. This affects coil design. Circular coils induce no electric field at the exact center of the coil, resulting in an unfocused stimulation field. Butterfly or figure–eight designs produce more focal electrical fields where the coils meet. Coil caps have been designed to allow most motor cortex to be exposed to an induced magnetic field for electrical current induction (Figure 13.2).

Disadvantages and Reservations

The most significant disadvantages of TcmMEPs are that (1) good signals are difficult to obtain in the operating room; coil designs other than circular may improve on this to some degree; (2) TcmMEPs are susceptible to suppression with most anesthetic agents; and (3) coil application and positioning may be unwieldy.

As with TceMEPs, the final common pathway for magnetic transcranial stimulation is neural excitation by an electrical current. Potential complications include (1) electrical neural injury, which is unlikely since the maximum current produced in the brain is about 0.25 A. (2) Tissue heating is related to charge and charge density, which are considered insufficient with TceMEPs. (3) Kindling is unlikely.

As with TcmMEPs, many relative contraindications must be assessed from a risk-benefit perspective. As with TceMEPs, calvarial defects, epilepsy, and implanted metal must be considered. Other devices that may be affected by transcranial stimulation include implanted drug pumps or dorsal column stimulators, cardiac pacemakers, and intracranial monitors.

DIFFERENCES BETWEEN TRANSCRANIAL ELECTRICAL AND MAGNETIC STIMULATION

TceMEP and TcmMEP monitoring are examples of evolving innovative technology and instrumentation used to monitor spinal cord functional and electrical integrity. Differences between these two monitoring modalities include the following:

1. TcmMEP is painless in application, unlike the "jolting" of TceMEP.
2. TceMEP is more resistant to anesthetic suppression.
3. Responses obtained with TcmMEP vary with the direction of current within the coil. For example, inside a circular coil, a clockwise current induces a counterclockwise current, activating the left hemisphere.
4. CMAPs induced by TcmMEP have a 2- to 4-ms longer latency than those from TceMEP. It is likely that TceMEP directly activates corticospinal pathways and TcmMEP produces an indirect stimulation. The major differences appear to be in the physiological aspects of the CMAPs produced.

NEUROGENIC MOTOR EVOKED POTENTIALS

Neurogenic motor evoked potentials (NMEPs) were developed in part to decrease the anesthetic limitations imposed by motor tract monitoring after transcranial stimulation. NMEP monitoring was originally developed in the early 1980s using surgically placed epidural stimulating electrodes. Variations with blind epidural electrode placement and development and testing of other techniques have led to use of other stimulating sites. Spine-to-spine and spine-to-peripheral nerve monitoring can be done.

Spinal cord stimulation for elicitation of NMEPs has required some elucidation of neuronal tracts. Because the cord is compact, the activated neuronal tissue might include both ascending and descending tracts, interneurons, anterior and posterior spinal roots, or a combination of any of these anatomic and functional entities. A study in a canine model studied spinal cord stimulation at T1–2 with a constant voltage-stimulating electrode applied to the spinal cord midline after laminectomies and response recordings from the cord at L2 and dorsal nerve roots. They concluded that descending spinal cord evoked potentials travel on multiple ascending and descending tracts. The potential waveform consists of an earlier motor tract wave followed by multiple smaller waves that may be potentials "backfiring" down the ascending tracts. Although NMEP amplitude is low, often 1–2 mV, and background electrical interference can often be noted in the recording, the waveform is usually clearly delineated (Figure 13.3). We record from needle electrodes either in the popliteal fossa or over the posterior tibial nerve. The prominent orthodromic motor component of the NMEP is relatively large. The antidromic waves forming the possible sensory component are smaller and not reliably found.

Technical Aspects

For recording NMEPs, we usually use a Nicolet Viking (Nicolet Biomedical Instruments, Madison, WI). Because NMEPs have a small amplitude, a sensitive amplifier setting allows a reliable response recording at the lowest–intensity stimulation possible. A constant voltage signal set to 100 V in single pulses for 0.3 ms at 4.7 Hz is usually used to start, and intensity is gradually increased as needed for maximal response recording. The fewest number of samples possible are obtained for averaging, at times less than 20, always less than 100 stimulations. A 100-µV full-scale sensitivity is usually used, with a 10-Hz low-frequency filter and 3,000-Hz high-frequency filter setting.

NMEPS are stimulated by two 0.5-inch, Teflon-coated, tip-exposed, stimulating needle electrodes (JO-5, The Electrode Store, Yucca Valley, CA) placed in close proximity to the spinal cord. The anode is placed rostral to the cathode; otherwise a form of "anode block" occurs, resulting in lower–amplitude recordable potentials. These needle electrodes are separated by one vertebral body and can be inserted translaminarly in the superior margin of the surgical incision, into the vertebral corpus so that the needle tip is within 1 cm of the cord, or through a percutaneous site rostral to the surgical field onto lamina. The upper cervical cord can also be stimulated by the anode electrode placed in the retropharynx with the cathode placed on the skin over the upper cervical cord.

Advantages of Neurogenic Motor Evoked Potentials

Cord stimulation from stimulating electrodes inserted into the vertebral body has particular advantages. These include (1) avoidance of the not yet fully delineated potential effects of cortical stimulation, (2) avoiding the spinal canal

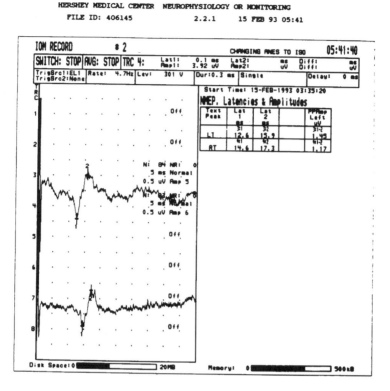

Figure 13.3 A baseline neurogenic motor evoked potential recorded from the popliteal fossa of each lower limb after stimulation at the C6/C7 level. The orthodromic motor component is clearly visible; the antidromic sensory waves are buried in the electrical artifact.

for stimulation, and (3) allowing use of muscle relaxants intraoperatively, since myogenic potentials can be altered by muscle relaxants. (4) Furthermore, NMEPs are resistant to suppression by anesthetic agents.

Technical Problems with Neurogenic Motor Evoked Potentials

Not all changes in or disappearances of NMEPs are secondary to spinal cord injury. Technical problems sometimes occur.

1. When cervical or high thoracic stimulation is used, artifact appears on the electrocardiograph monitor screen. It may appear as a paced tachycardia of 300 beats per minute (Figure 13.4).
2. After insertion of hardware, such as Harrington rods during scoliosis surgery, if the instrumentation is near the stimulating electrodes, a "shorting-out" effect may occur with a marked decrease in response amplitude or complete loss of the NMEP. Careful electrode placement

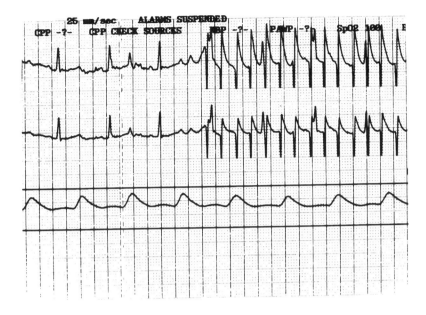

Figure 13.4 Cervical or high thoracic stimulation for neurogenic motor evoked potential monitoring may result in artifactual changes in the electrocardiograph without changes in actual heart rate.

away from the hardware is preferable to increasing amplitude intensity in order to again record the NMEP.

3. The stimulating current can be shunted away from the spinal cord by irrigation fluids or blood collecting around the needle electrodes placed within the bone. A dry stimulation site is vital.
4. Unless the patient is receiving muscle relaxants, with a minimum loss of 2 (or preferably more) of 4 twitches, there is paraspinous muscle contraction that can at times be severe enough to displace electrodes and be an unnecessary irritant within the surgical field.

Reliability and Sensitivity of Neurogenic Motor Evoked Potentials

NMEPs are viewed by those using them clinically as being more reliably obtained than SSEPs, TceMEPs, or TcmMEPs. Baseline NMEPS were obtained intraoperatively in approximately 93% of patients when NMEPs were initially introduced at our institution. In this same patient group, baseline SSEPs were recorded in 88%. Other clinical studies have found easy NMEP elicitation in greater than 90% of patients. Repeatability of cortically recorded SSEPs is reduced by anesthetic agents administered, but NMEPS are relatively unaffected if muscle relaxation is maintained. This has proven to be particularly important in patients in whom cortically recorded SSEPs are not recordable and in whom potentials from the cervical spinal cord are often difficult to obtain.

Both animal and clinical studies suggest that NMEPs are more sensitive and specific for detection of spinal cord compression, distraction, and ischemia than SSEPs. In swine, both disappeared approximately 14 minutes after aortic cross-clamping. With spinal cord distraction, SSEP degradation required at least 15% distraction, whereas NMEPs changed at 5–10% spinal cord distraction. In 300 patients monitored intraoperatively, NMEPs proved more indicative of postoperative motor tract function than SSEPs.

Time to loss of NMEPs and SSEPs can be either slow (approximately 20 minutes) or fast (approximately 3.5 minutes). The mechanism of injury for slow loss of the potential is diffuse cord ischemia. Fast loss occurs with mechanical injury and structural changes or localized ischemia.

MEPs are one of several methodologies available to clinicians for monitoring intraoperative spinal cord function. The varieties of motor tract monitoring available for assessing functional integrity of the motor system make decisions about stimulation site, response recording site, and types of responses necessary. As a monitoring group, we have decided on electrical stimulation of the spinal cord to elicit a NMEP as the most consistently reliable while providing adequate sensitivity to pathophysiologic changes along with resistance to anesthetic effects. Further research and technological development may alter this in the future. At present, spinal cord stimulation avoids clinically significant anesthetic suppression. Electrical stimulation of the spinal cord is technically easy and initiates recordable potentials, whereas magnetic stimulation of the cord, unlike transcranial stimulation, may not induce a flow of electrical current to induce a response potential. We have found that the neurogenic response is obtained more reliably than a myogenic response. For more complete monitoring of spinal cord integrity, NMEPS are always combined with SSEPs, when they are recordable, and sometimes with Stagnara "wake-up" tests as well. However, as is the case for many new developments in medicine, although those of us who use them are convinced of this benefit and utility, their full clinical value and cost-effectiveness are not yet fully clarified.

KEY REFERENCES

Barker AT, Jalinous R, Freeston I. Noninvasive magnetic stimulation of human motor cortex. Lancet 1985;1:1106. *This paper describes the initial use of transcranial magnetic stimulation of the motor tracts with recording of MEPs.*

Machida M et al. Spinal cord monitoring. Spine 1985;10:407–413. *This was one of the early studies describing spinal cord electrical stimulation and peripheral recording of evoked responses at both muscles and nerves.*

Merton PA, Morton HB. Stimulation of the cerebral cortex in the intact human subject. Nature 1980;285:227.

Merton PA et al. Scope of technique for electrical stimulation of human brain. Lancet 1982;1:597–600. *These two papers describe the initial development of transcranial electrical stimulation for elicitation of MEPs.*

Osenbach RK, Yamada T, Traynelis VC. Transcranial Magnetic Stimulation of the Motor Cortex. In CM Loftus, VC Traynelis (eds), Intraoperative Monitoring Techniques in Neurosurgery. New York: McGraw-Hill, 1994;239–250.

Owen JH et al. Sensitivity and specificity of somatosensory and neurogenic-motor evoked potentials in animals and humans. Spine 1988;13:1111–1118.

Owen JH et al. Relationship between duration of spinal cord ischemia and postoperative neurologic deficits in animals. Spine 1990;15:618–622.

Owen JH et al. The clinical application of neurogenic motor evoked potentials to monitor spinal cord function during surgery. Spine 1991;16:S385. *Much of the development and initial studies of neurogenic motor evoked potentials was done by Dr. Owen and his colleagues. These papers, read as a unit, give a full understanding of the basis of NMEPs and their clinical potential with operating room use.*

RECOMMENDED READING

Ben-David D, Holler G, Taylor P. Anterior spinal fusion complicated by paraplegia: a case report of a false–negative SSEP. Spine 1987;12:536–539.

Lesser RP et al. Postoperative neurological deficits may occur despite unchanged intraoperative somatosensory evoked potentials. Ann Neurol 1986;19:22–25. *These two papers provide examples of intraoperative mishaps that make a good case for motor tract monitoring.*

Edmonds H, et al. Transcranial magnetic motor evoked potentials (tcMMEP) for functional monitoring of motor pathways during scoliosis surgery. Spine 1989;14:683–686.

Owen JH, Naito M, Bridwell KH. Relationship among level of distraction, evoked potentials, spinal cord ischemia and integrity, and clinical status in animals. Spine 1990;15:852–857.

Owen JH et al. Effects of spinal cord lesioning on somatosensory and neurogenic-motor evoked potentials. Spine 1989;14:673–683.

Penfield W, Boldrey E. Somatic motor and sensory representation in the cerebral cortex of man as studied by electrical stimulation. Brain 1937;60:839, 1937. *This paper provides much of the background for understanding motor–cortex function and the basis on which monitoring motor pathways was developed.*

14

Intraoperative Electromyography

Patrick M. McQuillan, M.D.
Nanette Newberg, M.S.

This chapter focuses on electromyographic monitoring during surgical procedures for (1) selective dorsal rhizotomy (SDR), used in the treatment of spasticity; (2) release of tethered cords; and (3) the evaluation of pedicle screw position in spinal fusion surgery.

Selective dorsal rhizotomy is used to treat spasticity in carefully selected patients. The purpose of intraoperative monitoring during this procedure is to preserve sensory innervation and allow motor retraining of the affected muscle group during subdivision and sectioning of portions of dorsal nerve roots.

The tethered cord syndrome may result from any form of spinal dysrhaphism in which the conus medullaris of the spinal cord is prevented from normal upward movement during development. The purpose of cord-releasing operations is to eliminate tightness of the spinal cord, cauda equina, and spinal nerves tethered by anomalous tissue. For that reason, monitoring for tethered spinal cord syndrome must detect whether the tight tissue contains nerve elements before the surgeon cuts the tissue for cord release.

Pedicle screw fixation of the lumbar spine has become an accepted technique in spinal fusion surgery. This technique provides rigidity for fixation of the vertebral segment. Neurologic deficits due to inaccurate pedicle screw placement have been documented, and recent evidence supports the use of electromyography (EMG) as a more sensitive electrophysiologic means for detecting malpositioned pedicle screws.

SELECTIVE DORSAL RHIZOTOMY
Background

The purpose of SDR is to reduce debilitating spasticity. The most common application is in children with cerebral palsy, although the operation has also been used to reduce spasticity in patients with multiple sclerosis, spinal cord injury, and brain trauma.

Cerebral palsy is a motor disorder caused by a perinatal insult to the developing brain. Associated disorders such as hydrocephalus, seizures, and impairment of cognition, speech, vision, and hearing may occur in cerebral palsy, but its primary manifestation is disturbance of motor function. The disorder is usually classified as spastic, dystonic-athetoid, ataxic, or mixed, with the spastic type being most common. The spastic type has become more common due to improved survival rates among low-birth-weight premature infants, who are prone to develop spastic cerebral palsy.

While the use of SDR to relieve spasticity in human patients was first reported over 80 years ago, and nonselective partial SDRs have been performed, it was not until recently that a selective procedure using electrophysiologic techniques was developed. Fasten and colleagues described the basic technique and the results for a series of patients with cerebral palsy in the late 1970s. In 1983, Laitinen and colleagues reported use of a similar technique on a small series of patients with spasticity from various causes, and Peacock and colleagues reported on a series of 60 patients with cerebral palsy that they treated in South Africa. Currently, groups are actively performing the procedure in about 15 centers in the United States, and recently a number of these centers have begun to use electrophysiologic monitoring in the operating room in a novel way.

This procedure involves a lumbar laminectomy performed to expose the dorsal roots of the second lumbar to second sacral spinal nerves—those roots that serve the lower limbs. At each level, subsets of dorsal root fibers (rootlets) are stimulated using single pulses or pulse trains ranging in frequency from 20–50 per second, thereby activating the stretch reflex and producing motor responses in the lower limbs. Rootlets associated with an abnormal motor response, as judged by EMG recordings from various muscle groups and observation of lower-limb movement, are sectioned, leaving intact rootlets associated with normal responses. This select-and-cut approach minimizes the number of rootlets sectioned and, in so doing, preserves sensory input that is also transmitted to the central nervous system via the dorsal roots.

Many patients with cerebral palsy can apparently benefit from this procedure, and the results have been remarkably good. Patient selection, however, is critical. The available evidence indicates that the spastic form of cerebral palsy is most amenable to treatment with SDR. According to Peacock and colleagues, "patients whose function improved most dramatically following rhizotomy were purely spastic, were intelligent, and had some degree of forward locomotion. Their lower limbs were more affected by spasticity than the upper limbs." To be considered for surgery, the patient must have spasticity that has reached a point where it does not respond to physical and occupational therapy. Patients with the other forms have benefited only to the extent that coexisting spasticity was relieved.

In the spastic form of cerebral palsy, the motor cortex is primarily affected. Patients with lower-limb spasticity typically walk on their toes with their knees bent in a jerky, scissoring motion. The patient's arms are usually held up for balance, and there may be pronounced compensatory motions of the trunk. The muscles in the affected areas are continually stiff due to increased muscle tone. The upper limbs may also be affected. The basal ganglia are primarily affected in the dystonic form. In such patients, muscle movements are smooth and writhing in nature. In the ataxic form, there is damage to the cerebellum, resulting in clumsiness and lack of balance. For such patients, the results have been quite gratifying, with muscle tone reduced to normal or near normal; with intensive rehabilitative training, they could learn more normal patterns of movement. The postoperative rehabilitation program is a critical element in achieving a good outcome. For a number of patients, there were also initially unexpected improvements in upper-limb function and even speech. These could be explained subsequently by examining the presumed mechanism by which the procedure relieves spasticity.

Mechanisms of Selective Dorsal Rhizotomy

The mechanism of spasticity is thought to be a lack of central inhibitory influences on motor nerves. Normally, there is a balance between inhibitory and excitatory influences on motor nerves. Facilitation is normally provided via afferent fibers from muscle spindles as part of the stretch reflex. Inhibition, on the other hand, is provided via descending tracts from higher centers involved in motor control. These influences are modulated to maintain proper muscle tone and allow for appropriate movement and posture. When the inhibitory component is insufficient due to damage to brain motor centers, the excitatory influences prevail, resulting in a continuous level of abnormal muscle tension in the affected muscles and resistance to movement.

The purpose of the SDR is to decrease the level of facilitory input to motor nerves of the legs by cutting a portion of the posterior root afferent fibers, thereby bringing about a more normal balance of excitatory and inhibitory input. The potential problem of such an approach is that the posterior roots also contain afferent fibers carrying information necessary for normal cutaneous sensation and proprioception. These sensory modalities are clearly beneficial in the rehabilitory process and clearly should be spared as much as possible. Since the rootlet fibers carrying muscle spindle input are in appearance indistinguishable from those carrying desirable sensory input, the functional measure of motor response to electrical stimulation was adopted as a means for selecting rootlets for sectioning.

Rootlet selection is based on the observation that in patients with spasticity there are several modes of muscle activity in response to electrical stimulation of posterior roots or rootlets. On the basis of studies in animals, one type of response was assumed to be the result of a normal nerve circuit and the others were assumed to be the result of circuits in which the normal inhibitory influences were reduced or absent.

The normal response is a brief twitch of the appropriate muscles (as recorded by EMG) in response to the first stimulus in a pulse train of 30–50 Hz. (At stimulus rates above 10 Hz, inhibitory influences apparently come into play, resulting in suppression of muscle response to subsequent stimuli.) There are several types of putatively abnormal response, including repetitive responses to each pulse in the appropriate muscles, dissemination of the response to inappropriate muscle groups (sometimes at quite a distance, such as in the contralateral limb or the arms), and continued muscle responses after the cessation of the stimulus train.

Abnormal circuits are typically irregularly scattered among the lumbar and sacral roots. A single root can contain fibers connecting to both normal and abnormal circuits of various types. In such cases, the roots must be divided into rootlets (5–15 per root) to determine which are the sources of the abnormal responses. The normal rootlets are then spared and the abnormal rootlets are sectioned. Typically, less than 50% of lumbar and sacral rootlets are sectioned in the procedure.

Results of Selective Dorsal Rhizotomy

In almost all cases reported, there has been an improvement in spasticity postoperatively. The most successful results were obtained in patients in whom spasticity was the primary problem. Depending on the patient, there were improvements in muscle tone, mobility, posture, balance, and mass reflexes. In many cases, there was improvement in upper limb function, and in some, in speech and breath control as well. These improvements were explained by Peacock and colleagues, "on the basis that dorsal root neurons are involved not only in their respective spinal cord segmental reflex, but have collaterals that ascend giving branches that synapse with spinal anterior horn cells at many levels and with brainstem motor nuclei. By dividing lumbar posterior rootlets, not only would facilitory influences be reduced in the lumbar segments of the cord, but also on motor neurons at higher levels. Where upper limb function and speech are interfered with because of increased tone in the relevant muscle groups, decreasing facilitory input would reduce tone and may improve function."

Anesthetic Considerations

The anesthetic technique for SDR must allow muscle contraction in response to direct electrical stimulation of the dorsal nerve rootlets. The electrophysiologist's main requirement for adequate EMG recording is that muscles not be paralyzed.

Children undergoing SDR often have exaggerated pain and muscle spasm postoperatively, probably from severe hyperesthesia and dysesthesia in combination with polysynaptic flexion reflexes. Intrathecal morphine acts in the dorsal horn to inhibit polysynaptic nociceptive input and to decrease the severity of reflex spasm. The therapeutic range of intrathecal morphine for SDR pain is 7–35 µg/kg.

Hyperthermia is a potential concern in children having SDR during electrical stimulation. It is necessary to use light draping, lower room temperatures after draping, high fresh gas flows, no heating blanket or fluid warmer, and no heat and moisture exchanger. The potential for hyperthermia during stimulation may be related to increased metabolic demands secondary to muscle activity from stimulation. If so, this increased metabolic demand may account for the relatively high anesthetic requirements seen in children undergoing SDR.

The observations of increasing temperature and muscle spasms in children having SDR leads us to consider issues related to malignant hyperthermia. We believe that succinylcholine is relatively contraindicated in children having SDR.

Propofol has proved to be an unacceptable anesthetic because of muscle spasms seen during stimulation. Although there are reports that laryngoscopy and intubation are possible after propofol, probably secondary to depressed pharyngeal and laryngeal reactivity, there are other reports that propofol has poor muscle relaxation properties, and its use to facilitate intubation is not always acceptable.

While either deep inhalation anesthesia or intermediate-acting nondepolarizing muscle relaxants can be used for intubation, any level of muscle relaxant at the time of stimulation interferes with electrophysiologic monitoring signal quality. Isoflurane, halothane, and narcotics do not interfere with electrophysiologic monitoring, even if rapid changes or bolus doses are administered. Inhalation anesthetic requirements and narcotic doses can be high. Isoflurane may be preferred to halothane, as lower concentrations are needed during stimulation.

Methods
Presurgery Muscle Selection
Selection of the muscle groups to be monitored is completed during the presurgery assessment to optimize the information gained during the surgical procedure. Although the muscles selected for monitoring may vary depending on the clinical status of the child, muscles are chosen to ensure that L2–S1 nerve roots are represented. Problems in the adductor longus, medial gastrocnemius, a medial hamstring, and gluteus maximus muscles often lead to the greatest functional deficits in children with cerebral palsy. We believe the gluteus maximus muscle is very important for walking and is often weak in these children. Thus, it is monitored to avoid sectioning many rootlets that, when stimulated, lead to electrical activity in this muscle.

Selection of Abnormal Responses During Surgery
The decision to transect or preserve specific rootlets is made on the basis of several factors. The first is the observed muscle contractions in the legs. They are observed to confirm the electrical response pattern, to define contractions in unmonitored muscle groups, and to assist with troubleshooting if no electrical response is observed. Second, the electrophysiologic responses monitored are carefully observed through eight-channel recordings (Figure 14.1A and B). Third, medical facts based on presurgery assessment, desired outcome, the number of rootlets severed at previous levels, the strength and quality of responses, and the agreement among all pieces of information must all be considered together.

Definition of Abnormal and Normal Responses
Electrophysiologic and Behavioral Responses to Dorsal Root Stimulation
Normal electrophysiologic responses recorded following stimulation of the ventral portion of the root do not exhibit inhibition and therefore appear similar to the abnormal sensory root response. A normal behavioral response to ventral root stimulation appears as a 1-second sustained contraction with complete relaxation following stimulation. This is frequently used to help localize the spe-

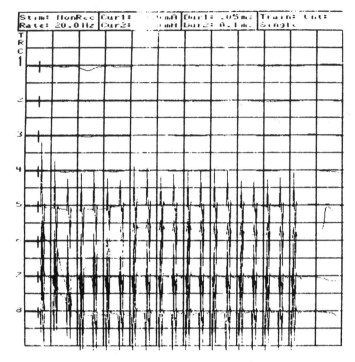

A

Figure 14.1 A. A normal electrophysiologic response to S1 nerve root. Root stimulation is shown. There is no spread to contralateral muscle groups. (Traces 1–4 represent the right lower limbs—gastrocnemius, anterior tibialis, hamstrings, and quadriceps. Traces 5–8 represent the same muscles on the left lower limb.) B. An abnormal response to root stimulation. There is a diffuse response in contralateral muscles unrelated to segmental distribution of the root. (Traces are from the same muscles as Figure 14.1A.)

cific nerve root before beginning the procedure. The difference between the abnormal sensory rootlet and the normal motor rootlet appears to be in the intensity of stimulation necessary to activate the action potentials. A normal motor rootlet can exhibit a strong electrophysiologic and motor response at 0.1–0.5 mA of current. Sensory rootlets generally require 2.5–5.0 mA to activate an electrophysiologic response.

TETHERED SPINAL CORD
Background

An abnormal "tethering" of the spinal cord can result in vascular compromise through mechanical stretching and distortion, causing progressive neurologic deficit, orthopedic deformity, and bladder dysfunction. It most commonly occurs as a result of pathology in the lumbosacral region, but can develop in other regions of the spinal canal. It is common in a variety of conditions (Table 14.1).

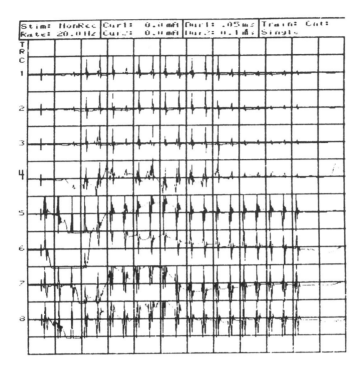

B

Figure 14.1 *(continued)*

Pathophysiology

The pathophysiologic changes associated with a tethered cord are thought to be caused by a combination of three factors:

1. Mechanical distortion of the cord with tethering has been shown experimentally to cause tearing of neuronal membranes.
2. Impaired oxidative metabolism has been demonstrated experimentally in animals with both acute and chronic traction of the spinal cord. Similar studies have been performed on patients undergoing surgical release of a tethered cord. Improved oxidative metabolism after surgical release of the tether has been shown.
3. Impaired blood flow within the tethered spinal cord causes ischemia of the spinal cord. Blood flow is improved with release.

Diagnosis

Tethered cord syndrome can be diagnosed from a combination of both clinical and radiologic or imaging findings. Physical findings include progressive neurologic deficits, orthopedic deformities, and physiologic disruptions of function and clinical signs (Table 14.2).

Table 14.1 Conditions Associated with Tethered Cord

Myelomeningocele	Spina bifida occulta
Lipomyelomeningocele	Syringomyelia
Lipoma of the filum terminale	Thickened filum terminale
Diastematomyelia	Neuroectodermal appendage
Myelocystocele	Dermal sinus
Neurenteric cyst dermoid	Previous surgery

Table 14.2 Signs and symptoms of spinal cord tethering

A. Progressive neurologic deficit
   1. Muscular weakness
   2. Sensory loss
   3. Change in bladder function (perhaps the most sensitive indicator)
   4. Change in bowel function
   5. Change in gait
   6. Development of or increase in spasticity
B. Orthopedic deformity
   1. Scoliosis
   2. Kyphosis
   3. Equinovarus or (rarely) equinovalgus
   4. Recurrent hip dislocation
C. Back or leg pain
D. Tenderness on palpation over the tether
E. Neurocutaneous stigmata suggesting dysraphism
   1. Capillary hemangioma
   2. Hypertrichosis
   3. Subcutaneous lipoma
   4. Midline color change
   5. Midline dimple
F. Acute change after mechanical stress
   1. Lithotomy position
   2. Trauma
   3. Hyperflexion of the spine
   4. Flexion at the hip (e.g., kicking a ball)
G. A change in urodynamics, specifically leak pressure measurements and sphincter and detrusor electromyography
H. A history of diminished activity or exercise intolerance

Radiographic Diagnosis

Magnetic resonance imaging can demonstrate a posterior, caudally displaced cord. Scar, lipoma, dermoid, and a tight filum may be seen. Ultrasonography can determine the presence or absence of cord pulsations. A tethered cord does not pulsate normally. This test is only useful in infants and in children with a bony defect overlying the region in question. It is important that the most terminal portions of the cord be visualized, since pulsations can dissipate caudally with tethering.

Myelogram and postmyelographic computed tomography may define a tether by demonstrating bony, lipomatous, or soft-tissue encroachment on the spinal cord. The subarachnoid space will not extend circumferentially around the cord. Again, in cases involving the lumbosacral region, the cord can be displaced posteriorly and caudally (below L2). The filum can be observed to be "tight" and thickened. Dermoids and lipomas may be the source of the tether.

Management

A laminectomy for the release and resection of the structures (filum terminale, lipoma, dermoid, or scar tissue) causing the tether should be performed.

Monitoring

Monitoring for tethered spinal cord syndrome must detect whether the tight tissue contains nerve elements before the surgeon cuts the tissue for cord release. Palpation of muscle contraction evoked by stimulating the tight tissue has been widely used to detect the presence or lack of neural elements. However, it is difficult to feel muscle contraction of the lower leg muscles correctly through drapes; it is also difficult to diagnose the remaining weak contractions of muscles partially deteriorated due to tethered spinal cord syndrome during surgery. Monitoring bowel and bladder function during surgery is important because the operating level is usually in the lumbosacral region. Evoked muscle action potentials of the external anal sphincter have been used to monitor bowel and bladder function. However, recording only from the external anal sphincter appears to be insufficient to monitor bowel and bladder function. Monitoring sensory function is another important problem. Considering these characteristics of tethered spinal cord syndrome, we have developed the monitoring system described herein.

Monitoring systems fundamentally consist of recording evoked muscle action potentials. As recording sites, we chose lower-extremity muscles for monitoring of lower-limb function. We also chose the external anal sphincter and external urethral sphincter for bowel and bladder function. The muscle action potentials of the tibialis anterior and triceps surae muscles were recorded in most of our cases. The quadriceps femoris muscle also was chosen when the operative field was extended to the upper lumbar region. The muscle action potentials of the external anal sphincter and external urethral sphincter were extremely sensitive. Nevertheless, since these two sphincter muscles are innervated by the pudendal nerve, it is better to also monitor the detrusor function, which is innervated by the pelvic nerve. The vesical pressure measurement method appeared to indicate the detrusor function. However, this intraoperative monitoring method showed a few problems: high-frequency stimulations of over 10–20 per second were needed for sufficient evaluation of vesical pressure elevation, and vesical pressure elevation reacted slowly to the stimulations.

Monitoring Adequacy

At present, somatosensory evoked potentials (SSEPs) are widely used for spinal cord monitoring of spinal disorders in Japan. In the monitoring system using SSEPs, disturbance of spinal cord function between the recording and stimulating electrodes can be observed as changes in the SSEP. Therefore, spinal cord injuries already inflicted or being inflicted can be monitored by SSEP. Unfortunately, this monitoring system appears to be inadequate for tethered spinal cord syndrome, as neural elements must be detected before cutting or releasing in these cases. Evoked spinal cord potential wave changes can be observed only just after cutting or exactly while injuring neural elements.

The most adequate monitoring method for tethered spinal cord syndrome is to monitor myogenic evoked potentials following stimulation of the tissues to be cut. Muscle action potential recording is an easy method, and wave amplitudes are high enough to be understood easily and are also promptly evoked following stimulation. In one series eight spinal dysraphism cases were without adequate monitoring systems. Compared to the recovery of 60% of patients reported in the monitored series, the former results showed an absence of cases of neurologic recovery. The investigators were convinced that an adequate monitoring system not only prevents neurologic deterioration but ensures satisfactory surgical results.

Monitoring Bowel and Bladder Function

Since the operative field is usually in the lumbosacral area, bowel and bladder function must be monitored carefully. Pang and Casey reported a monitoring system using a double-lumen polyethylene balloon catheter that was inserted into the anus to record pressure of the external anal sphincter. Usually it is difficult to record anal pressure in cases of severe neurologic dysfunction. On the other hand, muscle action potentials of the external anal sphincter can be recorded easily.

Because the muscle action potential system is a sensitive and easy technique, it is superior to the balloon system for monitoring tethered spinal cord syndrome. For monitoring bladder function, both voiding and storage functions must be checked. Routinely, voiding function is evaluated by vesical pressure recording and storage function by muscle action potentials of the external urethral sphincter. With regard to the muscle action potential monitoring of the external urethral sphincter, correct insertion of an electrode needle into the external urethral sphincter is quite difficult in infant girls. According to James et al., muscle action potentials of the external anus sphincter might be able to substitute for those of the external urethral sphincter as both the external urethral sphincter and anal sphincter are innervated by the pudendal nerve from the S2–S4 segments. For monitoring the voiding potentials of the detrusor muscle, which is innervated by the pelvic nerve originating from the S2–S4 segments, we have been using the vesical pressure method because monitoring of muscle action potentials of the detrusor muscle are not available yet in our hospital. Although vesical pressure recording creates problems for intraoperative monitoring, as responses are slower and less sensitive than those from muscle action potentials, doubtful tissues can be evaluated by this method.

Postoperative Management

Postoperative pain is optimally managed by an intradural injection of morphine sulfate (0.01 mg/kg) at the time of surgery in patients over 1 year of age. Additional analgesia may not be required for 12–24 hours. The patient should be kept with the head of the bed at a 20-degree angle to avoid respiratory depression. When necessary, adjunctive intravenous narcotics are effective.

The prone position is most comfortable initially, and it allows the spinal cord to fall anteriorly (intended to prevent retethering) until the patient is ambulatory. Early mobilization is preferable. Physical therapy for ambulation should be initiated if the patient does not ambulate well independently. Adequate pain control is helpful in improving mobilization.

Temporary urinary retention can be managed with intermittent catheterization. This will usually return to the preoperative status within 10 days to 3 months. New, permanent urinary dysfunction is an infrequent complication.

Spinal fluid leaks occur infrequently. They can be managed with positioning the head downward, pressure dressings, oversuturing the wound, or continuous subcutaneous catheter drainage if necessary. Surgical reexploration is rarely required. There is a high incidence of retethering with a postoperative cerebrospinal fluid leak.

Prognosis

The purpose of operative intervention is to prevent continued neurologic deficit and orthopedic deformity. Some improvement in function and scoliosis may occur, particularly in cases with symptoms of short duration. Surgery is primarily prophylactic. Improvement may not occur, which should be made clear to the patient and parent. In most cases, pain will completely resolve.

Retethering remains a risk, and at least 10% of patients retether and require reexploration. The exact incidence of retethering is not known. Intervention should be sooner rather than later, since the natural history of the disease is a progressive decline in function.

ELECTROMYOGRAPHY FOR PEDICLE SCREW PLACEMENT

Spinal instrumentation systems that use the pedicle as a point of fixation have become increasingly popular adjuncts to spinal stabilization in patients with diagnoses of spondylolisthesis, spinal stenosis, segmental instability, failures of previous spinal surgery, and scoliosis. The pedicle provides the most rigid site for fixation of the vertebral segment. Transpedicular instrumentation does not depend on the presence of posterior elements and thus can be used in the patients after laminectomy. Successful use of the pedicle for fixation requires proper placement of the pedicle screw. Incorrect placement can compromise the fixation or produce a neurologic deficit or radiculopathy.

Various techniques to verify correct placement have been proposed, including radiographs and direct inspection of the pedicle. Radiographs are not foolproof, and direct inspection results in additional cost and potential morbidity to the patient.

Intraoperative SSEPs have been used to monitor lumbosacral nerve root function as a means of preventing neurologic deficits, determining adequacy of decompression, and predicting outcome. Since multiple nerve roots contribute to the cortical SSEP, it is possible to damage one nerve root without changing the cortical potential significantly. Dermatomal SSEPs have been used to improve the sensitivity and specificity for detecting single nerve root dysfunction. However, it is possible for a pedicle screw to broach the cortex and lie next to a nerve root without compressing it, potentially leading to irritation and postoperative radiculopathy.

Evaluation of pedicle screw placement using evoked EMG has been reported in both animal and human models. Constant voltage stimulation of a probe placed in the pedicle was combined with monitoring of evoked EMG activity from the hindlimb muscles. The rationale for this monitoring approach is that a correctly placed screw should be fully surrounded by bone, which has high impedance to electrical current. If the cortex of the pedicle has been broached, current flow through the defect leads to excitation of the adjacent nerve root with resulting evoked EMG activity at a stimulation intensity of ≤20 V (Figure 14.2). EMG activation at 20–30 V may be perceived as suspicious. Recent research has suggested that this technique may be a more sensitive electrophysiologic means for detecting malplaced pedicle screws in a clinical setting.

CASE STUDY

A 3-year-old boy required SDRs for relief of spasticity. After evaluation and planning, the operation was performed under general anesthesia with halothane, without long-acting muscle relaxants, which would interfere with the recordings and visible motor response. The patient was placed in the prone position. After induction and prior to surgery, monopolar EMG needles were inserted into appropriate muscles. For each lower limb, needles were placed in the following muscle groups: gastrocnemius, tibialis anterior, quadriceps, and hamstring. Reference needles were inserted in the side of each foot. Needle pairs were also placed in the left and right forearms (extensor carpi ulnaris). A ground plate was positioned on the buttocks.

Preoperative Baseline Recordings

A. Multichannel surface EMG recordings
   1. 200 mV, 200 ms, free running, eight (or four) channel
   2. Filters: 30 low, 8,000 high
   3. G1-G2 1 cm apart over end plate
   4. Bilateral
   5. Medial gastrocnemius; anterior tibial; vastus medialis, adductor longus
   6. Multiple runs

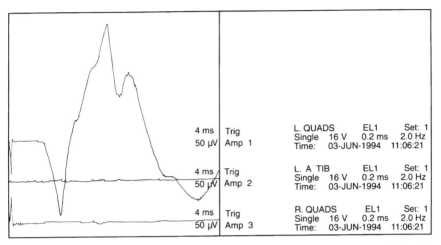

Figure 14.2 An electromyographic response to pedicle screw stimulation. Of the three traces, the top trace from the left quadriceps (L. QUADS) shows a large evoked response at 16-V stimulation—a positive response. No response is noted from the left anterior tibialis (L. A TIB) at the right quadriceps (R. QUADS).

  a. Resting
  b. Selective muscle contraction
  c. Startle
  d. Mechanical tap (arm and leg)
  e. Passive motion (knee and ankle)
  f. Clonus
  g. Patellar reflex (hammer)
B. H reflexes
  1. Tibial at knee: recording two-channel (soleus and anterior tibial)
  2. Peroneal at knee: recording two-channel (soleus and anterior tibial)
  3. 1-cm G1-G2 distances—use electrodes placed for multichannel surface EMG recordings.
  4. Stimulate peroneal knee and tibial knee separately to define recording electrodes selectively
  5. 1 and 2 bilaterally
  6. Repeat twice for reproducibility
C. Standard nerve conduction studies on weakest or atrophic leg
  1. Peroneal/extensor digitorum brevis with F waves
  2. Tibial/abductor hallucis with F waves
  3. Sural with velocity
D. Tonic vibration reflex bilaterally when available

Preoperative Wiring

A. Surface EMG: Bilateral gluteus medius to gluteus maximus, rectus femoris

to internal hamstring, abductor hallucis to abductor digiti minimi, anterior tibial to medial gastrocnemius
B. Monopolar needle electrodes for stimulation of tibial nerve in popliteal fossa
C. Cathode-proximal, anode-distal
D. Handheld, sterile, bipolar stimulator for direct root stimulation
E. Stimulator box setups (only one used at a time)
   1. Rhizotomy box
      a. Stimulator No. 1 plugged into "single" input
      b. Stimulator No. 2 plugged into "train" input
      c. Output to handheld bipolar stimulator in surgical field
      d. Switch to single and train to get single root stimulation
   2. Standard box
      a. Stimulator No. 1 plugged into "left" input
      b. Left tibial knee into "left median" output
      c. Right tibial knee into "left tibial" output
      d. Switch between median and tibial to get single shocks for H reflex testing on left and right legs
F. Viking stimulation setup
   1. Stimulator No. 1: single shocks, 0.05 ms, no delay, nonrecurrent
   2. Stimulator No. 2: train of shocks, 50 Hz, 28 stimuli, 0.05 ms, no delay, nonrecurrent
G. Viking amplifier setup
   1. All channels (amp 1–8): triggered, 1 K, LF-100, HF-10,000
   2. Sweep speed: single shocks at 5 ms; train at 20 ms

Late Response Testing with Surgery

Test H reflex to medial gastrocnemius and F wave to abductor hallucis bilaterally:

1. Preoperative awake in induction room
2. Immediately after induction is completed before neuromuscular block
3. After neuromuscular block clears
4. Ten minutes; any change in agent or depth

Rootlet Testing

A. After laminectomy and initial dissection
B. Single shocks (0.05 ms) at slowly increasing voltage with handheld surgical bipolar stimulator
   1. Identify ventral root (stimulus threshold below 1.0 mA)
   2. Identify dorsal root (higher threshold, wider distribution)
C. For each dorsal rootlet stimulated with single shocks at 0.5-ms duration:
   1. Determine threshold for movement of leg (5–80 mA)
   2. Determine distribution of motor response at threshold

Table 14.3 Positions of electromyography needles for selective dorsal rhizotomy

Channel	Negative Input	Positive Input
1	Ipsilateral gastrocnemius	Ipsilateral foot
2	Ipsilateral tibialis anterior	Ipsilateral foot
3	Ipsilateral quadriceps	Ipsilateral foot
4	Ipsilateral hamstring	Ipsilateral foot
5	Ipsilateral arm proximal	Ipsilateral arm distal
6	Contralateral gastrocnemius	Contralateral foot
7	Contralateral gastrocnemius	Contralateral foot
8	Contralateral quadriceps	Contralateral foot

3. Stimulate with train of 18 at 50 Hz, at threshold
   a. Determine distribution
   b. Determine persistence
4. Note size of rootlet
5. Note all of above aspects of rootlet testing on worksheet for each rootlet

TESTING PATIENTS

During the stimulation and recording part of the procedure, the EMG needles were connected to the eight channels of the Viking amplifiers as shown in Table 14.3.

The contralateral lower-limb channels and upper-limb channels (i.e., channels 6–8) are varied according to the particular patient.

Extended cables are usually required for the upper limb and upper leg electrodes to connect with the Viking input box. The Viking was positioned at the foot of the operating table so as not to interfere with the sterile field and anesthesiologist.

The Viking was set to produce a 20-Hz stimulus train lasting 1 second. The recording epoch was 2 seconds in duration (100 ms/div), beginning 50 ms prior to the first stimulus. This allowed the operator to view the EMG responses to stimuli during the train, plus activity for nearly a second after the train ceased. In determining whether the muscle responses are normal or abnormal, activity in both segments of the epoch was judged. The filter settings were set for a bandpass of 2–2,000 Hz. The display amplitude was set to 1 mV/div.

The surgery consisted of a limited laminectomy and opening of the dura to expose the L2–S2 roots. At each level, the posterior root was isolated for stimulation. Each root was divided into 10–15 rootlets, each of which was stimulated using two unipolar probes separated by approximately 1 cm. An ascending progression of stimulus intensities beginning at 2–3 mA was used to determine the threshold for a response. Stimulus intensities of 10–15 mA were commonly used, and in the absence of a response at lower intensities, intensities of 20 mA were occasionally necessary.

The response to stimulation was judged from (1) the Viking display on a slave monitor, and (2) leg movements noted both visually and by touch. Rootlets

Table 14.4 Criteria used for judging the nature
of the muscle response during dorsal rhizotomies

A. Observed muscle contractions
  1. Normal: initial contraction of appropriate ipsilateral muscle groups with immediate release.
  2. Sustained: muscle contraction is sustained.
  3. Diffuse: contraction is noted in other muscle groups or other leg (i.e., bilateral response).
  4. Other: varying patterns are described.
B. EMG recordings
  1. Normal: initial ipsilateral action potential is noted without further response.
  2. Abnormal: a series of action potentials in response to each pulse in the stimulus train. Additional responses in poststimulus period may be seen.
  3. Absent: no EMG activity is noted. Regarded to be a normal response.

---

judged to produce an abnormal response were sectioned, and rootlets associated with a normal response were left intact (Table 14.4).

The procedure was followed at each of the six levels on both sides. Once the sequence had been completed, it was repeated at all levels, and again selectively at certain levels. This repetition is routinely done since abnormal responses occasionally do not show up on the initial pass. The mechanism of this phenomenon is hypothesized to be refractoriness caused by manipulation or initial stimulation.

It should be noted that throughout the procedure the motor roots were stimulated as necessary at low stimulus intensities (2 mA) to ensure that the anatomy was correct, that the pathway was intact, and that the instrument was working.

In the procedure observed, 0–100% of the rootlets were severed at each level depending on the electrophysiologic or observational responses obtained. In total, 43% of the rootlets were cut. The stimulation and recording portion of the surgery lasted approximately 1 hour and 15 minutes.

KEY REFERENCES

Newberg N, Cooch J, Walker M. Intraoperative monitoring in selective dorsal rhizotomy. J Pediatr Neurosurg 1991;17:124.

Peacock W, Staudt L. Selective posterior rhizotomy: evolution of theory and practice. J Pediatr Neurosurg 1991;17:128.

Shinomiya K et al. Intraoperative monitoring for tethered spinal cord syndrome. J Spine 1991;16:1290.

RECOMMENDED READING

Abbott R, Forem SL, Johann M. Selective posterior rhizotomy for the treatment of spasticity: A review. Childs Nerv Sys 1989;5:337.

Aminoff MJ et al. Electrophysiologic evaluation of lumbosacral radiculopathies: Electromyography, late responses, and somatosensory evoked potentials. Neurology 1985;35:1514.

Cohen BA, Huizenga BA. Dermatomal monitoring for surgical correction of spondylolisthesis. Spine 1988;13:1125.

Cohen BA, Major MR, Huizenga BA. Predictability of adequacy of spinal root decompression using evoked potentials. Spine 1991;16(Suppl):S379.

Fasano VA et al. Electrophysiological assessment of spinal circuits in spasticity by direct dorsal root stimulation. J Neurosurg 1979;4:146.

Fasano VA et al. Surgical treatment of spasticity in cerebral palsy. J Childs Brain 1978;4:289.

Gepstein R, Brown MD. Somatosensory evoked potentials in lumbar root decompression. Clin Orthop 1989;245:69.

Herron LD, Trippi AC, Gonyeau M. Intraoperative use of dermatomal somatosensory-evoked potentials in lumbar stenosis surgery. Spine 1987;12(4):379.

James HE et al. Use of anal sphincter electromyography during operations on the conus medullans and sacral nerve roots. Neurosurgery 1979;4:521.

Kanev PM, et al. Management and long-term follow-up review of children with lipomeningocele. J Neurosurg 1990;73:48.

Keim HA et al. Somatosensory evoked potentials as an aid in the diagnosis and intraoperative management of spinal stenosis. Spine 1985;10(4):338.

Laitinen LV, Nilsson S, Fugl-Meyer AR. Selective posterior rhizotomy for treatment of spasticity. J Neurosurg 1983;58:895.

Matsuzaki NH et al: Problems and solutions of pedicle screw plate fixation of lumbar spine. Spine 1990;15:1159.

Peacock WJ, Arens LJ, Berman B. Cerebral palsy spasticity. Selective posterior rhizotomy. Pediatr Neurosci 1987;13:61.

Peacock WJ, Arens LJ, Berman B. Cerebral palsy spasticity: Selective posterior rhizotomy. Pediatr Neurosci 1987;62:119.

Peacock WJ, Arens LJ. Selective posterior rhizotomy for the relief of spasticity in cerebral palsy. S Afr Med J 1982;62:119.

Weinstein JN et al. Spinal pedicle fixation: Reliability and validity of roentgenogram-based assessment and surgical factors on successful screw placement. Spine 1988;13:1012.

West JL III, Ogilvie JW, Bradford DS. Complications of the variable screw plate pedicle screw fixation. Spine 1991;16(5):576.

15

Intraoperative Facial Nerve Monitoring

David A. Wiegand, M.D.

Intraoperative facial nerve monitoring is used during a variety of surgical procedures in which the facial nerve is at risk: excision of posterior fossa tumors (such as acoustic neuromas), vestibular neurectomy, mastoid and temporal bone procedures, and others. Facial nerve monitoring during such cases has gained wide acceptance but is not established as the standard of care. Preliminary data suggest that such monitoring may, if appropriately used, improve outcomes in certain procedures, reducing the incidence of facial nerve injury.

MONITORING METHODS

Facial nerve monitoring involves the continuous intraoperative assessment of facial muscle activity. Monitoring devices either sense the electromyographic activity of facial muscles or detect facial muscular contraction and movement. Electromyography (EMG) monitors are quite sensitive but are affected by electrical artifacts and interference from various sources within the operating room. Motion sensors may be somewhat less sensitive but provide reliable and specific detection of facial muscle contraction with fewer signal artifacts.

Electromyographic Detection of Facial Muscle Activity

EMG activity (evoked or spontaneous electrical discharge of motor unit groups) is detected using either skin surface electrodes placed over the facial muscles of expression or by percutaneously placed intramuscular electrodes. Bipolar electrode arrays of this type are usually placed over the orbicularis oculi and the orbicularis oris (Figure 15.1). These broad, flat muscles allow easy placement of electrodes, which remain outside the surgical field. In general, intramuscular electrodes are preferable, using individual 2-cm needle electrodes placed percutaneously and taped in place (Figure 15.2). Alternatively, Teflon-coated wire electrodes may be used. The connecting leads of a given electrode pair should be braided to reduce unwanted noise artifacts. A third, reference electrode is placed at another site. Typically this is an electrocardiograph electrode patch on the skin of the neck or shoulder. Since the electrical signals from active muscle motor units

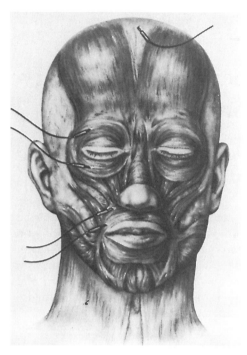

Figure 15.1 Placement of electrodes for facial nerve monitoring. The author uses a reference electrode on the shoulder, rather than a vertex electrode. This montage provides for two channels of electromyographic monitoring (of the orbicularis oculi and orbicularis oris muscles). *Reproduced with permission from JM Kartush. Electroneurography and intraoperative facial monitoring in contemporary neurotology. Otolaryngol Head Neck Surg 1989;101:496.*

are in the microvolt amplitude range, sensing electrodes are connected to a differential instrumentation amplifier with a high common-mode rejection ratio. This provides sensitive detection of muscle motor unit discharges while rejecting much of the stray electrical interference arising from electrocautery units, fluorescent lighting, and other sources of electrical noise within the operating room. Depending on the monitoring system used, the electromyographic signal may be presented as a waveform on a liquid crystal display, shown as a waveform on a computer monitor, displayed on a bar graph indicator panel, or presented as an audio signal. If monitoring personnel are available, a continuous silent waveform display on a bright, easily visible computer monitor is preferable. Monitoring personnel can then comment on periods of activity, leaving the operating room free of background noise. However, many surgeons prefer to listen to the continuous EMG waveform on a speaker, which allows them to hear muscle activity without the need to look away from the surgical field. Most instruments provide both options, as well as adjustments for sound volume and overall sensitivity. (See Chapter 14 for more information on intraoperative EMG.)

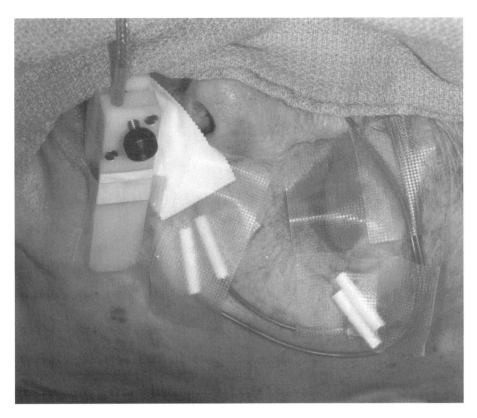

Figure 15.2 Intraoperative placement of needle electrodes for electromyographic recording and oral commissure "clip" for strain gauge motion detection. Electrodes and the strain gauge clip are secured with tape to prevent intraoperative dislodgment. A protective shield is subsequently placed over the strain gauge clip to minimize artifacts from contact with surgical drapes.

Electromyographic Discharge Patterns

During intraoperative facial nerve monitoring, a variety of facial muscle EMG discharge patterns may occur. The facial muscles should be (1) electrically silent during surgical manipulations that don't affect the nerve. If the nerve is exposed during surgery, periods of increased (2) random spike discharges may occur. These may be related to drying of the nerve, to irrigation or heating effects, or to variation in the levels of anesthetic and paralytic agents used during the procedure. (3) Bursts of activity may accompany nerve irritation; these may be caused by traction on the nerve, dissection or drilling near the nerve, or heating of the nerve by laser or other means. Use of a pulsed nerve stimulator produces discharges that are synchronized with the stimulus. None of these patterns can be observed during periods of electrocautery use, which causes spike discharge artifacts that obliterate the EMG signals.

Facial Motion Detection

The second class of facial nerve monitors uses sensitive strain gauge detectors to directly sense the motion of facial muscle contraction. One such instrument (the Silverstein monitor, W.R. Medical Electronics, Stillwater, MN), uses a strain gauge built into a plastic clip, which is placed in the oral commissure and adjusted to be in firm contact with the buccal region. Regional muscle contraction causes physical displacement of the strain gauge, which acts as a variable resistor in the detection amplifier. A contraction waveform is generated with each muscle contraction event. This arrangement is extremely sensitive and detects even small facial muscle contractions. However, precautions must be taken to avoid extraneous motion, such as the movement of surgical drapes and placement of instruments near the monitor clip. It is helpful to place a mechanical shield over the clip to isolate the strain gauge from these other influences as much as possible.

The output signal from motion detection monitors is an analog representation of the strain gauge displacement. Each muscle contraction causes a discrete pulse in the output signal. Since the strain gauge senses motion, not electrical discharge, the output signal is free of electrical interference under most circumstances. The presence or absence of muscle contraction is therefore fairly easy to interpret.

INTRAOPERATIVE MONITORING

In practice, either of the above systems or both may be used with success for intraoperative monitoring. Figure 15.3 shows the monitoring equipment we use, which combines EMG and motion detectors with a computerized display and alarm system. Although some authors indicate that facial nerve monitors function effectively in the presence of partial muscle motor unit blockade, paralytic agents (which abolish facial motion) must be used with caution in these procedures. The anesthesiologist and the surgeon must be continuously aware of the patient's level of paralysis to correctly interpret the clinical data from the monitors.

During surgery, the surgeon may monitor both spontaneous and evoked activity in the facial muscles. Spontaneous activity often provides an indication that surgical manipulation is near the facial nerve. For instance, during mastoid surgery, spontaneous discharge of the facial nerve may indicate that the surgeon is drilling near the facial nerve before the nerve can actually be seen. Similarly, spontaneous facial nerve activity may occur during excision of tumors, such as acoustic neuromas, when surgical dissection is near the facial nerve fibers. Since tumors may grossly distort the normal path of the facial nerve, this information can be helpful in guiding the progress of tumor dissection.

In cases in which the surgeon is able to visualize and isolate the facial nerve, facial nerve monitors may be used to detect evoked facial muscle activity. A nerve stimulator can be used, for instance, to stimulate various areas of the capsule surrounding an acoustic neuroma, allowing the surgeon to attempt mapping the course of the facial nerve. At the end of tumor resection, stimulation of the facial nerve at the brain stem can be used to verify that the entire facial nerve remains intact. Some

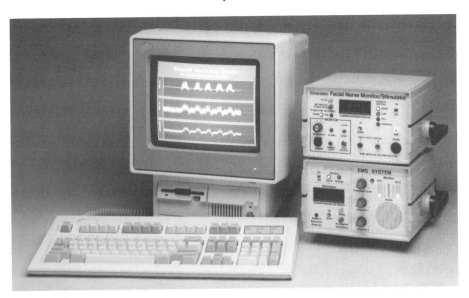

Figure 15.3 The monitoring system used by the author (Wiegand Monitoring System, W.R. Medical Electronics, Stillwater, MN) combines a two-channel electromyographic monitor (Brackmann EMG Monitoring System) and a single-channel strain gauge motion detector (Silverstein Facial Nerve Monitor) with a computerized display and alarm system. The system includes nerve stimulator circuitry and provisions for continuous stimulation using insulated surgical instruments.

authors indicate that electrical stimulation of bone overlying the facial nerve in the mastoid region can allow the surgeon to estimate the amount of bone overlying the facial nerve and have provided approximate guides for the amount of stimulus current required for each millimeter of bone thickness. Surgical instruments have been designed that can be connected to surgical stimulator circuits. Thus, a single instrument can serve both as a dissector and a continuous stimulus probe during surgery.

The utility of intraoperative facial nerve monitoring depends on the correct interpretation of the data provided by the monitor. For instance, a period of electrical silence may occur when the facial nerve is intact and no evoked activity is being produced. However, the same electrical silence may result from a cut facial nerve or from an electrode array that has become disconnected. Similarly, a motion signal from a strain gauge detector circuit may represent facial muscle contraction or simply movement of drapes across the surgical field. Activity sensed in an electromyographic circuit may represent either facial muscle activity or electrical interference, such as that produced by an electrocautery unit. The monitor, by itself, can neither protect the facial nerve nor provide the correct interpretation of its signals. It is only through experience that the physician—neurologist, anesthesiologist, or surgeon—learns to correctly correlate the monitor data with the surgical reality. For this reason, frequent use of intraoperative facial nerve monitoring, even on routine cases, can be quite useful.

Cautions

In practice, facial nerve monitoring often provides imperfect data. During long procedures, the facial nerve may become increasingly difficult to stimulate, and spontaneous activity may stop. The results of facial nerve evoked response testing at the end of an 18-hour surgical procedure may be equivocal even though the nerve is intact, because of this degradation in the ability of the nerve to respond to electrical stimuli. The same process may make it impossible for the surgeon to identify the facial nerve and to distinguish it from other nerves or from tumor during the later hours of a prolonged surgical procedure. It is not uncommon for the surgeon at the end of a such a case to visualize the facial nerve as being anatomically intact but incapable of evoked electrical or mechanical response. Precise localization of the facial nerve, even when it can be successfully stimulated, can also be difficult. The spread of stimulus current through cerebral spinal fluid, for instance, can make it possible to evoke a facial nerve response from many points along the circumference of a tumor, and some of these may be quite remote from the actual course of the facial nerve. The use of bipolar rather than unipolar stimulus probe configurations can reduce this effect to some extent, but precise localization of the facial nerve remains an intraoperative problem in many cases. For all these reasons, the facial nerve monitor must be regarded as a helpful but imperfect adjunct to surgical experience and judgment.

Facial nerve monitoring is possible using a variety of commercially available devices. This monitoring appears to improve surgical outcome in some instances and can be provided with little increase in operative time. For facial nerve monitoring to succeed, the surgeon and the monitoring team must be well acquainted with the high variability of the data quality and with its interpretation. The routine use of facial nerve monitoring can be expected to become more frequent and to become more helpful as monitoring and nerve-stimulating systems improve and as monitoring teams themselves become more experienced.

KEY REFERENCES

Kwartler JA et al. Facial nerve monitoring in acoustic tumor surgery. Otolaryngol Head Neck Surg 1991;104:814.

Leonetti JP, Brackmann DE, Prass RL. Improved preservation of facial nerve function in the infratemporal approach to the skull base. Otolaryngol Head Neck Surg 1989;101:74.

Lennon RL et al. Effect of partial neuromuscular blockade on intraoperative electromyography in patients undergoing resection of acoustic neuromas. Anesth Analg 1992;75:729.

RECOMMENDED READING

Kartush JM. Electroneurography and intraoperative facial monitoring in contemporary neurotology. Otolaryngol Head Neck Surg 1989;101:496.

Silverstein H, Rosenberg S. Intraoperative facial nerve monitoring. Otolaryngol Clin North Am 1991;24:709.

16

Intraoperative Cortical Stimulation and Recording

Ralph A.W. Lehman, M.D.

The prospect of brain resection causes great concern for the function of the areas being considered for excision. This is especially true for excision of an epileptic focus and surgery in or about areas of obvious gross functional importance. In the case of an epileptic focus, the region responsible for abnormal brain activity must be located for removal, whereas for surgery in areas normally of functional importance, the regions responsible for normal brain activity must be located and preserved. These two concerns often conflict and can try the judgment of the patient and physician.

Many techniques are used to localize cortical areas of abnormal and normal function. These include clinical evaluation as well as anatomic, metabolic, and neurophysiologic studies, particularly those provided by neuroimaging. In the case of epilepsy surgery, electrophysiologic studies are almost invariably included and are usually a major guide to the area of primary abnormality. Localization of normal function is often carried out by a variety of methods, but with lesions in areas close to those recognized to control motor, sensory, or language function, electrophysiologic localization studies are often done. Similar tests for other brain functions are rarely carried out.

Electrophysiologic testing for normal and abnormal cortical activity can take one of two forms: cortical recording or cortical stimulation. Normal functions can be localized from sensory evoked responses recorded at the cortex or from the functional effects produced by stimulation of the cortex; an epileptic focus can be localized from abnormal activity seen on recordings or from seizure activity induced by stimulation. These methods become possible and achieve increasing validity, precision, and freedom from artifact if intracranial rather than extracranial electrodes are used, and this can be done at open craniotomy.

INDICATIONS, ISSUES, AND AIMS OF INTRAOPERATIVE STUDY

Patients with intractable epilepsy, typically with complex or simple partial seizures, whose evaluation provides an unsatisfactory degree of localizing information may undergo intracranial electrode implantation and recording to further localize the source of seizure onset. Intracranial electrode studies are advised for patients whose noninvasive studies leave sufficient doubt among the investigating team members that a decision for surgical resection or about its extent is not possible. Such recordings may take one of two forms: chronic recordings from implanted electrodes or acute intraoperative electrocorticographic recordings (IECoG). Both methods are sometimes used in the same patient. Some centers think that preoperative chronic invasive recording is preferable to IECoG since the latter is restricted to a unilateral interictal recording and limited in duration, whereas chronic study permits bilateral recording during actual seizures and on repeated occasions. However, chronic invasive recording requires an additional operation and a monitored hospital stay prior to the resection. IECoG is used (1) to confirm the preoperative localization in further detail, (2) to determine the extent of the epileptic focus, and (3) to permit a tailored resection of as much of the region at issue as can safely be removed.

Often mapping of normal brain function is carried out at the same time as IECoG to help determine the approach to and limits of safe cortical manipulation. For the same reason, brain mapping is often carried out during resection of nonepileptic lesions such as a tumor or vascular malformation. Since even the classically described motor and sensory areas can be hard to recognize from purely anatomic landmarks and because wide individual variation makes functional localization on this basis only approximate, electrical brain mapping has become recognized as a helpful technique.

As with invasive recording for epilepsy, both chronic intracranial recordings or acute studies on the operating table can be used. As with IECoG, mapping done at the operating table has the advantages of a single operation and reduced hospital stay but is limited by time constraints and the effects of a general anesthetic or the cooperation of an awake but sedated patient. Advantages of intraoperative study with the patient awake rather than under general anesthesia include a greater likelihood of obtaining a satisfactory study and particularly the ability to test language and other cognitive functions.

ELECTROCORTICOGRAPHY AND BRAIN MAPPING
Preoperative Patient Preparation

If intraoperative stimulation and recording are to be carried out under general anesthesia, informing the patient is relatively straightforward and no additional preparation is required. If the patient is to be awake during at least part of the operation, extra discussion with the surgeon and preparation are needed; these are detailed in the remainder of this section. Some matters might be discussed on more than one occasion. Information should be offered regarding the reasons for an awake craniotomy and what will be done during that portion of the procedure.

The patient should realize that it will be possible to discuss any needs or discomfort with the surgeon and anesthesiologist at any time during the course of the procedure. It should be mentioned that some pain may be experienced but that it can and will be controlled and that the patient should feel free to let the surgeon and anesthesiologist know if the procedure is becoming intolerable in some way. It should be stated that throughout surgery the anesthesiologist will be sitting in front of the patient and accessible while the surgeon will be at the head of the table on the other side of the drapes but able to converse with the patient. Clearly assuring the patient that he or she will be able to communicate with the operating team helps provide the confidence and preparation necessary to recruit the patient's active cooperation for and during the operative procedure. If this is not possible or acceptable, the patient should have surgery under a general anesthetic or forego resection. Awake craniotomy is usually not feasible in children younger than 12 years of age.

Details should be provided with respect to position and the need to move only within established limits. The patient also should be made aware that during functional brain mapping or even IECoG, sedation will be diminished and that on awakening some disorientation may occur but that the patient will be called by name by the surgeon and asked if he or she hears himself or herself being called. As the patient responds, he or she will be reminded that he or she is undergoing surgery in the operating room. The patient should also be told that he or she will be asked about pain and additional injections of local anesthetic will be used to control it. Patients should be forewarned that they should not shake their heads to answer yes or no questions but should make all such responses and other communications verbally. These instructions will be repeated at the time the patient is awakened in the operating room.

Additional instructions should include the nature of any motor or sensory testing that will be carried out, along with a very general description of some things the patient might expect to experience as a result and the need to report such experiences in as much detail as possible. The possible unintended or deliberate induction of a seizure by stimulation should be included in the discussion. Specific preparation for intraoperative testing is necessary. If language or other cognitive testing is to be done, preoperative trials offer the opportunity to establish a baseline for intraoperative testing as well as the chance to be sure that the test procedure and the responses desired and permitted are understood. It is helpful to have the person who will administer and record the test at surgery perform the preoperative training and testing.

Clearly all of these details must be discussed and mutually understood by the surgeon and anesthesiologist so that each can take into account the other's requirements for the safe and effective conduct of the operative procedure.

Initial Operative Preparation and Procedure

Preoperative medications include antibiotics and may include steroids as well. Seizure medications are not discontinued but are often reduced to levels at which preoperative monitoring has demonstrated interictal spikes. Sedation prior to patient delivery to the operating room is avoided. Vascular lines and a urinary catheter are placed.

Patient Positioning

If the patient is to have an awake craniotomy, the operating table must be unusually well padded. The patient then can place himself or herself on the appropriate side in a position of comfort. Additional foam rubber cushions and pillows at potential pressure points as well as a cushioned horizontal support for the upside arm are repositioned until the patient affirms them as comfortable. Both arms are positioned so that they can be readily viewed by the anesthesiologist. A support that will hold the surgical drapes out of the way is then attached to the head of the operating table in front of the face. This support creates a corridor under the drapes through which the anesthesiologist can gain a view of the patient's face as well as access to the airway. The patient, in turn, should be able to view the anesthesiologist and any test apparatus. Portions of a bar-based retractor system such as the right angle support bars of a Thompson spinal retractor are a helpful means of constructing the frame for such a window. Two mobile intravenous poles are steadied and positioned against the operating table in front of the chest and knees. These support the surgical drapes and permit visualization and access to the rest of the body by the anesthesiologist.

Anesthesia for "Awake" Craniotomy

The two popular anesthetic techniques for "awake" craniotomy are both intravenous: a purely neuroleptanalgesic technique or, alternatively, anesthesia with propofol supplemented by neuroleptics (see Chapter 8). Even though craniotomy is to be done under general anesthesia, muscle relaxants probably should be avoided. Even when reversed, such agents may prevent responses to motor cortex stimulation for some time after twitches to peripheral stimulation reappear.

The anesthetic can be gently increased after the patient is comfortably positioned. With anesthesia deeper but not compromising respiration, the head may be fixed to the operating table with point fixation if so desired. The head is shaved, the incision marked, and the field draped. The proposed incision is then slowly and thoroughly infiltrated at all depths with a mixture consisting of equal parts 1% lidocaine with 1:200,000 epinephrine and 0.5% bupivacaine. Meticulous circumferential full-depth infiltration is carried out just beyond the proposed incision and scalp flap to create a field block. Incision and craniotomy are then performed with additional infiltration to the deep layers, including the proximal underside of the reflected temporalis muscle.

Prior to any bone work, the anesthesiologist is asked to begin to awaken the patient. The bone flap is created and removed. The dura is then infiltrated with a fine needle using the same local anesthetic, especially in the region of any meningeal vessels. Surgery is then halted awaiting the fuller awakening of the patient. Once the patient responds to being called by name and is reoriented to the operating room and the need to avoid head movement, inquiry is made with respect to pain and discomfort. The patient is informed of operative manipulations as they occur.

Recording and Stimulation Sequence

After any positional readjustments and further infiltration of local anesthetic, the dura is opened and intracranial studies are begun. If IECoG is to be done, it is usually done first. Functional brain mapping should be done after IECoG. If evoked recordings are planned, these should be done before any stimulation study to reduce the chance of seizure and its possible interference with further testing. In the uncommon case that stimulation is used purposefully to induce seizures, this is done after all other studies since it is difficult to obtain patient cooperation after a seizure, and any medication given to control it interferes with further electrophysiologic study. Should a seizure occur, it is stopped with a short-acting intravenous barbiturate or benzodiazepine.

Following any recording and stimulation studies, anesthesia is deepened so that the patient will tolerate resection and wound closure. On occasion this is not done at this point and the patient is left awake for testing during the brain resection as described below.

INTRAOPERATIVE CORTICAL RECORDING
Electrocorticography

IECoG can be carried out with flexible cotton-wick or carbon-tipped electrodes, which are pressed gently against the cortex at regular intervals. Periodic spray of saline solution from a nebulizer moistens the interface between each electrode tip and the brain surface and between the electrodes and their holder. An electrode array in a Silastic sheet (grid) can be used for the same purpose. Subdural grids and especially strips may be slipped beyond the margins of the craniotomy if so desired. Sometimes depth electrodes are also used. A separate ground is placed in the soft tissues.

Interpretation of the IECoG requires the presence of an experienced electroencephalographer, who reports the findings as the recordings are made. IECoG is almost invariably limited to interictal activity, including abnormalities of the background and epileptiform activity (spikes and sharp waves). Since spikes may be recorded from both abnormal areas in which they originate as well as areas to which they propagate, interpretation of the pre- and postresection IECoG is difficult and its usefulness has long been a matter of debate. This difficulty is compounded by the effects of anesthesia. A useful atlas of intraoperative recording has been published.

While there is debate about the value of IECoG in determining the extent of cortical resection for intractable seizure problems, this debate is even more intense when a structural lesion such as a tumor or arteriovenous malformation is also present. Data have been presented both supporting and refuting the claim that resection of cortex displaying epileptiform IECoG activity increases the chance of postoperative relief of seizures beyond that obtained by excision of the lesion alone.

Cortical Recording: Evoked Responses

Cortical evoked response recordings are especially valuable for patients for whom awake anesthesia is not an acceptable option but functional mapping is considered desirable. Functional mapping is usually limited to stimulation rather than recording if the patient is undergoing awake anesthesia. Repetitive sensory stimulation produces a recordable average evoked response from the cerebral cortex in the region of primary sensory inputs. Such recordings permit mapping of primary somatosensory, visual, and auditory cortex. Most commonly, somatosensory cortex is mapped and the median nerve is stimulated, producing a negative (N1 peak at 20 ms or more) to positive wave sequence over the sensory, postcentral gyrus with reversal anterior to the fissure of Roland. Stimulation of other somatic nerves, the optic, and the auditory is also used.

Evoked response recording during awake or selected forms of general anesthesia is possible, and agents making this possible should be chosen in advance. Electrodes may be either multiple–contact Silastic strips or grids in fixed arrays or individually mobile electrodes mounted on a common holding device. These are usually the same electrodes as were used for IECoG if the operation is for epilepsy. Mapping beyond the cortical surface exposed by craniotomy can be accomplished by sliding subdural electrode strips to the area of interest. When a mass lesion is to be operated, recordings can be obtained epidurally before dural incision. This permits functional mapping without exposing any more of a potentially swollen brain than necessary. The dural incision can then be limited to the region of safest approach as suggested by the functional mapping.

As with stimulation mapping of the cortical surface, functional mapping by recording evoked cortical responses is significant when positive responses are obtained. Absence of response does not necessarily prove absence of function, even with respect to the specific stimulus being applied. This is especially true if no positive responses have been obtained from any of the other areas tested.

Cortical Stimulation: Functional Responses

Cortical stimulation is an excellent method of functional localization. However, this technique requires awake anesthesia and a cooperative, informed patient. A handheld stimulating probe or grid electrode permits stimulation of the exposed cortex. Mapping usually is carried out with bipolar stimulation. Parameters often consist of a biphasic square pulse at 50 Hz of 0.3 ms (as low as 0.1 or even as high as 1.0 ms) duration per phase over 1–12 seconds, with the longer stimuli being reserved for cognitive testing. Under general anesthesia and in young children, increasing the pulse duration up to 0.5 or even 1.0 ms in combination with increases in current amplitude may be helpful.

Peak-to-peak currents of 1 mA are gradually increased in increments of 0.5–1.0 mA until there is a functional response, a cortical afterdischarge (AD), or peak-to-peak current reaches 10–15 mA. For this reason a recording electrode array is left in place during stimulation so that ADs can be detected. Such discharge indicates the potential for inducing a seizure and also makes the localization of any observed functional change suspect since other areas of the brain demonstrate induced activity. If the stimulation is being delivered with a grid consisting of electrode contacts embedded in a sheet of material, stimulation can be delivered through varying pairs of adjacent contacts while the stimulating pair and a dozen nearby contacts are used to check for AD. If a stimulating probe is being used, a set of flexible electrodes mounted on a common holder permits stimulation between its contacts and the recording of any AD. Often the threshold of AD is determined at only a few sites in the region under study and stimulation is then limited to currents less than this. It should be realized, however, that the threshold stimulus necessary to produce a functional response or AD can vary considerably in adjacent cortical sites. Both functional and AD threshold are usually lowest in the sensory motor cortex and should be redetermined in different cortical regions. Pulse duration should not be changed without redetermining the AD threshold. Routine mapping is done subdurally, but if a structural lesion and a swollen brain are present, an epidural study may be preferable for the reasons given in the previous section. However, careful infiltration of the dura with local anesthetic is necessary if stimulation rather than evoked response studies are being done since dural stimulation can be quite painful.

During stimulation mapping, inadvertent cueing of the patient with respect to the onset or occurrence of cortical stimulation or excessive details of the expected response should be avoided. Two types of response to cortical stimulation are possible—positive (elicitation) and negative (disruption). The former is characteristic of the results obtained during most sensory and motor mapping, while the latter characterizes the effect of stimulation on tests of language and other cognitive function. Though report of sensations experienced or visible motor responses are obtained readily with the aid of the anesthesiologist or other experienced observer, language testing requires more active participation by the patient. In its simplest form, the patient reads a presented script and speech arrest is noted. More sophisticated testing is possible. The effects of cortical stimulation are quite focal if AD does not occur and stimulation a few millimeters away may produce a different or no response. No response to stimulation is considered reliable unless it can be reproduced from the same site on more than one occasion. Repeated stimulation of the same site should be separated by at least enough time to stimulate at another location unless there has been an AD, in which case a longer delay of 2 minutes is advisable if false-negative responses are to be avoided.

If no functional effects are elicited by stimulating the exposed cortex, there can be no assurance that the exposed brain is not necessary to the functions being tested. In such cases, slipping a subdural strip beyond the exposed area and eliciting an effect from more distant stimulation provides an indication that the critical cortical regions are indeed located elsewhere. When operation comes within 2 cm of the functionally determined site, functional deficit is apt to result. The only clear exception to this rule appears to be an area of language functioning in the basal aspect of the dominant temporal lobe. The converse, however, is not true. Failure to elicit function from an area of cortex does not offer any certainty that that region can be excised with impunity. Mapping is far more effective at revealing what is best left intact than it is at indicating what can be removed without ill effect.

On rare occasions it is judged advisable to resect brain in sites demonstrated to be of functional importance. In such instances stimulation of each segment of cortex and of white matter prior to its removal can help guide the surgeon. Alternatively or in addition, the patient may be asked to continuously perform a functionally relevant task and observed by the anesthesiologist for any weakening of performance. Resection is then halted in any regions where surgical manipulation has altered performance.

Cortical Stimulation: Seizure Induction

Cortical stimulation to induce seizures has been used by a few centers in an attempt to localize seizure origin and direct subsequent excisional surgery. Underlying this method is the assumption that the site of seizure origin will be sampled and that it will be activated with the stimuli being used. Since the patient is awake, subjective and objective observations of the induced seizure can be compared to those usually experienced as a further check on the validity of seizure localization. Such seizure induction, however, risks propagating electrical seizure activity to the site responsible for the patient's clinical seizure manifestations and can result in false localization. This technique cannot be used safely during craniotomy and has been used only with implanted electrodes on a subacute or chronic basis in the few centers that value it. It has, however, been employed intraoperatively to induce ADs and even mild clinical symptoms for similar purposes in the past.

Acknowledgment *The author expresses his gratitude to Dr. George Ojemann for the opportunity to learn many of the lessons expressed here.*

KEY REFERENCES

Berger M, Ojemann GA. Intraoperative brain mapping techniques in neuro-oncology. Stereotact Funct Neurosurg 1991;58:153. *A clear exposition of technical factors in functional brain mapping.*

Fried I, Cascino GD. Lesional Surgery. In J Engel (ed), Surgical Treatment of the Epilepsies (2nd ed). New York: Raven, 1993;501–509. *Presents the arguments for and against the importance of IECoG in cases in which tumor or vascular malformation is associated with epilepsy.*

Gloor P. Contributions of Electroencephalography and Electrocorticography to the Neurosurgical Treatment of the Epilepsies. In DP Purpura, JK Penry, RD Walter (eds), Neurosurgical Management of the Epilepsies. Advances in Neurology 8. New York: Raven, 1975;59–106. *A classic description of theoretical and practical considerations in IECoG and electroencephalography in general.*

Jayakar P. Physiological Principles of Electrical Stimulation. In O Devinsky, A Beric, M Dogali (eds), Electrical and Magnetic Stimulation of the Brain and Spinal Cord. New York: Raven, 1993;17–27. *An excellent review of practical considerations and their theoretical underpinnings.*

Luciano D, Devinsky O, Pannizzo F. Electrocorticography During Cortical Stimulation. In O Devinsky, A Beric, M Dogali (eds), Electrical and Magnetic Stimulation of the

Brain and Spinal Cord. New York: Raven, 1993. *A comprehensive review of cortical stimulation for functional localization.*

Sperling MR. Intracranial Electroencephalography. In MR Sperling, RR Clancy (eds), Atlas of Electroencephalography. Vol. 3. Amsterdam: Elsevier, 1993. *A rare comprehensive atlas of intracranial recording largely based on chronic invasive electrodes but applicable to IECoG as well.*

Weber JP, Silbergeld DL, Winn RL. Surgical resection of epileptogenic cortex associated with structural lesions. Neurosurg Clin North Am 1993;4:327. *Presents a metaanalysis of the literature that evidences greater seizure relief when IECoG-identified epileptiform cortex is also excised in cases in which tumor or vascular malformation is associated with epilepsy.*

RECOMMENDED READINGS

Berger MS et al. Low-grade gliomas associated with intractable epilepsy: Seizure outcome utilizing electrocorticography during tumor resection. J Neurosurg 1993;79:62.

Cendes F et al. Increased interictal spiking and surgical outcome after selective amugdalo-hippocampectomy. Can J Neurolog Sci 1993;20(Suppl 2):S11.

Fiol ME et al. The prognostic value of residual spikes in the post-excision electrocorticogram after temporal lobectomy. Neurology 1991;41:512.

Jasper HH, Arfel-Capdeville G, Rasmussen T. Evaluation of EEG and cortical electrographic studies for prognosis of seizures following surgical excision of epileptogenic lesions. Epilepsia 1961;2:130.

Jayakar P et al. A safe and effective paradigm to functionally map the cortex of childhood. J Clin Neurophysiol 1992;9:288.1992.

Kraemer DL, Spencer DD. Anesthesia in Epilepsy Surgery. In J Engel (ed), Surgical Treatment of the Epilepsies (2nd ed). New York: Raven, 1993;527–538.

McBride MC et al. Predictive value of intraoperative electrocorticograms in resective epilepsy surgery. Ann Neurol 1991;30:526.

Ojemann GA, Dodrill CB. Verbal memory deficits after left temporal lobectomy for epilepsy. J Neurosurg 1985;62:101.

Ojemann GA, Whitaker H. Language localization and variability. Brain Lang 1978;6:239.

Ojemann GA. Intrahemispheric Localization of Language and Visuospatial function: Evidence from Stimulation Mapping During Craniotomies for Epilepsy. In H Akimoto et al (eds), Advances in Epileptology: XIIIth Epilepsy International Symposium. New York: Raven, 1982;373–388.

Ojemann GA. The intrahemispheric organization of human language, derived with electrical stimulation techniques. Trends Neurosci 1983;6:184.

Rasmussen T. Cortical Resection in the Treatment of Epilepsy. In DP Purpura, JK Penry, RD Walter (eds), Neurosurgical Management of the Epilepsies. Advances in Neurology 8. New York: Raven, 1975;139–153.

Silbergeld DL. A new device for cortical stimulation mapping of surgically unexposed cortex. J Neurosurg 1993;79:612.

Silbergeld DL. Intraoperative transdural functional mapping. J Neurosurg 1994;80:756.

17

Combining Somatosensory and Motor Evoked Potentials for Posterior Spine Fusion

Lee S. Segal, M.D.

Modern posterior spinal instrumentation systems greatly enhance the spine surgeon's ability to address complex deformities, posttraumatic instabilities, and other vertebral column disorders. Evolving from the Harrington distraction rods introduced three decades ago, the newer implant systems permit application of a combination of corrective forces in all three dimensions. With instrumentation systems such as Cotrel-Dubousset, TSRH, and Isola, we can now simultaneously distract, compress, derotate, and translate the spine to restore normal vertebral column alignment.

But the same corrective forces that permit us to normalize skeletal alignment can potentially cause deleterious effects on the spinal cord and nerve roots. Before the use of internal fixation of the spine, the risk of major neurologic injury after posterior spine fusion for scoliosis was almost nonexistent. The incidence of spinal cord injury dramatically increased with the application of internal spinal implants, ranging from 0.72–4.0% in a number of studies.

The devastating complication of spinal cord injury (SCI) after posterior spine fusion (PSF) with instrumentation may occur directly from mechanical injury to the spinal cord or indirectly from ischemia. There is increasing evidence that vascular embarrassment to the spinal cord is the primary cause of SCI. Dommisse identified a critical watershed area of the thoracic cord in which the blood supply to the anterior two-thirds of the spinal cord in the majority of patients is provided without collaterals by the artery of Adamkiewicz. Corrective maneuvers during surgery, such as distraction or derotation of the spine, may result in occlusion or arterial spasm, increasing the risk of neurologic injury. Direct mechanical injury to the spinal cord can occur with passage of sublaminar wires or the insertion of sublaminar hooks and pedicle screws.

It is against this background that the use of spinal cord monitoring has become, according to Nash and Brown, the "standard of practice when performing spinal operations associated with a high risk of neurologic injury."

Since the introduction of the Stagnara wake-up test in 1973, spinal cord monitoring has progressed from clinical to electrophysiologic methods.

By using both somatosensory and motor evoked potentials, we can now continuously monitor anterior and posterior spinal cord function throughout our operative procedures. We are thus able to more effectively identify and avoid potentially reversible injury to the spinal cord, and to prevent major neurologic complications.

PREOPERATIVE CONSIDERATIONS

It is critical in the preoperative period to identify patients at high risk for neurologic injury and to be aware of operative procedures that increase the potential for spinal cord injury (Tables 17.1 and 17.2). A recent study noted that patients with kyphotic deformities accounted for 85% of their neurologic complications.

Patients at Increased Risk for Neurologic Injury

Particularly at risk are (1) patients with short segmented kyphotic deformities, as frequently seen in congenital kyphosis, neurofibromatosis, and skeletal dysplasias, such as diastrophic dysplasia. Children with (2) congenital scoliosis are at risk for neurologic injury, and they must be preoperatively evaluated for intraspinal anomalies such as diastematomyelia, syrinx, and tethered cord. Patients with (3) severe scoliosis, (4) postradiation deformity, and (5) preexisting neurologic deficit have an increased risk of neurologic injury. In a survey by the Scoliosis Research Society reported in 1975, 35% of the patients sustaining neurologic complications had a neurologic deficit preoperatively.

Operative Treatment of Spinal Deformities

The operative treatment of neuromuscular scoliosis in diseases such as cerebral palsy, muscular dystrophy, and myelomeningocele carries an increased risk of neurologic complications because many of these patients have severe curves or preexisting neurologic deficits (Figure 17.1). Segmental spinal instrumentation (SSI) that invades the spinal canal is more likely to be used in this group of patients, and these techniques pose risk of direct cord or nerve root injury.

Numerous procedures performed in conjunction with posterior spine fusion increase the risk of neurologic injury. The passage of sublaminar wires can directly traumatize the spinal cord. Meticulous attention to technique of wire passage can reduce the risk of injury to the underlying spinal cord, particularly in the thoracic and thoracolumbar spine. Delayed neurologic complications of sublaminar wires have been reported as well. These injuries are thought to result from slow epidural bleeding, cord edema, or inflammation caused by the epidural position of the wires.

Neurologic injury is more likely when intraoperative correction exceeds the correction obtained on preoperative bending radiographs. Excessive distraction or derotation places the spinal cord at risk for ischemic injury. Experimental and clinical studies have demonstrated decreased blood flow to

Table 17.1 High-risk conditions for intraoperative spinal cord injury

Kyphosis
Preexisting neurologic deficit
Congenital scoliosis
Neuromuscular scoliosis
Scoliosis of a severe degree

Table 17.2 High-risk surgical procedures

Sublaminar wire passage
Distraction and derotation maneuvers
Spinal osteotomies
Segmental vessel ligation

the spinal cord after distraction and derotation, causing differential ischemic injury to the motor and sensory tracts. A high rate of neurologic injury from spinal osteotomies performed after previous posterior spine fusion is reported.

In complex spinal deformities such as kyphoscoliosis, anterior spine release and fusion are often performed as a preliminary staged procedure to allow increased correction of the deformity and enhance the rate of successful arthrodesis. Paraplegia can occur following anterior spine fusion for congenital kyphoscoliosis, with complete loss of somatosensory evoked potentials after ligation of the segmental arteries at the apex of the deformity. Patients with delayed paraplegia after segmental artery ligation and anterior spine fusion followed by posterior fusion with SSI have also been reported. Spinal cord monitoring (somatosensory evoked potential [SSEP] monitoring) in these patients was uneventful, and the delayed paraplegia was thought to be due to progressive ischemia and edema in the postoperative period. Sequential clamping of critical segmental vessels before ligation in conjunction with spinal cord monitoring has been recommended to prevent ischemic injury to the spinal cord.

CRITICAL PERIODS DURING POSTERIOR SPINE FUSION

The successful use of spinal cord monitoring requires the surgeon to identify those critical periods during a posterior spine fusion when the spinal cord is at particular risk for neurologic injury. These periods depend on both the deformity being addressed and the spinal instrumentation used. The newer spinal instrumentation systems may use hooks, wires, and pedicle screws alone or in combination.

Pedicle Screw Placement

Pedicle screw placement is the first critical period of the procedure. The risk of neurologic injury increases the more cephalad the vertebral level, as the

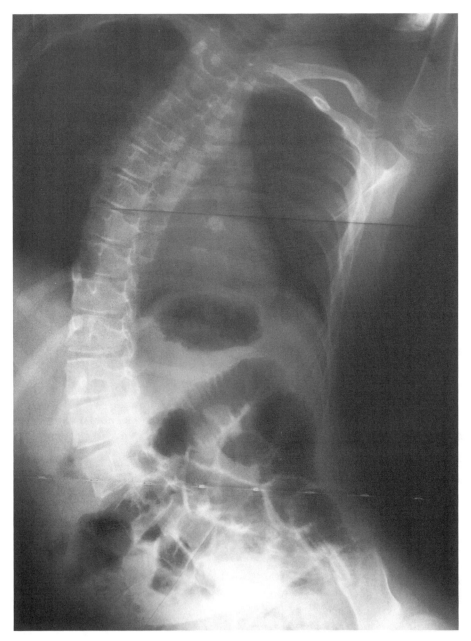

Figure 17.1A Preoperative posteroanterior radiograph of a 13-year-old spastic quadriplegic cerebral palsy patient with a 94-degree scoliosis and a severe pelvic obliquity.

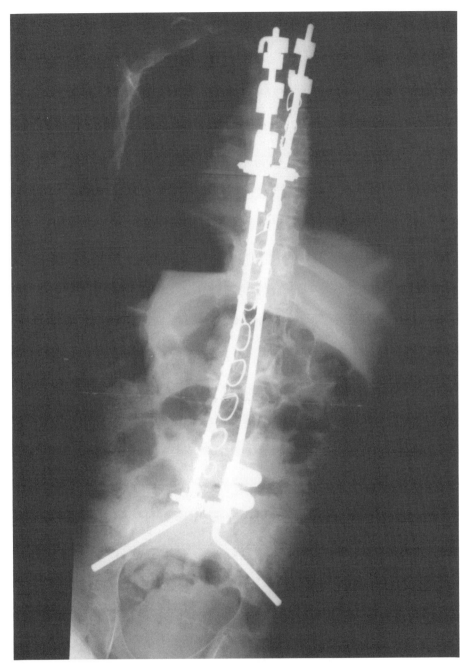

Figure 17.1B   Postoperative posteroanterior radiograph following posterior spine fusion with segmental spinal instrumentation to the pelvis. Somatosensory evoked potential and neurogenic motor evoked potential monitoring remained unchanged throughout the procedure.

pedicle diameter and the spinal canal become smaller. Deformities associated with significant rotation distort pedicle anatomy and the landmarks for the pedicle screw entry become more difficult to determine.

Insertion of Laminar and Pedicle Hooks

The second critical period involves insertion of laminar and pedicle hooks. The spinal cord can be directly injured as the inferior surface of the lamina is contoured with an osteotome. The shoe portion of the hook is then placed underneath the lamina and into the epidural space, where the spinal cord is also at risk for direct contusion.

Placement of Sublaminar Wires

Sublaminar wires provide translational correction of a spine deformity and distribute forces over multiple sites along the instrumented spine. SSI with sublaminar wires is used most often in the surgical management of neuromuscular scoliosis, but its applications are increasing. Techniques that have been described to minimize the depth of wire penetration and potential cord injury include (1) careful midline laminotomies, (2) resecting portions of the overlying spinous processes if the posterior elements are overlapped, (3) contouring the wire to the largest possible radius, and (4) meticulous technique in wire passage. Spinous process wire fixation was developed to minimize the risk of cord injury. The risk of neurologic injury is greater in the thoracic spine than the lumbar spine. This holds true for sublaminar wires, laminar hooks, and pedicle screws (Figure 17.2). The decreased canal size and osseous anatomy contribute to this increased risk. The increased stiffness of the thoracic spine may lead to a greater potential risk for ischemic injury.

Application of Corrective Forces The final critical period is the application of corrective forces, particularly distraction and derotation (Figure 17.3). The spinal cord must be monitored for at least 30 minutes after the final spine maneuver to detect the possible development of delayed neurologic complications.

To effectively monitor the spinal cord, the spine surgeon, the anesthesiologist, and the neuroelectrophysiologist must maintain a continuing dialogue. The spine surgeon must alert the others when a critical phase of the PSF is about to occur. The anesthesiologist must inform others present in the operating room of changes in the patient's body temperature, blood pressure, and other nonsurgical variables that may affect spinal cord monitoring. The neuroelectrophysiologist must report significant changes in the evoked potentials as soon as they occur.

Two mechanisms of injury are associated with either a rapid or a more gradual change in evoked potentials. Rapid loss of evoked potentials is believed to result from gross structural changes and decreased perfusion to a limited segment of the spinal cord. A gradual loss of signal is thought to be due to ischemia over a longer span of the spinal cord.

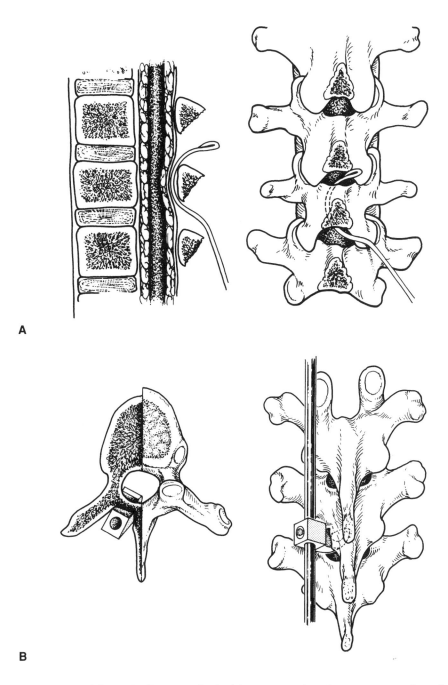

Figure 17.2 Schematic diagram of spinal instrumentation that may cause direct injury to the spinal cord. A. Passage of sublaminar wire. B. Placement of sublaminar hook. C. Insertion of pedicle screw.

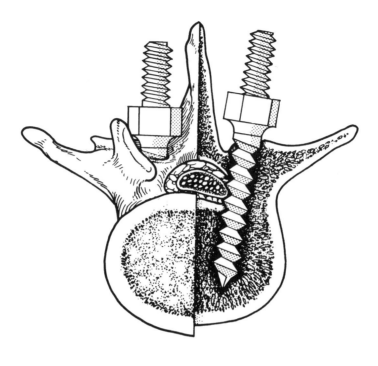

c

Figure 17.2 *(continued)*

The surgeon's response should be governed by circumstances and the pattern and rate of signal degradation. The team should be alert to technical problems that may cause false-positive alarms. It may be appropriate to observe for a time to see if signals return. It may be necessary to stop the procedure and perform a "wake-up" test. If signal loss directly follows application of the corrective force, the surgeon may need to decrease the correction achieved or remove the instrumentation.

SPINAL CORD MONITORING

Advances in spinal cord monitoring have paralleled those made in our understanding and treatment of complex spine disorders. As the potential for neurologic injury has increased with more sophisticated spinal instrumentation, the ability to evaluate the functional integrity of the spinal cord and detect injury early on a continuing basis have dramatically improved.

Wake-Up Test

The "gold standard" of spinal cord monitoring has been the Stagnara "wake-up" test. It was initially described in 1973 as a clinical method of assessing spinal cord motor function. In a report on 124 patients treated with

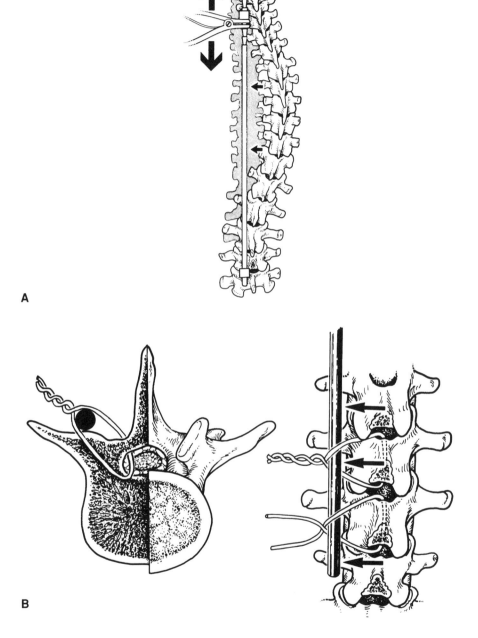

Figure 17.3 Schematic diagram of corrective forces used during spinal instrumentation that may cause ischemic injury to the spinal cord. A. Distraction. B. Translation. C. Derotation.

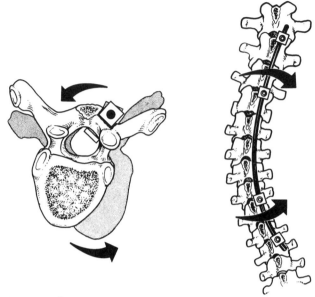

C

Figure 17.3 *(continued)*

Harrington distraction instrumentation, motor activity not present with awakening returned within 5 minutes of rod removal. Subsequent reports indicated that neurologic injury could be decreased or reversed if distraction of the spinal cord was removed soon after a neurologic deficit was detected.

Advantages of the wake-up test include (1) the ease of administration and the fact that (2) there is no requirement for extra equipment. Furthermore, (3) a patient's blood pressure increases when the patient is awakened, improving spinal cord perfusion and thus protecting against potential ischemic injury. The test may function as a dual protector, monitoring the motor activity of the cord and inhibiting overdistraction of the spine by the Harrington rod.

Disadvantages of the wake-up test include (1) the inability to monitor the spinal cord throughout the procedure. Because the test does not provide an ongoing assessment of cord function, the duration between the onset of injury and recognition may be prolonged, increasing the risk of permanent injury. (2) False-negative results are possible since motor deficits may be delayed. (3) Injury to the sensory tracts and nerve root injuries may also remain undetected, because the wake-up test only monitors gross motor function through the corticospinal tracts. (4) The wake-up test cannot be applied to patients who are unable to cooperate. Patients with cerebral palsy and other neuromuscular diseases, who may be at high risk for spinal cord injury, cannot use the wake-up test. The "wake-up" test presents significant risks including accidental extubation, dislodgment of spinal instrumentation, and air embolism. During the test, the thoracic wound should be flooded with saline to prevent air from entering open veins should the patient drop intrathoracic pressure with spontaneous inspiration.

Somatosensory Evoked Potentials Monitoring

Monitoring of SSEPs was developed to provide continuous real-time monitoring of spinal cord function. Although its limitations should be recognized, SSEP can play an important role in identifying potential problems and preventing catastrophic postoperative neurologic complications.

Numerous authors have noted that SSEPs are highly sensitive to physiologic and technical variables, including halogenated anesthetic agents, the patient's body temperature and blood pressure, and the use of electrocautery and other sources of electrical interference in the operating room. SSEP amplitudes and latencies may change from preoperative baseline to postinduction recordings. When nonsurgical variables are controlled and adequate postinduction baselines are obtained, SSEPs are a reliable and reproducible method of spinal cord monitoring. Subcortical monitoring increases the accuracy and reproducibility of SSEPs and may allow the use of halogenated anesthetic agents.

The major disadvantage of SSEPs is the inability to consistently detect injury to the motor tracts of the spinal cord. Case reports have described postoperative neurologic complications despite unchanged SSEPs throughout the operative procedure. In a combined survey of the Scoliosis Research Society and the European Spinal Deformity Society, a 28% incidence of neurologic deficit undetected by SSEPs was reported. The high rate of false-negative results was attributed to (1) an increased kyphotic correction, (2) not monitoring both amplitude and latency, and (3) an inadequate number of recording leads.

The assumption that significant motor tract injury must result in changes in dorsal column activity and SSEPs is incorrect. A disassociation between motor and sensory evoked potential monitoring was demonstrated in 3 of the 30 patients evaluated after derotation maneuvers for scoliosis. Ischemic injury to the anterior spinal cord, with preservation of the posterior column circulation, resulted in unchanged SSEPs.

SSEPs may be even less reliable in patients with neuromuscular disease. There is a high variability in SSEPs in patients with paralytic scoliosis, congenital scoliosis, and other neurologic disorders. There is an unacceptable 28% incidence of unreliable tracings in the neuromuscular population.

Motor Evoked Potentials

Monitoring techniques for motor evoked potentials (MEPs) were developed to overcome the inherent limitations of SSEPs. With the translaminar technique originated by Owen, obtaining neurogenic MEPs avoids the problems of cortical stimulation and epidural electrode placement associated with other methods of MEP monitoring and allows use of muscle relaxants.

Because of the anatomic separation of the motor and sensory spinal cord tracts and their blood supplies, MEPs are more reliable predictors of anterior spinal cord integrity and motor function than SSEPs. Neurogenic MEPs (NMEPs) are more sensitive and specific to the damaging effects of ischemia, distraction, and compression than SSEP spinal cord monitoring. Neurogenic

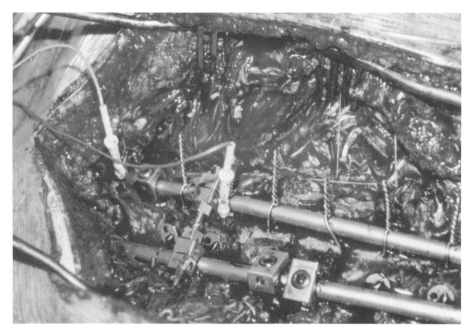

Figure 17.4 Intraoperative placement of stimulating electrodes into the spinous process-es at the proximal levels of the spine exposure and instrumentation.

MEPs consistently degraded at lower levels of distraction than SSEPs, demon-strating a differential sensitivity of the motor and sensory tracts to ischemia. There can be MEP and SSEP disassociation during distraction and derotation maneuvers, reflecting the two independent neural pathways and separate blood supplies within the spinal cord. In a clinical study of more than 300 patients, NMEPs were a more valid predictor of postoperative motor status. Greater than 90% reliability in NMEP monitoring can also be obtained.

The major limitation of NMEP is its inability to provide continuous moni-toring of the sensory tracts. There are also problems with the translaminar tech-nique of NMEP monitoring. Pooling of blood and other fluids around the proxi-mal stimulating leads and the presence of the metal instrumentation itself can interfere with the signal by shunting current away from the spinal cord (Figure 17.4). Percutaneous stimulating electrodes, placed in the spinous processes prox-imal to the incision, may solve this problem.

Combining Somatosensory Evoked Potentials and Motor Evoked Potentials Monitoring

Combining somatosensory and motor evoked potential spinal cord monitoring during PSF enhances our ability to detect spinal cord injury while the ischemic insult is still reversible. Selected patients and procedures at high risk for neurologic injury should have combined SEP and MEP monitoring if

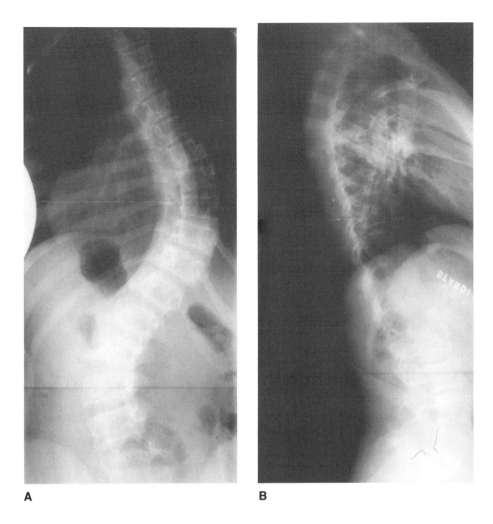

A   **B**

Figure 17.5 A, B. Preoperative posteroanterior and lateral radiographs of a 12-year-old girl with a double major idiopathic scoliosis and a grade 1 spondylolisthesis. C, D. Postoperative posteroanterior and lateral radiographs following posterior spine fusion and segmental spinal instrumentation and pedicle screw fixation distally. Somatosensory evoked potential and neurogenic motor evoked potential monitoring were stable throughout the procedure. A "wake-up" test was performed after the instrumentation was completed.

available (Figure 17.5). In particular, combined monitoring should be considered for high-risk procedures and high-risk patients such as those with neuromuscular scoliosis.

We have used combined SSEP and MEP monitoring for posterior spine fusions in a series of 27 patients. The most common preoperative diagnosis in

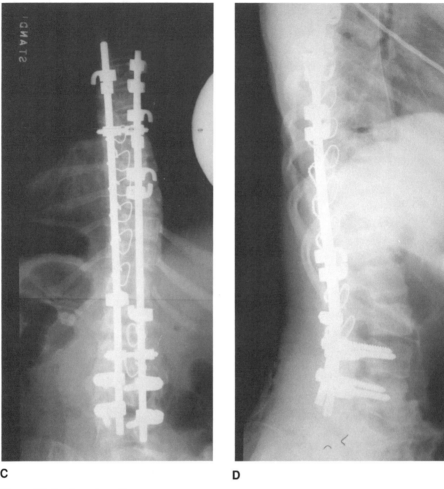

C   D

Figure 17.5 *(continued)*

these patients is neuromuscular scoliosis, reflecting a clinic population that includes large numbers of children with cerebral palsy, muscular dystrophy, and myelomeningocele. In 85% of patients monitored, reproducible SSEPs and MEPs were obtained. Three patients (11%) had unsuccessful SSEP monitoring but reproducible MEP monitoring that remained unchanged throughout the procedure. Two of these patients had spastic quadriplegic cerebral palsy and the other child had Down syndrome with spastic hemiplegia. Our experience agrees with other series reporting difficulties with SSEP monitoring in neuromuscular scoliosis and confirms the merit of combined SSEP and MEP monitoring for these patients. In one patient, with a diagnosis of ataxia telangiectasia, we could obtain neither SSEPs nor MEPs, although the wake-up test was successful at the completion of the instrumentation. We cannot explain the failure of electrophysiologic monitoring in this patient. Failure of SSEP monitoring in five patients with Charcot-Marie-Tooth disease, a progressive hereditary sensorimotor neuropathy, has also been reported. Failure of SSEP monitoring was attributed to demyelination of the peripheral nerves, degeneration of the dorsal columns, and disruption of the anterior horn cells. In cooperative patients, we continue to perform the wake-up test after SSEP and MEP spinal cord monitoring, whether or not there have been changes have in the evoked potentials.

CASE STUDY

An 11-year-old girl with a severe kyphoscoliosis secondary to diastrophic dysplasia, a rare autosomal recessive skeletal dysplasia, required surgical correction of her deformity. To address the magnitude and rigidity of her scoliosis and kyphosis, we performed a preliminary anterior spine release and fusion. The short segmented kyphoscoliosis placed the child in a high-risk category for neurologic injury. During PSF we obtained satisfactory postinduction baselines for both SSEPs and MEPs. After placing a thoracic laminar hook, both the somatosensory and MEPs were lost (Figure 17.6). The hook was promptly removed. After the evoked potentials failed to return, a successful wake-up test was obtained. The procedure was completed with an in situ fusion without instrumentation, followed by immobilization in a halo vest. In the postoperative period, the child had sensory dysesthesias and motor weakness, which gradually resolved with no long-term sequelae. In this case, spinal cord monitoring combining SSEPs and MEPs played a significant role in altering the preoperative surgical plan and preventing catastrophic neurologic complications.

Acknowledgement   *The author thanks Edwards P. Schwentker, M.D., for his suggestions and assistance in preparing this chapter.*

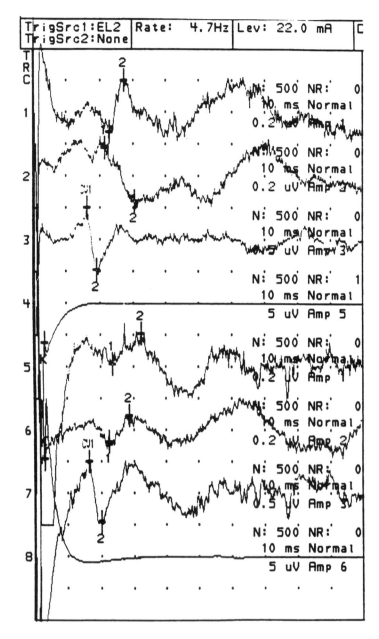

A

Figure 17.6 Spinal-cord monitoring in an 11-year-old patient with diastrophic dysplasia undergoing a posterior spine fusion for a severe kyphoscoliosis. A. Baseline intraoperative somatosensory evoked potential in response to posterior tibial nerve stimulation. B. Loss of somatosensory evoked potential after thoracic hook placement. C. Baseline intraoperative neurogenic motor evoked potential. D. Loss of intraoperative neurogenic motor evoked potential after thoracic laminar hook placement.

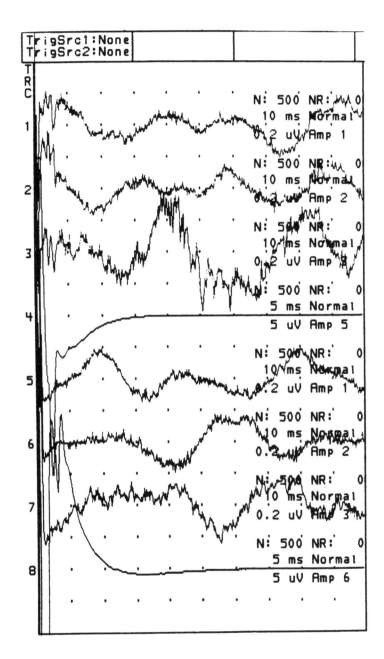

B

Figure 17.6 *(continued)*

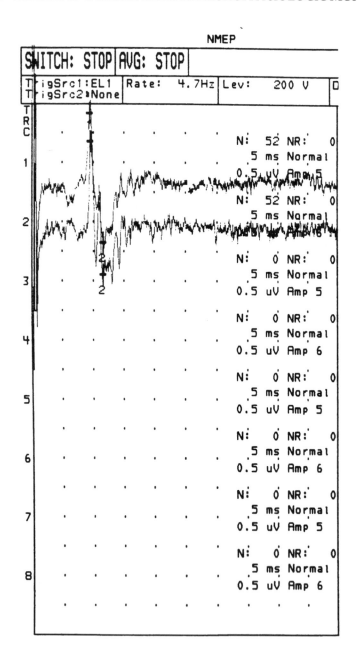

C

Figure 17.6 *(continued)*

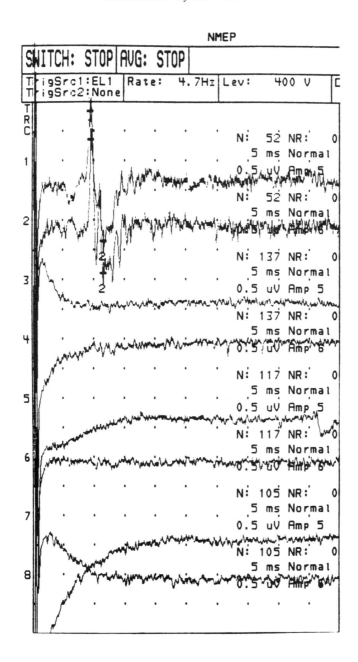

D

Figure 17.6 *(continued)*

KEY REFERENCES

Ashkenaze D et al. Efficacy of spinal cord monitoring in neuromuscular scoliosis. Spine 1993;18(12):1627. *A reliable tracing could not be obtained in 28% of the procedures in this review, and two postoperative neurologic deficits were missed with somatosensory cortical evoked potential (SCEP) spinal cord monitoring. SCEP monitoring for neuromuscular scoliosis proved unreliable and nonspecific.*

Engler GL et al. Somatosensory evoked potentials during Harrington instrumentation for scoliosis. J Bone Joint Surg [Am] 1978;60:528. *Describes the technique of anesthesia and SSEP spinal cord monitoring used during Harrington distraction instrumentation for scoliosis in 55 patients. No complications or neurologic complications were noted.*

Hall JE, Levine CR, Sudhir KG. Intraoperative awakening to monitor spinal cord function during Harrington instrumentation and spine fusion. J Bone Joint Surg [Am] 1978;60:533. *Detailed description of the wake-up test. Three patients in a consecutive series of 166 patients were found to have a neural deficit on awakening, which resolved on release of the distracting force.*

Lubicky JP et al. Variability of somatosensory cortical evoked potential monitoring during spinal surgery. Spine 1989;14(8):790. *Intraoperative variability of SCEP monitoring was found to correlate with patient diagnosis, age, neuromuscular status, and procedural factors. Patients with neuromuscular disorders such as cerebral palsy and myelomeningocele had high SCEP variability, which may limit the reliability and usefulness of spinal cord monitoring in detecting spinal cord injury before irreversible changes occur.*

Machida M et al. Monitoring of action potentials after stimulation of the spinal cord. J Bone Joint Surg [Am] 1988;70:911. *Experimental animal and clinical studies by these authors demonstrated that motor action potentials and SSEPs reflected two independent functions of the spinal cord.*

Owen JH, et al. The clinical application of neurogenic motor evoked potentials to monitor spinal cord function during surgery. Spine 1991; 16(8s):s385. *Clinical study of concomitant use of SSEP and NMEP spinal cord monitoring during spinal surgery (300 procedures). SSEP demonstrated greater variability than NMEP. NMEP was found to be a more valid indicator of postoperative motor status than SSEP. The authors recommend that both SSEP and NMEP be used together to monitor spinal cord function during surgical procedures that place the spinal cord at risk.*

Owen JH, Naito M, Bridwell KH. Relationship among level of distraction, evoked potentials, spinal cord ischemia, and integrity, and clinical status in animals. Spine 1990;15(9):852. *Experimental animal study demonstrating increased sensitivity of NMEP to the effects of overdistraction. Compared to SSEPs, NMEPs were more valid predictors of spinal cord function in the more flexible regions of the spine.*

Vauzelle C, Stagnara P, Jouvinroux P. Functional monitoring of spinal cord activity during spinal surgery. Clin Orthop 1973;93:173. *Initial report describing the wake-up test in 124 procedures with Harrington instrumentation.*

Wilber RG et al. Postoperative neurological deficits in segmental spinal instrumentation. J Bone Joint Surg [Am] 1984;66:1178. *Review of 137 patients with scoliosis who underwent PSF and SSEP spinal cord monitoring. Twelve patients (17%) had neurologic complications. Passage of sublaminar wires, intraoperative correction exceeding preoperative bending correction, and lack of surgical experience were factors increasing the risk of spinal cord injury.*

RECOMMENDED READING

Abel MF et al. Brainstem evoked potentials for scoliosis surgery: a reliable method allowing use of halogenated anesthetic agents. J Pediatr Orthop 1990;10:208.

Apel DM et al. Avoiding paraplegia during anterior spinal surgery. The role of somatosensory evoked potential monitoring with temporary occlusion of segmental spinal arteries. Spine 1991;16(8S):S365.

Ben-David B, Haller G, Taylor P. Anterior spinal fusion complicated by paraplegia. A case report of a false-negative somatosensory-evoked potential. Spine 1987;12(6):536.

Ben-David B, Taylor PD, Haller GS. Posterior spinal fusion complicated by posterior column injury. A case report of a false-negative wake-up test. Spine 1987;12(6):540.

Ben-David B. Spinal cord monitoring. Orthop Clin North Am 1988;19(2):427.

Bieber E, Tolo V, Uematsu, S. Spinal cord monitoring during posterior spinal instrumentation and fusion. Clin Orthop 1988;229:121.

Bradshaw K, Webb JK, Fraser AM. Clinical evaluation of spinal cord monitoring in scoliosis surgery. Spine 1984;9(6):636.

Dawson EG et al. Spinal cord monitoring. Results of the Scoliosis Research Society and the European Spinal Deformity Society survey. Spine 1991;16(8A):S361.

Dinner DS et al. Intraoperative spinal somatosensory evoked potential monitoring. J Neurosurg 1986;65:807.

Dommisse GF. The blood supply of the spinal cord: a critical vascular zone in spinal surgery. J Bone Joint Surg [Br] 1974;56:225.

Drummond DS et al. Interspinous process segmental spinal instrumentation. J Pediatr Orthop 1984;4:397.

Forbes HJ et al. Spinal cord monitoring in scoliosis surgery. J Bone Joint Surg [Br] 1991;73:487.

Ginsburg HH, Shetter AG, Raudzens PA. Postoperative paraplegia with preserved intraoperative somatosensory evoked potentials. J Neurosurg 1985;63:296.

Johnston CE II et al. Delayed paraplegia complicating sublaminar segmental spinal instrumentation. J Bone Joint Surg [Am] 1986;68:556.

Jones ET, Matthews LS, Hensinger RN. The wake-up technique as a dual protector of spinal cord function during spine fusion. Clin Orthop 1982;168:113.

Keim HA, Hilal SK. Spinal angiography in scoliosis patients. J Bone Joint Surg [Am] 1971;53:904.

Keith RW, Stambough JL, Awender SH. Somatosensory cortical evoked potentials: A review of 100 cases of intraoperative spinal surgery monitoring. J Spinal Disorders 1990;3(3):220.

Krishna M et al. Failure of somatosensory evoked potential monitoring in sensorimotor neuropathy. Spine 1991;16(4):479.

Lesser RP et al. Postoperative neurological deficits may occur despite unchanged intraoperative somatosensory evoked potentials. Ann Neurol 1986;19:22.

Letts RM, Hallenberg C. Delayed paresis following spinal fusion with Harrington instrumentation. Clin Orthop 1977;125:45.

Levy WJ. Spinal evoked potentials from the motor tracts. J Neurosurg 1983; 58:38.

Loder RT, Thomson GJ, LaMont RL. Spinal cord monitoring in patients with nonidiopathic spinal deformities using somatosensory evoked potentials. Spine 1991;16(12):1359.

Lonstein JE et al. Neurologic deficits secondary to spinal deformity: A review of the literature and report of 43 cases. Spine 1980;5:331.

MacEwen GD, Bunnell WP, Sriram K. Acute neurological complications in the treatment of scoliosis. A report of the scoliosis research society. J Bone Joint Surg [Am] 1975;57:404.

Machida M et al. Dissociation of muscle action potentials and spinal somatosensory evoked potentials after ischemic damage of spinal cord. Spine 1988;13(10):1119.

Machida M et al. Spinal cord monitoring. Electrophysiologic measures of sensory and motor function during spinal surgery. Spine 1985;10(5):407.

Machida M, Yamada T. Spinal Cord Monitoring. In SL Weinstein (ed), The Pediatric Spine. New York: Raven, 1994; 851–860.

Moe JH. Complications of scoliosis treatment. Clin Orthop 1967;53:21.

Mustain WD, Kendig RJ. Dissociation of neurogenic motor and somatosensory evoked potentials. A case report. Spine 1991;16(7):851.

Naito M et al. Effects of distraction on physiologic integrity of the spinal cord, spinal cord blood flow, and clinical status. Spine 1992;17(10):1154.

Nash CL Jr, Brown RH. Current concepts review. Spinal cord monitoring. J Bone Joint Surg [Am] 1989;71:627.

Owen JH et al. Effects of spinal cord lesioning on somatosensory and neurogenic motor evoked potentials. Spine 1989;14(7):673.

Owen JH et al. Relationship between duration of spinal cord ischemia and postoperative neurologic deficits in animals. Spine 1990;15(7):618.

Owen JH et al. Sensitivity and specificity of somatosensory and neurogenic-motor evoked potentials in animals and humans. Spine 1988;13(10):1111.

Owen JH. Evoked Potential Monitoring During Spinal Surgery. In KH Bridwell, RL DeWald (eds), The Textbook of Spinal Surgery. Philadelphia: Lippincott, 1991;31–66.

Roy EP III et al. Intraoperative somatosensory evoked potential monitoring in scoliosis. Clin Orthop 1988;229:94.

Segal LS, Schwentker EP. Wire holding frame for sublaminar segmental instrumentation. A technical note. Spine (in press), (1994).

York DH, Chabot RJ, Gaines RW. Response variability of somatosensory evoked potentials during scoliosis surgery. Spine 1987;12(9);864.

Zindrick MR et al. Factors influencing the penetration of wires into the neural canal during segmental wiring. J Bone Joint Surg [Am] 1989;71:742.

18

Pharmacologic Effects of Anesthesia on Intraoperative Neurophysiologic Monitoring

Garfield B. Russell, M.D., FRCPC
Gregory C. Allen, M.D., FRCPC
Jeffry L. Jones, M.D.

Anesthetics depress cerebral metabolism and alter the neuroelectric activity of the brain, which is recorded on the electroencephalograph (EEG) and with evoked potentials. Metabolism may be altered through (1) inhibition of transmitter substance synthesis (acetylcholine, catecholamines), (2) inhibition of glycolysis, and (3) changes in citric acid cycle intermediates and amino acids. The variations in anesthetic effects produced on the EEG and evoked potentials are influenced by the greater effect agents have on synaptic transmission as compared to axonal conduction. This difference explains why cortically recorded evoked potentials are more suppressed than evoked potentials recorded subcortically after stimulation at the same site. The interaction between anesthetic states and EEG and evoked potentials recorded intraoperatively makes it imperative that those caring for patients having surgery with intraoperative neurophysiologic monitoring be aware of potential interactions.

ANESTHESIA AND THE ELECTROENCEPHALOGRAPH

Awake patients have a dominant alpha (8–13 Hz) frequency 75–90% of the time, with a less frequent dominant fast beta frequency (>13 Hz). For 20% of patients, there is an intermittent delta (0–3 Hz) or theta (4–7 Hz) irregular rhythm of varying amplitude.

Anesthetic agents produce EEG changes related to anesthetic depth, although not all agents affect the EEG similarly. Anesthetic induction is usually associated with alpha activity spreading from the occiput anteriorly, then decreased alpha and increased low-amplitude (<30 µV) beta activity during cortical excitation. With increasing anesthetic depth, theta and delta activity become dominant. These may be high-amplitude (>100 µV). Fast waves may be superimposed on dysrhythmic slow waves. Depending on the anesthetic agent and the dose, this type of pattern may continue, a theta and delta rhythm may predominate, or a period of burst suppression may develop. For the most part, the degree of electrical suppression on EEG caused by anesthetics correlates with the effects on cortically recorded evoked responses as well. However, not all anesthetics cause a similar dose response. Other factors may be related to anesthesia (such as hypothermia or hyperventilation of neurosurgical patients) and may also exert an effect.

Halogenated Anesthetics and the Electroencephalograph

All volatile anesthetics produce a dose-related depression of cerebral metabolism (CMR). This metabolic depression is primarily suppression of synaptic activity (which is responsible for 60% of the cellular consumption of metabolic substrates) rather than effects on neuronal homeostatic function (which is responsible for 40% of the metabolic rate). The CMR is reduced more by isoflurane and enflurane than by halothane; 1.0 MAC decreases CMR 45%, 50%, and 30%, respectively. Maximum CMR suppression (EEG isoelectricity) is seen with isoflurane at about 2 MAC. EEG isoelectricity with halothane occurs at 4 MAC, but this may be secondary to interference with neuronal oxidative phosphorylation. Both halothane and enflurane cause dominant high-amplitude theta and delta activity at surgical levels of anesthesia. Three percent enflurane reduces cerebral oxygen consumption ($CMRO_2$) by 50%; the onset of seizure activity during hypocapnia returns $CMRO_2$ to baseline.

Sevoflurane and desflurane are two new halogenated ethers. Desflurane was recently released into clinical practice, while sevoflurane is still undergoing clinical trials in North America, with clinical release probable. In rabbits, sevoflurane has similar CMR depressant effects to isoflurane. In dogs, desflurane at 0.5–2.0 MAC decreased $CMRO_2$ approximately 20%, again similar to isoflurane. Electroencephalographic depression occurs at equipotent dosages of desflurane and isoflurane.

Nitrous Oxide

Nitrous oxide (N_2O) is commonly used in combination with intravenous and volatile anesthetics. Published studies have demonstrated differing neurophysiologic effects because of (1) interspecies differences for anesthetic susceptibility, (2) increased catecholamines from associated sympathetic stimulation, and (3) the comparison of different anesthetic regimens. When N_2O is given along with intravenous sedation or other anesthetic agents, no changes or slight decreases (about 15%) in $CMRO_2$ are seen.

The EEG of subjects exposed to N_2O alone can be difficult to distinguish from the awake state. The diffuse 10-Hz alpha activity seen during room-air breathing decreases in frequency and amplitude with N_2O breathing. A fast oscillatory activity at approximately 35 Hz develops predominately over the frontal lobes and later over the occipital lobes. The amplitude and the relative

EEG quantity consisting of this fast activity correlate positively with N_2O concentrations. Other EEG changes are similar to those produced by volatile agents. Low doses of N_2O result in EEG activation with low-amplitude fast-wave activity, changing into high-amplitude slow waves as the inspired partial pressure increases. Although sudden discontinuation has resulted in seizures in mice, seizure activity is not found in humans.

Intravenous Anesthetics

Most intravenous anesthetic agents cause a dose-related decrease in $CMRO_2$ as well as associated neuroelectric depression. Intravenous anesthetics vary widely in their pharmacologic type and relative potency, so some variations in dose-response relationships are expected.

Induction Agents

The barbiturates (thiopental, methohexital, thiamylal) produce a maximum $CMRO_2$ decrease of 50–55% at concentrations associated with EEG isoelectricity. Like volatile agents, the metabolic effect is secondary to neurophysiologic depression, not altered cellular homeostasis. EEG changes are similar to those induced by other anesthetic agents. After low doses, low-voltage, fast EEG activity is seen, followed by increasing waveform amplitude. This leads to generalized slowing with delta and theta activity. Burst suppression or isoelectricity occurs at higher doses. The transition through these phases is more rapid with speedy administration.

Etomidate, an imidazole derivative used for anesthetic induction, is associated with stimulation of central gamma amino butyric acid (GABA) inhibition. $CMRO_2$ is reduced 50%, also coincident with isoelectricity. Low doses of etomidate activate the EEG and may increase epileptiform activity detected with depth electrodes in epileptic patients. With deepening anesthesia, high-amplitude delta waves supervene. Higher doses can result in burst suppression along with relative hemodynamic stability (Figure 18.1).

Ketamine produces both cerebral excitation and depression. Activation of thalamic and limbic structures has been demonstrated in humans who have ketamine-induced seizure activity. Human studies have shown no change in CMR, despite 60% increases in cerebral blood flow. High-amplitude theta activity with background beta activity is present after induction doses of ketamine.

Propofol, also a CMR depressant, given as a bolus of 2 mg/kg followed by a continuous infusion (0.2 mg/kg/minute), decreased CMR 36%. Low doses can produce EEG activation with fast-wave activity that may obscure epileptic foci. Although there have been concerns about physical seizure-like activity after sedation or anesthesia with propofol, and after withdrawal when it has been used for sedation in intensive-care patients, EEG monitoring has not documented seizure activity.

EEG depression and isoelectricity are easily attained with induction doses of propofol. In a study of 17 patients, 15 showed synchronous burst suppression within

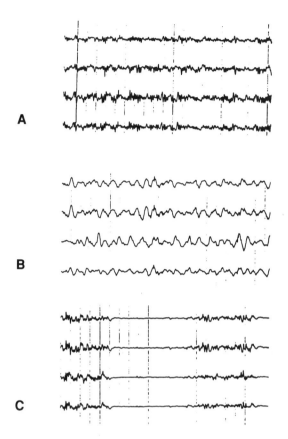

Figure 18.1 Electroencephalograph in a 32-year-old woman for a giant basilar artery aneurysm clipping. A. A baseline EEG after general anesthetic with a thiopental induction followed by fentanyl (3 μg/kg bolus and 0.5 mg/kg 1-hour infusion) and 70% nitrous oxide. B. Diffuse EEG slowing is demonstrated as thiopental loading is begun for cerebral protection prior to application of temporary clips. C. Burst suppression resulted. *Courtesy of the Intraoperative Neurophysiological Monitoring Service, Departments of Anesthesia and Medicine (Division of Neurology), Penn State University College of Medicine, Hershey, PA 17033.*

3 minutes of induction, with a median duration of 9.3 minutes. Activity bursts after propofol are characterized by spindle generation, whereas bursts with volatile agents or barbiturates include low-amplitude, mixed-frequency activity with rhythmic theta waves. Recovery after propofol is associated with increased beta activity.

Sedatives
The benzodiazepines are most frequently used as sedatives but also can be used for anesthetic induction. Sedation with diazepam, lorazepam, or midazolam occurs after binding to the GABAergic receptor complex, enhancing GABA

inhibitory activity. Benzodiazepines decrease $CMRO_2$ 20–35%. This decrease is less than that seen with barbiturates. The EEG is activated with sedation but is suppressed with decreased frequency and increased amplitude at higher doses of benzodiazepines.

Narcotics

Most patients receive narcotics as part of their anesthetic regimens. The narcotics as a group seem to either not effect CMR or to slightly reduce it. With 70% N_2O, CMR has been shown not to change in humans. Clinically, morphine appears to depress CMR in the stimulated brain but to have minimal effects when there is no arousal. Effects of fentanyl on CMR have been studied primarily in animal models. Although some investigations have documented large reductions in CMR in animals, fentanyl, 25 mg/kg, with background pentobarbital anesthesia has also been shown to have no effect. EEG slowing along with increased amplitude can occur without changes in consciousness. Significant EEG suppression is not apparent. Seizure activity has been demonstrated in rats secondary to narcotic administration. Clinical seizure activity after synthetic narcotic administration has also been reported in humans.

Adjunctive Agents

Droperidol is commonly used as an antiemetic or in combination with a narcotic for neuroleptanesthesia. The vasodilator properties tied to its mild alpha-blocking activity may decrease systemic blood pressure. Even when this occurs, 0.25 mg/kg of droperidol with fentanyl 5 µg/kg does not change CMR. EEG slowing does occur, but effects are similar to those when narcotics are administered alone.

The benzodiazepine receptor antagonist flumazenil is used to antagonize residual sedation from agents such as diazepam or midazolam. In a canine model with background general anesthesia and without benzodiazepines, CMR was stable. When midazolam was given, CMR, intracranial pressure (ICP), and cerebral blood flow (CBF) decreased; with administration of flumazenil CMR returned to baseline, but CBF and ICP measured 50% and 200%, respectively, above baseline. Flumazenil can result in seizure activity when given in excessive doses.

Lidocaine is given both intratracheally by spray and intravenously to attenuate hemodynamic stimulation and ICP increases secondary to laryngoscopy. It causes a dose-dependent decrease in $CMRO_2$, but unlike thiopental, lidocaine depresses $CMRO_2$ beyond isoelectricity by affecting ionic homeostatic function. Blood levels greater than 5–10 µg/ml can cause cerebral toxicity with grand mal seizures and increased $CMRO_2$. Mild EEG slowing may be seen at less than toxic levels.

Neuromuscular Blockers

Depolarizing and nondepolarizing neuromuscular blockers do not alter EEG. Most questions have been raised about the depolarizing agents. Succinylcholine administered to head-injured patients did not change the EEG (two channels recorded), Doppler-determined middle cerebral artery blood velocity, or ICP.

ANESTHESIA AND EVOKED POTENTIALS

Anesthetic agents depress the cortical response to administered stimuli whether the stimuli are surgical or controlled, as in somatosensory evoked potential (SSEP) monitoring. The relative potency of agents on SSEPs is similar to that on EEG, with specific exceptions. Motor evoked potential recording quality varies with the type of stimulation and the stimulation site used.

Somatosensory Evoked Potentials

Most anesthetic agents have similar effects on SSEPs and EEG. Agents that quickly produce EEG slowing and isoelectricity have relatively more potency to decrease SSEP amplitude and increase latency. However, there are specific exceptions to this. SSEPs are responses to specific stimuli whereas the EEG exhibits spontaneous activity. This factor may result in some difference in each monitor's responses to anesthetics.

The Volatile Anesthetics

All the volatile anesthetic agents depress cortical somatosensory responses to stimulation. There are some differences in their specific disruptive effects. Some investigators consider halothane less and enflurane most suppressive, whereas others consider enflurane least and halothane most depressive. Clinically, we find all agents to have similar effects. Concentrations of each above 0.5 MAC prolong latency and decrease amplitude enough to interfere with monitoring. Equipotent concentrations of N_2O do suppress SSEPs but generally less than the halogenated agents. A mix of N_2O and a volatile anesthetic appears to have a greater depressant effect on SSEPs compared to an equipotent administration of a single agent.

Intravenous Agents: Differences in Effects

Barbiturates may decrease evoked potential amplitude, but potentials can be recorded (even though amplitude is reduced and latency is increased) after doses sufficient to cause EEG burst suppression.

Etomidate may increase the amplitude of somatosensory evoked responses even though it does result in some prolongation of SSEP latency. Doses of 0.1 and 0.2 mg/kg augment the evoked waveform amplitude, but typical induction doses (0.3 mg/kg) result in amplitude reduction (Figure 18.2). The exact mechanism is unclear.

Ketamine can also be "SSEP friendly." It may either significantly not alter or potentiate SSEP amplitude.

Narcotics (fentanyl, sufentanil, alfentanil, morphine) may mildly decrease SSEP amplitude, but in usual therapeutic doses, do not interfere with SSEP monitoring. In rabbits, a dose-dependent and naloxone-reversible effect of 100 µg of fentanyl was noted on both evoked spinal and cortical potentials after posterior tibial nerve stimulation. The effect was less at more intense levels of stimulation.

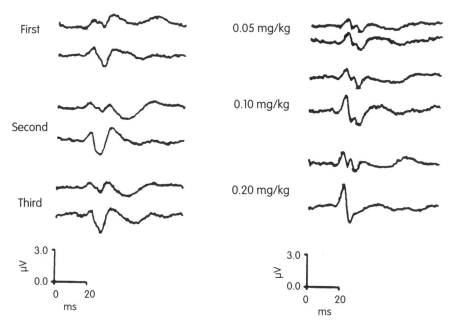

Figure 18.2 Etomidate increases somatosensory evoked potential amplitude. On the left, repeated doses of etomidate 0.1 mg/kg had a similar effect. On the right, different doses (0.05, 0.10, and 0.20 mg/kg) produced a dose-dependent increase in amplitude. Negative waves are upward. *Reprinted with permission from RW McPherson, R Levitt. Effect of time and dose on scalp-recorded somatosensory evoked potential wave augmentation by etomidate. J Neurosurg Anesthesiol 1989;1:16.*

Benzodiazepines decrease SSEP amplitudes with minimal effect on latency. However, we have noticed a wide variation in individual susceptibility. In some patients the common practice of giving a small dose of midazolam at the beginning of anesthesia results in marked interference with SSEP recording.

Neuromuscular Blockers

Muscle relaxants themselves have no significant effect on SSEP generation or conduction. However, by decreasing spontaneous and induced muscle activity, better-quality recordings are often made with muscle relaxation present. Physical artifact is decreased.

Brain Stem Auditory Evoked Responses

Brain stem auditory evoked responses (BAERs), particularly the earlier waveforms from subcortical generators, are much more resistant to changes induced by anesthetic agents than are EEGs and SSEPs.

Waveform latency and amplitude are affected by volatile anesthetics with similar effects reported for halothane, enflurane, and isoflurane. This effect is greater than any effect from N_2O. Dose-dependent decreases in amplitude and prolonged latency can be demonstrated for waves III–V. However, the effects are not sufficient to interfere with clinical monitoring quality. Latency is usually prolonged less than 1 ms and amplitude decreases are minimal.

The subcortical BAER is not altered by intravenous anesthetics, including barbiturates, etomidate, or the narcotics. Barbiturate doses three times that required to produce cortical EEG isoelectricity may increase subcortical latencies slightly. Etomidate can result in slight increases of the latencies of waves I and III. Both racemic ketamine and the S(+) ketamine isomer have been shown not to alter midlatency auditory evoked potentials in humans.

Motor Evoked Potentials

Motor evoked potentials (MEPs) can be produced by transcranial magnetic or electrical stimulation or spinal cord electrical stimulation. The recorded responses can be either neurogenic or myogenic. Anesthetics have greater effects on evoked responses that are transmitted through pathways with the greater number of synapses, as well as those resulting from less than supramaximal stimulation.

Neurogenic Motor Evoked Potentials

Of the potentials used to monitor the motor tracts, neurogenic motor evoked potentials (NMEPs) are most resistant to anesthetic-induced changes. The peripheral responses are recorded from muscle or nerve after spinal cord electrical stimulation. Cortical synaptic transmission is bypassed and axonal transmission within the spinal cord motor tracts and the peripheral nerves is tested for integrity of conduction. We have recorded good NMEPs from the popliteal fossa using nitrous oxide–narcotic techniques, balanced techniques with volatile agents, and anesthesia administered primarily with volatile agents. However, volatile anesthetics have been shown to have a depressant effect on spinal-sciatic evoked responses in swine (Figure 18.3). No differences were demonstrated between equipotent doses of isoflurane, enflurane, and halothane. In our laboratory, NMEPs were maintained in rats at isoflurane concentrations sufficient to cause burst suppression (Figure 18.4).

Transcranial motor evoked potentials from either electrical (TCeMEPs) or magnetic (TCmag-MEPs) stimulation are more susceptible to anesthetic suppression. Of all types of MEPs, the TCmag-MEPs appear to be most depressed by anesthesia. Cortical synaptic transmission is not bypassed; therefore anesthetic-induced cortical depression can occur. The greater depressant effects on transcranial magnetic stimulation may also be influenced by the higher incidence of less than supramaximal stimulation with stimulating magnets. Anesthetic agents do not significantly affect peripheral nerve impulse transmission. Although the volatile agents can depress some neuromuscular junction transmission at concentrations of 1.5–2 MAC, this effect is not large. Myogenic responses to TCeMEPs are less suppressed by fentanyl and etomidate than by propofol or

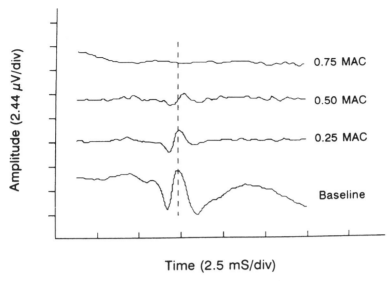

Time (2.5 mS/div)

Figure 18.3 The attenuation of the spinal-sciatic evoked responses to increasing concentrations of isoflurane. (MAC = minimum alveolar concentration.) *Reprinted with permission from LH Short, RE Peterson, PD Mongan. Physiologic and anesthetic alterations on spinal-sciatic evoked responses in swine. Anesth Analg 1993;76:263.*

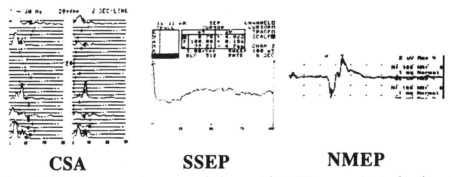

CSA   **SSEP**   **NMEP**

Figure 18.4 The neurogenic-motor evoked potential (NMEP) was maintained in this rat model despite general anesthesia with isoflurane concentrations sufficient to completely eliminate the somatosensory evoked potential (SSEP) waveform and result in burst suppression on the compressed spectral array (CSA).

midazolam. The suppressive effect of propofol and midazolam on TCmag-MEPs is also greater (Figure 18.5). The depressant effects of isoflurane, enflurane, and halothane are marked and similar (Table 18.1). Sevoflurane and desflurane are likely to have similar effects. Although ketamine can increase TCmag-MEP latency and decrease amplitude, reliable recordings can be made. In baboons, amplitude depression occurred after ketamine 15–20 mg/kg; latency delay

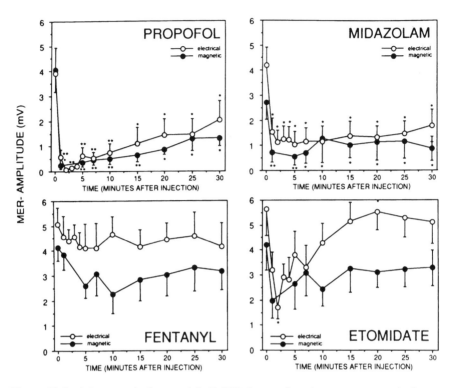

Figure 18.5 Motor evoked potentials (MEP), here referred to as motor-evoked responses or MERS, after transcranial electrical or magnetic stimulation over time. The MEP amplitudes (millivolts, mean ±SEM) are shown after administration of propofol, 2 mg/kg; midazolam, 0.05 mg/kg; fentanyl, 3 μg/kg; or etomidate, 0.3 mg/kg. *Reprinted with permission from CJ Kalkman et al. Effects of propofol, etomidate, midazolam, and fentanyl on motor evoked responses to transcranial electrical or magnetic stimulation in humans. Anesthesiology 1992;76:506.*

required 35–40 mg/kg. Although suppressant effects are present, ketamine is more "TC-MEP friendly" than most other intravenous agents.

Nitrous oxide produces significant amplitude depression at 75 vol% and a dose-dependent prolongation of latency (Figure 18.6). However, this effect is less than that seen with volatile agents, barbiturates, and other agents such as midazolam and propofol. Because of the difficulty involved in recording high-quality TC-MEPs intraoperatively, some anesthesia departments have developed protocols to maximize proficiency (Table 18.2).

While muscle relaxants themselves do not affect cerebral metabolism or synaptic activity, myogenic responses can be affected by neuromuscular blockade. Although good myogenic responses can be obtained with up to 80% blockade, many anesthesiologists avoid neuromuscular blockade if possible. Neuromuscular relaxants do not alter neurogenic potentials.

Table 18.1 Effects of the volatile anesthetic agents halothane, enflurane, and isoflurane on the compound muscle action potential from transcranial electrical stimulation.

Anesthetic	Latency (ms)	Amplitude (mV)	Duration (ms)
Halothane			
0 %	7.2±1.6	349±170	16±4.41
1 %	11.2±1.5	23±16	10±1.3
Enflurane			
0 %	7.3±2	501±219	19±3.7
1 %	10.8±1.7	215±217	12±2.3
Isoflurane			
0 %	10.0±2.5	194±148	17±6.4
1 %	11.2±1.9	103±89	9±2.8

Source: Derived from data in SS Haghighi, R Madsen, KD Green et al. Suppression of motor evoked potentials by inhalation anesthetics. J Neurosurg Anesthesiology 1990;2: 73–70. Latency, amplitude, and duration are given as mean ± standard deviation.

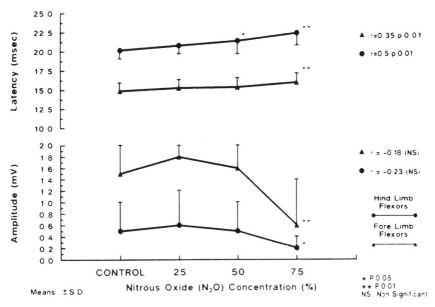

Figure 18.6 A dose-response curve of nitrous oxide (N_2O) on motor evoked potentials from transcranial magnetic stimulation at 1.5 tesla. *Reprinted with permission from RF Ghaly, JL Stone WJ Levy et al. The effect of nitrous oxide on transcranial magnetic-induced eletromyographic responses in the monkey. J Neurosurg Anesthesiol 1990;2:178.*

Table 18.2 An anesthetic protocol developed for intraoperative motor evoked potential recorded with transcranial magnetic stimulation and myogenic recording

Premedication	Avoid if possible or limit to a minimal dose
Induction	Use short-acting agents (i.e., thiopental, 2–4 mg/kg; etomidate, 0.2–0.4 mg/kg, propofol 1.0–2.5 mg/kg, or ketamine, 1–2 mg/kg). Supplemental agents may include alfentanil 0.005–0.02 mg/kg; lidocaine, 0.5–1.0 mg/kg; muscle relaxants (short-acting, i.e., succinylcholine, 1–3 mg/kg, or intermittent-acting, i.e., atracurium 0.4–0.5 mg/kg)
Maintenance	Inhalation agent(s): nitrous oxide ≤50 vol% and/or a volatile agent <0.25 MAC; use injectable agent(s) as a continuous infusion (etomidate, 0.01–0.02 mg/kg/minute; ketamine, 10–30 µg/kg/minute; propofol, 01.–0.2 mg/kg/minute; and alfentanil, 0.02–0.1 µg/kg/minute); constant muscle relaxant to maintain 2–3 twitches in a train of 4 with an atracurium infusion. Corticosteroid coverage will be needed for those administered etomidate infusions
Alternatives	Neuroleptanalgesia with droperidol and fentanyl
Hemodynamic	Use titratable intravenous agents (i.e., maintenance: esmolol, nitroglycerin)

Protocol is derived from a protocol in RF Ghaly, JL Stone, WJ Levy. A protocol for intraoperative somatosensory (SEP) and motor evoked potentials (MEP) recording [letter]. J Neurosurg Anesthesiology 1992;4:69.

Electromyography

Electromyography (EMG) depends on obtaining strong compound muscle action potentials (CMAPs) after nerve stimulation. Because they do not alter axonal transmission, anesthetic agents and sedatives are not significant factors in quality EMG recording. Anesthetic agents reduce artifact and active muscle activity that interferes with quality recording. As stated above, myogenic potentials are eliminated by complete blockade of the neuromuscular junction. Volatile anesthetics can increase neuromuscular blockade at concentrations of more than 1.5 MAC and can potentiate the effect of neuromuscular relaxants. However, good monitoring is possible with partial blockade and maintenance of a single twitch of the train-of-four.

ANESTHETIC AGENTS AND CEREBRAL PROTECTION

Analysis of animal and clinical research reveals that volatile anesthetic agents have shown no cerebral protective benefits, although tolerance to lower blood flow prior to EEG depression is seen with isoflurane. Sevoflurane and desflurane have not been studied. Benzodiazepines can potentiate GABAergic neurotransmission and decrease $CMRO_2$. This may allow neurons to resist incomplete ischemia and hypoxia. Propofol has been given to produce EEG burst suppression during carotid cross-clamping. In cat studies of propofol there is improved recovery of EEG activity, CBF, and ionic homeostasis, but no change in neuronal injury. Although etomidate has been used for cerebral protection (with EEG burst suppression) during temporary clipping of cerebral aneurysms, it has not been well studied.

The barbiturates have been the most extensively evaluated of all anesthetic agents as possible mediators of cerebral protection. As with other agents, no protection from global ischemia is seen. Permanent focal ischemia probably also does not benefit. Barbiturates may have a limited and situation-specific role in the treatment of brain hypoxia. They can be used to decrease refractory increased ICP and control posthypoxic seizures, and they may decrease neuropsychiatric complications of normothermic cardiopulmonary bypass.

KEY REFERENCES

Clark DL, Rosner BS. Neurophysiologic effects of general anesthetics. I. The electroencephalogram and sensory evoked responses in man. Anesthesiology 1973; 38:564. *This paper from more than 20 years ago gives a broad review of the effects of anesthetic agents on neuroelectric activity. Although many of the agents are of historical interest only, the concepts and general effects are unchanged.*

Martin JT, Faulconer A. Jr., Bickford RG. Electroencephalography in anesthesiology. Anesthesiology 1959; 20:359. *An historic and basic review of the effects of general anesthetic states on the EEG.*

McMeniman WJ, Purcell GJ. Neurological monitoring during anaesthesia and surgery. Anaesth Intens Care 1988; 16:358. *This short review gives a concise introduction to neuromonitoring during anesthesia.*

Schwartz DM, Bloom MJ, Pratt RE Jr, Costello JA. Anesthetic effects on neuroelectric events. Semin Hearing 1988; 9:99. *A thorough introduction to "the effects of anesthesia and systemic physiological aspects on the EEG and sensory evoked potentials." This is a broad-based and clinically oriented review.*

RECOMMENDED READING

Ebrahim ZY et al. The effect of propofol on the electroencephalogram of patients with epilepsy. Anesth Analg 1994;78:275.

Kalkman CJ, et al. Effects of propofol, etomidate, midazolam, and fentanyl on motor evoked responses to transcranial electrical or magnetic stimulation in humans. Anesthesiology 1992;76:502. *Propofol and midazolam are found to be more suppressive of motor evoked responses elicited by both magnetic and electrical transcranial stimulation than are fentanyl and etomidate.*

Madler C, et al. Sensory information processing during general anaesthesia: Effect of isoflurane on auditory evoked neuronal oscillations. Br J Anaesth 1991;66:81. *This paper and the one by Thornton et al. (see below) demonstrate that although early, brain stem–generated auditory evoked potentials are not altered by anesthetics. The midlatency components of the BAER do have a dose-dependent suppression, but not to the same degree as somatosensory evoked responses.*

McPherson RW, Sell B, Traystman RJ. Effects of thiopental, fentanyl and etomidate on upper extremity somatosensory evoked potentials in humans. Anesthesiology 1986;65:584. *Demonstrates somatosensory evoked potential amplitude potentiation by etomidate.*

Peterson DO, Drummond JC, Todd MM. Effects of halothane, enflurane, isoflurane and nitrous oxide on somatosensory evoked potentials in humans. Anesthesiology 1986;65:35.

Thornton C, et al. Effects of halothane or enflurane with controlled ventilation on auditory evoked potentials. Br J Anaesth 1984; 56:315.

Zenter J, Albrecht T, Heuser D. Influence of halothane, enflurane and isoflurane on motor evoked potentials. Neurosurgery 1992;31:298.

19

Special Problems in the Operating Room

Lawrence D. Rodichok, M.D.
Mary C. Schwentker, B.S.

The operating room (OR) presents a unique, largely unfamiliar, and at times intimidating environment for most clinical neurophysiology technologists and neurologists-neurophysiologists. And although the OR environment may be familiar to the anesthesiologist, neurophysiologic monitoring is relatively new territory for most. Likewise, surgeons are generally not accustomed to the intraoperative neurophysiologic studies being applied. Development of intraoperative neurophysiologic monitoring programs requires a successful interaction among several disciplines. Such programs succeed only when those involved are willing to learn as much as possible about the components of the system and to adapt to the needs of each person involved. This chapter addresses some issues that are important in the development and evolution of a neurophysiologic monitoring program for the OR.

PERSONNEL
Technologist

In the OR the neurophysiology technologist must be highly skilled and responsible. The studies involved are at least major modifications of those that the individual may have performed in the diagnostic laboratory, and in many cases they are unique to the OR. The OR presents several technical challenges not encountered in the diagnostic lab. In most intraoperative cases there is limited time to apply recording and stimulating electrodes, which must be secure enough to withstand patient movement and a prolonged procedure. There may be very few or no opportunities to modify these electrodes during the procedure. Leads must be routed around a variety of obstacles and secured so that they cannot be dislodged. Care must be taken that they do not come close to sources of electrical interference, such as heating blankets and fluid pumps. The recording instruments must be placed in a location that does not interfere with surgery (we prefer to be near the anesthesiologist). The technologist must be aware of other leads, tubing, and attachments, such as arterial lines, that are necessary to others caring for the patient. These may require modification of the usual setup, such as stimulating the ulnar nerve at the elbow if the median nerve is not accessible because of the presence of an arterial catheter.

The technologist must be prepared to tailor the study or studies planned to the clinical situation and the habits of the surgeon. Sometimes these decisions must be made on the spot. The technologist must therefore have a thorough working knowledge of the field to function well in the OR setting. During the procedure itself the technologist is required to interact with the anesthesiologist and the surgeon as well as the neurophysiologist, providing feedback on the neurophysiologic data. In the routine neurophysiology laboratory the technologist has been taught that he or she should not provide interpretation of a study to anyone. This is the responsibility of the neurologist or neurophysiologist. Although we feel that online supervision and interpretation by a qualified neurophysiologist are mandatory, the technologist will nevertheless be called on to provide much more interpretation than is customary in the neurophysiology lab.

Anesthesiologist

The anesthesiologist should be familiar with the factors within his or her purview that may influence the electroencephalograph (EEG) or evoked potentials being monitored. These include, but are not limited to, (1) choice of anesthetic, (2) systemic blood pressure, (3) body temperature, (4) hypercapnia or hypocapnia, and (5) neuromuscular blockade. A working knowledge of the various neurophysiologic studies is preferable and in some cases necessary. Effective communication between the technologist and anesthesiologist is very important. In many situations the first issue to be addressed if there is a change in the EEG or evoked response is whether a change in anesthetic technique or the patient's systemic parameters might be the cause.

Surgeon

The surgeon should understand the nature and purpose of the study being done. He or she needs to be aware of some of the technical aspects of the study so as not to have unrealistic expectations. For example, he or she needs to be aware of the effect of the Bovie or pneumatic drill on any neurophysiologic study. Also, the surgeon is often not aware of the time required to see EEG changes or to generate a reproducible average. In some studies, such as motor evoked potentials, the surgeon plays an active role in performing the study.

Neurophysiologist

A qualified neurophysiologist must be directly responsible for the studies being performed. This may be a properly trained anesthesiologist, neurologist, or nonphysician neurophysiologist. This individual must provide on-line supervision either in the OR or through a remote telemetry system that allows real-time transmission of the waveforms from the OR. In our institution this person is either in the OR or within the hospital at a remote monitoring site and capable of being in the OR within minutes. In many cases the neurophysiologist must be present during portions or the entirety of a case to properly direct and interpret the study.

TECHNICAL STANDARDS

We have found it useful to attempt to adhere to the usual technical standards for EEG and evoked potential monitoring as set by the American EEG Society for diagnostic studies. The society has also published standards for intraoperative monitoring. The latter are in very general terms at this time. Many of the techniques used in diagnostic testing must be modified for OR use, including electrode placements and filters. It is important that each center performing intraoperative monitoring have written guidelines for performing these studies. The performance and safety of all instruments used in the OR should be checked frequently and documented in a permanent record. In some cases each center needs to establish normative data for itself. Absolute latencies are of lesser value in the OR. Changes from baseline are critical. Each center must establish what it considers to be acceptable variability in amplitude, latency, or both in comparison to the preincision baseline that are compatible with a normal outcome. Those that fall outside that norm should be brought to the attention of the surgeon. Fortunately, it has been uncommon that a patient awakens with a new deficit. This has, however, made it difficult to establish rigid guidelines for evoked potentials in the OR.

INTERFERENCE

The diagnostic laboratory is usually specifically designed to minimize electrical interference. However, most ORs are not so designed, and even shielding does not eliminate artifacts due to instruments within the room. In general, sources of interference are of either physiologic or nonphysiologic origin.

Nonphysiologic Interference

The most common nonphysiologic types of artifact in the OR are:

1. The Bovie coagulator
2. Heating devices (blood warmer, heating blanket)
3. Operating microscopes
4. X-ray view boxes
5. X-ray devices, such as a C-arm
6. The operating table itself
7. Metal placed on or near the patient, such as spinal instrumentation or metal head holders

Each of these items may produce or amplify 60-Hz as well as slower-frequency interference. The interference can persist even when the instrument is not being used. It can only be eliminated by unplugging the offending instrument. Swaying of the leads or the jack box caused by movements of operative personnel can cause slower-frequency artifact. It is for this reason, among others, that the leads should be braided and the jack box secured in place.

For the most part, physiologic sources of interference are a much smaller problem in the OR than in the diagnostic lab. Electromyography interference is usually eliminated by neuromuscular blockade. Eye movements are not usually present in an anesthetized patient. Electrocardiogram artifact in the EEG may still be a problem.

Physiologic Interference

A number of physiologic variables are pertinent in the OR setting that are generally not important in the diagnostic laboratory. Most general anesthetics have some effect on EEG and evoked potentials. The same is true of most other agents acting on the central nervous system or affecting the blood pressure, temperature, oxygenation, or ventilation ($PaCO_2$). In general, both anesthetics and alterations in systemic variables have a much greater influence on potentials of cortical origin, including EEG, than those of subcortical origin. In fact it is unwise to be totally dependent on near-field cortical potentials to guide a case since it may become necessary to use levels of these agents that inevitably eliminate evoked potentials of purely cortical origin.

KEY REFERENCES

American EEG Society. Guidelines in electroencephalography, evoked potentials and polysomnography. J Clin Neurophysiol 1994;11(1):1. *Although the standards for diagnostic EEG and evoked potentials must be modified in the OR setting, they do serve as a useful starting point. Standards for the OR are in general terms but should be followed.*

20

Assessing and Responding to Detected Abnormalities During Intraoperative Neurophysiologic Monitoring

Gregory C. Allen, M.D., FRCPC

Before discussing specific scenarios where neurophysiologic monitoring is applied, some principles behind diagnostic testing must be noted. These may influence the results obtained from neurophysiologic monitoring as well as their interpretation. Diagnostic tests have certain stable properties that are independent of the prevalence or frequency of the abnormality to be detected. A test's *sensitivity* is the proportion of affected patients the test correctly identifies. An insensitive test gives a high false-negative result, which is disastrous for a monitored patient whose neurologic injury goes undetected.

A test's *specificity* refers to the proportion of unaffected patients correctly identified by the test. A nonspecific test leads to a high false-positive rate, with overcalling of potential injury. It is difficult to accurately calculate the specificity of monitoring, since adverse changes usually are acted on, sometimes with improvement, and the patient awakens neurologically intact. One cannot determine if the monitoring gave a true positive result, which led to the correction of a problem, or if the result was falsely positive and was unrelated to potential damage.

Other factors, such as technical considerations and anesthetic technique, can also affect the sensitivity and specificity of neurophysiologic monitoring. These factors affect the conditions under which a given patient is tested. However, when identical conditions are used, test sensitivity and specificity are independent of the prevalence of the abnormality detected.

Prevalence, or pretest probability of an abnormality, affects the predictive value of a test. Even a test with high sensitivity and specificity has low positive predictive value when disease prevalence is low. Predictive value is usually highest when prevalence is around 50%. When prevalence is lower—for example 1–3% risk of paraplegia—positive predictive value falls significantly. As prevalence decreases, negative predictive value rises, so that if changes are not detected, there is a very high probability that no neurologic injury has occurred. Here lies the greatest utility for neurophysiologic monitoring.

The reader should refer to the recommended readings for references on diagnostic test properties, the concept of the normal reference range, and the predictive value of tests.

NEUROPHYSIOLOGIC MONITORING: PRACTICAL PRINCIPLES

The following are some general principles that apply to neurophysiologic monitoring. Some of these principles seem obvious, but they are very important when determining the utility and limitations of these monitoring techniques.

1.   Monitors can assess only specific neurologic pathways, assuming they are intact. A pathway with a preoperative deficit may be difficult to monitor at best. For example, the electroencephalograph (EEG) does not assess the brain stem; a previous stroke may make the baseline preoperative EEG abnormal.

2.   Monitoring is "high-tech," so factitious changes can have multiple causes. These may be as simple as a displaced electrode or a disconnected wire.

3.   Monitoring tends to be oversensitive in an attempt to avoid false-negative results, and the changes noted may be nonspecific. There is uncertainty as to how much of a change is abnormal. For example, how much of an increase in latency is accepted before notifying the surgeon? Or is the rate of increase more significant?

4.   The brain stem and spinal cord are more resistant than the cerebral cortex to the effects of ischemia.

5.   The brain stem and spinal cord are more resistant to the effects of anesthetics than the cerebral cortex.

6.   Adverse neurologic outcome may not occur during the time of monitoring. The injury may occur after monitoring is discontinued; for example, a patient may have a stroke after carotid endarterectomy. Or there may be a time delay between the injury and a change detected by the monitor, as may occur with spinal cord injury and somatosensory evoked potentials (SSEPs).

7.   Monitors detect the effects of ischemia—that is, lack of oxygen delivery. Oxygen delivery depends on tissue perfusion (flow rather than pressure) and the oxygen content of the blood. Oxygen content depends in turn on hemoglobin content and oxygen saturation. This principle is the foundation for detecting the etiology of ischemia.

8.   Always consider the prevalence of the adverse outcome for which monitoring is being performed. In one study, for example, the prevalence of stroke after carotid endarterectomy was 9%; the positive predictive value of EEG monitoring was only 44%. However, most strokes occurred postoperatively, meaning that the prevalence of intraoperative stroke was much lower than 9%. Therefore, the positive predictive value of intraoperative EEG monitoring was approximately 7%.

CLINICAL SCENARIOS: MONITORING APPLICATIONS AND RESPONSES TO CHANGES
A 55-Year-Old Man for Acoustic Neuroma Resection

Patients with acoustic neuroma may present with hearing loss, headaches, unsteady gait, or tinnitus. As the tumor grows out of the internal auditory meatus into the posterior fossa, it may compress the facial or trigeminal nerve or the brain stem itself, producing hydrocephalus. Surgery may be performed to prevent further hearing loss or to decompress structures within the posterior fossa.

Indications for and Types of Monitoring

Neurophysiologic monitoring is performed during acoustic neuroma resection for the following reasons: (1) to prevent brain stem ischemia; (2) to preserve hearing, if still present; and (3) to prevent facial nerve injury leading to facial paralysis. Two modalities are used to monitor the acoustic (VIII) and facial (VII) nerve. The first is brain stem auditory evoked potentials (BAEPs), which monitor a very specific brain stem pathway and are very sensitive to ischemia. BAEPs do not monitor the cerebral cortex. Stimulation for BAEPs may be bilateral but independent if hearing is present in both ears, or contralateral to the lesion if the patient is already deaf on the ipsilateral side.

Facial nerves are monitored by monitoring myogenic responses through electromyography (EMG) in the muscles of facial expression, such as the orbicularis oculi. The surgeon uses a monopolar stimulating probe to identify the facial nerve in the surgical field. If it has been compressed, certain abnormal responses (autoexcitation, lateral spread response) are present; these abnormalities disappear with adequate facial nerve decompression.

Brain Stem Auditory Evoked Potentials

BAEPs are usually simple to record and interpret. They are not significantly affected by anesthetic agents, muscle relaxants, or mild hypothermia. Transient changes may be seen with hypotension or hypocarbia, but the majority of persistent or severe changes are due to surgical factors such as excessive retraction pressure, which alert the surgeon to the potential for neurologic injury. On the other hand, lack of significant BAEP changes allows surgeons to be more aggressive in their retraction and dissection and to resect as much of the tumor as possible.

Loss of ipsilateral waves I, V, or both is approximately 80% predictive of postoperative hearing loss. The surgeon may limit tumor resection to preserve hearing when transient EP changes begin to occur. If both ipsilateral waves I and V are intact at the end of surgery, the patient's hearing should be preserved (negative predictive value 95%).

Some BAEP changes are more serious (Table 20.1). Ipsilateral loss of waves III–V or bilateral or contralateral loss of evoked potentials (EPs) predicts severe neurologic injury. Loss of contralateral EPs appears relatively specific for

Table 20.1 Correlation Between Brain Stem Auditory
Evoked Potential (BAEP) Changes and Associated Clinical Events

BAEP Change	Associated Events
Transient latency increase	Drilling, irrigation, retraction, surgical irritation, hypocarbia and hypotension, positioning
Persistent latency increases	Retraction or pressure on auditory tract
Transient loss of EP	Retraction, pressure, surgical distention
Permanent loss of ipsilateral EP	Surgical interruption of auditory pathway
Loss of contralateral EP	Cerebellar edema

EP = evoked potential.
Source: Modified with permission from RD Miller (ed). Anesthesia (4th ed). New York: Churchill
Livingstone, 1994;1:333.

cerebellar edema; this potential EP change is the main reason for performing contralateral EPs in the presence of preoperative ipsilateral deafness.

Facial Nerve Monitoring

Facial nerve monitoring has not been assessed in any rigorous, controlled trial. As one source describes, surgeons are so convinced of its efficacy, based on their own experience, that it is virtually a standard of care for acoustic neuroma resection. Some outcome data suggest that monitored patients are less likely to have long-term facial weakness, but the number of patients in these studies is small.

Responding to Changes

How should one respond to changes in neurophysiologic function during acoustic neuroma resection? The anesthesiologist should provide a stable plane of anesthesia during times when monitoring is most important—that is, during approach to the tumor and tumor resection. One should react to significant BAEP changes by ruling out the various etiologies for ischemia (hypoperfusion, hypoxemia, anemia, severe hypocarbia) and take steps to correct any abnormalities detected. Evidence of prolonged brain stem retraction or cerebellar edema should be a warning not to extubate the trachea at the end of surgery. Further swelling may occur postoperatively, leading to airway obstruction, apnea, or cardiac arrest. Postoperative therapy with hyperventilation, diuretics, and steroids may be necessary.

The anesthetic management for facial nerve monitoring is similar to other procedures where EMG is used. Little or no neuromuscular blockade can be present for facial nerve EMG to be useful. The benefit to the patient of partial paralysis, using a muscle relaxant infusion, must be weighed against the risk of a false-negative response to facial nerve stimulation, with accidental damage or sectioning of the facial nerve.

Potent anesthetic agents, such as isoflurane, provide some muscle relaxation and do not significantly affect BAEPs or facial nerve EMG responses. However, some patients may not tolerate higher concentrations of potent anesthetic agents. For example, if a patient repeatedly became hypotensive with higher concentrations of isoflurane, or if isoflurane were contraindicated, as in malignant hyperthermia, how would one anesthetize the patient? How likely is it that the patient might become too light and move during the tumor resection, with the head secured by Mayfield headpins? Each choice has a measurable risk to the patient, and one must decide whether to use muscle relaxants on an individual basis.

Some centers use muscle relaxant infusions during facial nerve EMG monitoring. By using an endpoint of 2–3 twitches with train-of-four stimulation, accurate and reliable facial EMGs have been obtained, with no adverse patient outcomes. By using shorter-acting muscle relaxants, such as atracurium, the degree of neuromuscular blockade can be changed within minutes if there is any doubt about the facial EMG response.

A 5-Year-Old Boy for Tethered Cord Release

Tethered spinal cord syndrome may lead to progressive muscle weakness, gait disturbance, and sphincter dysfunction. Tethered cord release preserves or improves neurologic function by eliminating tightness of the spinal cord, cauda equina, and spinal nerves tethered by anomalous tissue. The goal of neurophysiologic monitoring is to prevent inadvertent damage by identifying nerve roots lying within the tissue being cut for cord release.

Monitoring Methods

In the past, surgeons have used nerve stimulators during cauda equina surgery and simply observed or palpated the leg muscles to detect a response to tissue stimulation. This method is insensitive and led to iatrogenic nerve injury. A more sensitive method is to use EMG to detect the response to stimulation in the operative field.

The advantage of EMG monitoring is its large-amplitude recordings that are easily understood. Neurotonic discharges warn that a nerve is within the operative field. Deliberate stimulation of neural tissues generates a compound action potential that will elicit a myogenic response. By performing multichannel recording—that is, three or four different muscle groups—all lumbosacral nerve roots can be monitored. Muscle groups that are commonly monitored include the quadriceps, tibialis anterior, hamstrings, gastrocnemius, and external anal sphincter.

Electromyography and Anesthesia

Anesthetic management during EMG monitoring for tethered cord release is straightforward. The neuromuscular junction must be relatively intact to allow myogenic responses to nerve stimulation. Therefore, no or only partial neuromuscular blockade is allowable during monitoring. The simplest plan is simply to avoid the use of muscle relaxants or use a short-acting relaxant for tracheal intubation. All patients who have received muscle relaxants should be checked to ensure they have recovered adequately for reliable EMG monitoring to be performed. If there is a clear benefit, a relaxant infusion technique with repetitive testing of the level of blockade is the most appropriate course.

Potent agents often can provide adequate clinical relaxation on their own, without interfering with EMG monitoring. Very deep inhalational anesthesia can reduce neuromuscular transmission slightly and may affect the response to tetanus or train-of-four stimulation.

During the procedure, if the surgeon is stimulating a structure he or she is certain is neural tissue and no myogenic response is recorded, technical factors related to both the stimulation and recording technique should be ruled out. The level of neuromuscular blockade should be checked, and if an infusion of muscle relaxant is being used, the infusion should be discontinued. Since the surgeon will not cut the tissues until certain they are not nerve roots, he or she can either wait to allow the patient to recover spontaneously or administer a reversal agent to achieve the desired level of neuromuscular blockade. If deep inhalational anesthesia is being used, the depth of anesthesia should be decreased to rule it out as a cause of the negative response.

Clinical Utility

The published experience with EMG monitoring for tethered cord surgery is limited. Case series have documented the utility of the technique, guiding surgeons in what tissues to preserve or cut, with favorable neurologic outcomes. The potential for injury during this procedure is high. The sensitivity and specificity of EMG monitoring appear to be quite acceptable. Therefore, the predictive value of monitoring should be quite high and clinically valuable.

A 65-Year-Old Woman for Clipping of a Middle Cerebral Artery Aneurysm

Cerebral aneurysm clipping is performed to prevent rebleeding following subarachnoid hemorrhage. Rebleeding is a major cause of morbidity and mortality in patients who survive the initial hemorrhage. Occasionally, aneurysm clipping is performed after an asymptomatic aneurysm is discovered (Figure 20.1).

Indications for Monitoring

Neurophysiologic monitoring is used during cerebral aneurysm clipping to detect ischemia during temporary clipping or induced hypotension, to decide if permanent vessel occlusion is feasible, to detect accidental vessel occlusion, and in the management of giant or multilobed aneurysms. It is questionable whether monitoring is helpful in the management of uncomplicated, small cerebral aneurysms.

Monitoring Used

The monitoring modality most often used in aneurysm clipping is SSEPs, with bilateral median nerve stimulation. This is adequate for most supratentori-

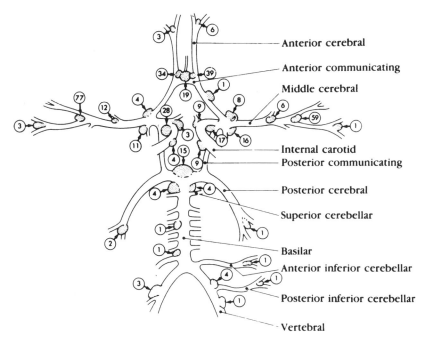

Figure 20.1 The location of 407 aneurysms in 300 consecutive patients classified by size and location. The numbers inside the circles reflect aneurysm indidence. *Reproduced with permission from SJ Peerless. Intracranial Aneurysms. In SP Newfield, JE Cottrell (eds), Neuroanesthesia Handbook in Clinical and Physiologic Essentials. Boston: Little, Brown, 1991.*

al aneurysms, except those of the anterior circulation, which require bilateral posterior tibial nerve stimulation. Aneurysms in the posterior fossa are monitored with both SSEPs and BAEPs, in an attempt to monitor a larger portion of the brain stem.

Besides measuring changes in latency and amplitude of cortical waveforms, SSEPs are used to detect increases in central conduction time (CCT). With median nerve stimulation, CCT is the difference in latency between the cervical waveform (N13) and the cortical waveform (N20). Some centers have determined normal reference ranges for CCT; a CCT more than 2.5 standard deviations above the mean is considered abnormal. Other centers consider a 1-ms increase in CCT as abnormal. With posterior tibial nerve stimulation, CCT can be determined by measuring the difference in latency between the lumbar root entry zone potential and the P37. However, the lumbar potential is not easily detected intraoperatively. The difference in latency between N34 and P37 can be employed. Generally, a significantly increased CCT, a decreased cortical waveform amplitude of 50% or greater, or disappearance of the EP are considered predictive of postoperative motor or sensory deficit.

Clinical Utility

In one study of internal carotid (ICA) and middle cerebral artery (MCA) aneurysms, SSEPs had a positive predictive value of 75% for detecting ischemia. Other centers have reported much lower values (19%) when all locations of aneurysms were considered. However, negative predictive values of 90% or more suggest that monitoring can provide evidence that no neurologic damage is developing. Monitoring for posterior circulation aneurysms is less reassuring, especially in the distribution of the basilar artery apex. In general, SSEP and BAEP monitoring may be predictive only 35–50% of the time, but they are considered unreliable at the basilar apex, and lack of change provides no reassurance to the surgeon. Monitoring may be unreliable for several reasons: (1) ischemia develops outside the monitored neurologic pathway, (2) collateral blood flow and general anesthesia produce protective effects, or (3) the diagnostic cutoff point is too high. In addition, if the neurologic deficit is not sensory or motor, as in the case of dysphasia or memory loss, then it will not be detected by neurophysiologic monitoring.

In the case of an MCA aneurysm, stable SSEPs allow the surgeon to work without urgency. The duration of temporary clipping can be extended, or the surgeon can consider intentional permanent occlusion of a vessel. In the case of a giant ICA aneurysm, the surgeon may choose to apply a ring clip. Thus, stable SSEP signals have a major effect on surgical management. The surgeon may use SSEP monitoring to guide the degree of tissue or vessel retraction that is tolerated during aneurysm dissection.

What if significant changes occur during aneurysm surgery? The surgeon now must work expediently, essentially as if he or she were working without neurophysiologic monitoring. It is important to remember that the false-positive rate for monitoring in aneurysm surgery is quite high, and many of the changes seen will be factitious. However, one must assume that the changes are real, seek a cause, and correct it. The surgeon may choose to readjust a clip, perform an extracranial-intracranial bypass, or even abandon the procedure.

How does the anesthesiologist respond to SSEP changes? The possible effects of anesthetic agents must always be considered. Preventive measures can be taken during the procedure, such as mild hypothermia, use of mannitol or spinal drainage to slacken the brain, or induced hypertension during temporary clipping. If changes do occur, adequate oxygenation and ventilation must be confirmed. Hypocarbia can decrease cerebral blood flow and may need to be reversed. Next, cerebral blood flow can be increased by volume expansion, hemodilution, and raising blood pressure and cardiac output. Finally, cerebral "protection" can be attempted with agents such as mannitol, nimodipine, lidocaine, barbiturates, or isoflurane. Some of those agents may cause the loss of SSEP signals and preclude further monitoring.

A good example of the utility of monitoring is during accidental aneurysm rupture. There is immediate loss of SSEP signals. The anesthesiologist induces hypotension and simultaneously expands the circulating blood volume, allowing the surgeon to see the operative field. The surgeon then places a temporary clip under direct vision, controls the bleeding, and releases the retractors. The anesthesiologist raises the blood pressure and the SSEP signal reappears. After a period of observation with stable SSEPs, the surgeon repositions the retractors and places a permanent clip on the aneurysm. The SSEPs remain unchanged and the patient awakens with no new neurologic deficit.

It is imperative that the anesthesiologist and surgeon stay in verbal contact throughout the dissection and clipping. The progress of the surgery also can be observed on a television monitor connected to the operating microscope. By maintaining visual contact with the operative field, the anesthesiologist can follow the surgeon's work when the surgeon must concentrate. If the aneurysm accidentally ruptures, the anesthesiologist can respond instantly, providing the surgeon with a bloodless field, allowing the surgeon to obtain hemostasis.

A 14-Year-Old Girl with Idiopathic Scoliosis for Posterior Spinal Instrumentation

Idiopathic scoliosis is managed surgically with posterior spinal fusion and instrumentation. The surgery attempts to halt the progress of spinal curvatures before significant cardiopulmonary dysfunction occurs. However, the surgical procedure itself is associated with a 1–3% risk of paraplegia, which is usually permanent. Neurophysiologic monitoring is used to reduce the risk of this complication.

Stagnara Wake-Up Test

First reported in 1973, the Stagnara wake-up test is still used to assess motor function during spinal surgery. It is a gross test of function, usually performed only once at the time of maximal distraction of the spine. No patient with a normal wake-up test has awakened with paraplegia.*

It may not always be possible to perform a wake-up test. The patient may be uncooperative (too young or developmentally delayed) or the procedure may preclude its use (as with an anterior spinal approach via thoracotomy). In addition, the wake-up test is not without risks, such as accidental extubation, venous air embolism, eye injuries, dislocation of the instrumentation, patient recall, or loss of vascular access.

Somatosensory Evoked Potentials

Because of the risks and limited utility of the wake-up test, more sophisticated monitoring techniques are used. The first technique advocated was monitoring of SSEPs, which allows repetitive testing of dorsal column function throughout the surgical procedure, not just at a single point in time. At the same time, spinal instrumentation systems have become more complex, with new

---

*One patient who had a normal intraoperative wake-up test has been reported to have awakened with an isolated dorsal column injury. Loss of proprioception resulted in severe gait impairment.

periods of increased risk identified, such as at sublaminar wiring. In 1991, 78% of the members of the Scoliosis Research Society (SRS) used SSEPs; 74% of that group also used the Stagnara wake-up test.

Although SSEP monitoring has reduced the risk of paraplegia in scoliosis surgery, case reports have appeared where SSEPs did not predict postoperative paraplegia. In the SRS survey, the sensitivity of SSEP monitoring was 87%, but its positive predictive value was only 39%. The prevalence of a major neurologic deficit was 1.2%. This result is not surprising, since SSEPs do not directly monitor the motor pathway or changes in anterior cord blood supply. Instead, SSEPs are considered to be a measure of overall spinal cord integrity.

The utility of SSEPs has been improved by use of subcortical recording electrodes (epidural, cervical, mastoids). General anesthesia attenuates the cortical responses, especially in patients with cortical disease such as cerebral palsy. Subcortical structures are more resistant to anesthetic agents. In one study of 1,168 patients, epidural recording increased the sensitivity of SSEP monitoring to 100%, but the positive predictive value was still only 38%. This was due to the relatively high number of false-positive responses, as well as the low prevalence of neurologic injury. There were no cases of paraplegia, but the incidence of motor deficit was 2.7%.

Motor Evoked Potentials

Because of the poor predictive value of SSEPs and the technical problems related to the wake-up test, attention has turned to monitoring the motor pathway directly. Motor-evoked potential (MEP) monitoring involves stimulation of the motor pathway (either cerebral cortex or spinal cord) and recording the neurogenic or myogenic response at a point caudal to the spinal instrumentation. Early reports have suggested MEPs are more specific than SSEPs and very sensitive for detecting motor deficits.

Stimulation for MEPs may be through the cerebral cortex, using transcranial electric or magnetic methods, or by direct electric spinal cord stimulation. Direct spinal cord stimulation bypasses cortical synaptic transmission, which may be attenuated by anesthetic agents and avoids the potential complications of transcranial stimulation, such as seizures and tissue burns. Responses to stimulation for MEPs are detected as neurogenic potentials over the sciatic nerve in the popliteal fossa, or as myogenic potentials from tibialis anterior electromyographic responses. Myogenic responses require minimal or no neuromuscular blockade, whereas profound neuromuscular relaxation allows low-amplitude NMEPs to be visualized by eliminating muscle artifact.

Responding to Changes in Somatosensory Evoked Potentials or Motor Evoked Potentials

How should one respond to significant changes in SSEP or MEP recordings? Both the surgeon and anesthesiologist must be notified, so both can review what has been done that might account for the changes (Table 20.2). Since changes in SSEPs may reflect an injury that occurred several minutes before,

Table 20.2 Scoliosis Surgery and Spinal Cord Monitoring

Monitoring options and changes seen	1. Stagnara wake-up test—inability to move one or both feet
	2. SSEPs—decreased amplitude, increased latency, loss of waveform
	3. MEPs— loss of neurogenic or myogenic response
Possible etiologies	Spinal cord ischemia, hypoxemia, hypoperfusion, hypothermia, hypocarbia, anesthetic agents, muscle relaxants, anemia
Times of increased risk	Spinal distraction, sublaminar wiring, during induced hypotension, inadvertent cord compression, trauma, use of certain instrumentations (e.g., Luque rods, Cotrel-Dubousset system), ligation of segmental arteries
Patient risk factors	Kyphosis, congenital or neuromuscular scoliosis, pre-existent neurologic deficit, preoperative use of spinal traction
Management options	Reduce spinal distraction; explore for cord compression; remove spinal instrumentation; remove test clamp on segmental artery; rule out hypoxemia, hypocarbia, hypothermia; raise blood pressure, discontinue induced hypotension, transfuse red cells (autologous, if available) to Hct ≥ 30

more than immediate activities should be considered as possible etiologies. The anesthesiologist must focus on treatable causes of spinal cord ischemia and on possible drug effects. Hypoxemia, hypotension, hypoperfusion, and anemia are serious problems that must be ruled out or treated. An appropriate response might be to confirm adequate ventilation, switch to 100% oxygen, reverse induced hypotension, and send blood samples for arterial blood gas and hemoglobin determination. If autologous blood is available, transfusion to a hematocrit of at least 30 may be a valuable intervention.

At this point, many surgeons would request an immediate Stagnara wake-up test to confirm the electrophysiologic changes warning of spinal cord ischemia. The anesthetic technique used must be reversible enough to allow this. At the beginning of surgery, the surgeon may have informed the anesthetic care team of his or her desire to do a planned wake-up test. With the increasing use of evoked potential monitoring, many surgeons will not do a wake-up test if the monitoring has been stable during the procedure. However, one should expect the need for an unplanned wake-up test in every case, especially in patients who are considered at high risk for spinal cord injury or who are undergoing higher risk instrumentations, such as the Cotrel-Dubousset system.

Injury can occur to the anterior or posterior spinal cord, or both, and SSEPs and MEPs monitor the two distinctly different pathways—that is, they complement each other. It is now recommended that both modalities be used when spinal cord function may be at risk. With more experience, such multimodal techniques may completely replace the use of the wake-up test, with its attendant risks.

A 72-Year-Old Man with Amaurosis Fugax for Carotid Endarterectomy

Carotid endarterectomy (CEA) is performed to prevent future strokes in high-risk patients. A major concern during CEA is adequacy of cerebral perfusion during carotid artery cross-clamp. The primary reason for neurophysiologic monitoring during CEA is to assess cerebral perfusion and to allow the surgeon to make an informed decision as to whether a surgical shunt is needed. Some surgeons either never or always use a shunt during CEA; in such cases monitoring may not influence surgical technique.

A minority of strokes occur because of inadequate cerebral perfusion after carotid clamping. Most strokes occur postoperatively and are embolic in origin. Intraoperative neurophysiologic monitoring will not have any influence on these strokes; there is little evidence that monitoring affects postoperative outcome. Studies of the benefits of shunting have shown no difference in outcome whether a shunt was used or not, or whether use was selective or nonselective, even in the presence of "major" EEG abnormalities. Meticulous surgical technique may be far more important. In the North American Symptomatic Carotid Endarterectomy Trial, surgeons were eligible to participate if their perioperative stroke rates were less than 6%; the use of shunts or neurophysiologic monitoring was not an entry criterion.

Cerebral Monitoring During Carotid Endarterectomy

What other indications are there for monitoring during CEA? Cerebral ischemia may be detected during other "at-risk" periods, such as neck hyperextension and rotation during positioning, tissue dissection, or during times of "relative" hypotension. For example, a patient with a high-grade carotid stenosis and contralateral carotid occlusion may require a high mean arterial pressure for adequate cerebral perfusion. Any drop in blood pressure may be deleterious. Monitoring has been advocated for detecting problems with shunts, such as thrombosis or kinking. It is also essential for inducing burst suppression or electric silence with barbiturates, providing a therapeutic endpoint.

Carotid Endartectomy During Regional Anesthesia

Some surgeons perform CEA under regional anesthesia, with the patient lightly sedated. Serial neurologic examinations are used to monitor the patient. This is relatively continuous and tests bilateral cerebral function. After carotid clamping, up to 10% of patients develop slurred speech or decreased grip strength; occasionally, loss of consciousness or seizures may occur. The neurologic deficit usually clears after a shunt is placed; in some cases, the blood pressure must be raised to reverse the deficit. Excessive sedation prevents adequate assessment of the patient. The anesthesiologist must also be prepared to manage serious complications, such as seizures or loss of the patient's airway. Both the patient and the surgeon must be comfortable with this technique. It is most frequently the surgeon who requests regional anesthesia for CEA.

Table 20.3 EEG Changes Associated with Anesthetic Drugs, PaO_2, $PaCO_2$ and Temperature

Increased frequency
    Barbiturates (low dose)
    Benzodiazepines (low dose)
    Etomidate (low dose)
    N_2O (30–70%)
    Inhalation agents (<1 MAC)
    Ketamine
    Hypoxia (initially)
    Hypercarbia (mild)
    Seizures
Decreased frequency/increased amplitude
    Barbiturates (moderate dose)
    Etomidate (moderate dose)
    Opioids
    Inhalation agents (>1 MAC)
    Hypoxia (mild)
    Hypocarbia (moderate to extreme)
    Hypothermia
Decreased frequency/decreased amplitude
    Barbiturates (high dose)
    Hypoxia (mild)
    Hypercarbia (severe)
    Hypothermia (<35°C)
Electric silence
    Barbiturates (coma dose)
    Etomidate (high dose)
    Isoflurane (2 MAC)
    Hypoxia (severe)
    Hypothermia (<15–20°C)
    Brain death

Source: Modified with permission from PG Barash. Clinical Anesthesia (2nd ed). Philadelphia: Lippincott, 1992;882.

Does serial clinical examination of the awake patient during CEA improve outcome? It seems implicit that it should, but there are no clinical trials to support that conclusion. There is good evidence that intraoperative neurologic changes identify patients who are at high risk for developing a postoperative stroke. These patients may benefit from antithrombotic therapy, intensive care admission, or early surgical reexploration.

Carotid Endartectomy and General Anesthesia

Most CEAs in North America are performed under general anesthesia. The airway and ventilation are controlled, and hemodynamic stability is maintained. If selective shunting is practiced, the surgeon requires some measure of the adequacy of cerebral perfusion, such as EEG monitoring. EEG monitoring is contin-

Table 20.4 Carotid Endarterectomy and Cortical Monitoring

Monitoring options	1. Neurologic exam/awake patient
	2. EEG, SSEPs, decreased amplitudes
Changes seen	1. Slurred speech, aphasia, focal weakness, loss of consciousness, seizures
	2. Increased latency, unilateral or bilateral EEG slowing
Possible etiologies	Hypoxemia, hypocarbia, hypothermia, anesthetic agents, metabolic changes, hypoperfusion, hyperperfusion (post-CEA)
Times of increased risk	Head positioning, tissue dissection, shunt placement/presence, complications-intimal dissection, "relative" hypotension on induction, carotid clamping, embolization, thrombosis, hemorrhage
Risk factors	Abnormal baseline EEG (e.g., previous stroke), contralateral carotid occlusion, diffuse intracerebral atherosclerosis, superimposed vertebrobasilar symptoms, poor collateral flow by cerebral angiography, cross-clamp times >30 min
Management options	Adjust head position, adjust retractors, unclamp artery, place shunt, adjust shunt, rule out hypoxemia, maintain normocarbia, raise blood pressure, check activated clotting time, administer heparin

uous, but assesses only the cerebral cortex. It is very sensitive to physiologic changes and to the effects of anesthetic agents (Table 20.3). A stable level of anesthesia is required for reliable EEG monitoring.

Carotid Endartectomy and Electroencephalography

How effective is the EEG as a monitor during CEA? Up to 20–40% of patients develop EEG changes after carotid clamping, but most do not awaken with a neurologic deficit. There is a correlation between regional cerebral blood flow and EEG changes during cross-clamping. In one study, 31% of patients developed EEG changes with carotid clamping; no intervention or shunting was performed. The postoperative stroke rate was 1%. The sensitivity of EEG monitoring for CEA was 70–90%, with a specificity of 75–90%. When the prevalence of postoperative stroke is 1% or less, the positive predictive value of EEG monitoring can be as low as 40%.

EEG monitoring is frequently used during CEA. Therefore, in the operating room, one must have a plan to respond appropriately to EEG changes with carotid clamping (Table 20.4). Should ipsilateral EEG slowing occur, the surgeon will probably place a shunt. The anesthesiologist should rule out hypoxemia and hypo- or hypercarbia and avoid significant changes in anesthetic depth at the time of vessel clamping. The activated clotting time also should be checked to confirm adequate anticoagulation. It may be helpful to lighten the anesthetic or to administer a vasopressor, such as phenylephrine, to increase blood pressure, in an attempt to increase cerebral perfusion.

If significant bilateral slowing occurs with carotid clamping, it implies that global cerebral perfusion has been compromised and that shunting with induced hypertension will be required. It may also be an indication for inducing EEG burst suppression for cerebral protection. Severe hypoxemia or hypotension may also cause bilateral slowing and must be ruled out. Bolus administration of intravenous anesthetic agents or an increase in volatile anesthetic concentration can also induce bilateral slowing and lead to inappropriate therapeutic decisions. The anesthesiologist must maintain communication with the surgeon, follow the progress of the procedure closely, and avoid making decisions in isolation.

KEY REFERENCES

Forbes HJ et al. Spinal cord monitoring in scoliosis surgery. J Bone Joint Surg [Br] 1991;73:487. *Report of author's experience in 1,168 consecutive patients using SSEPs during spinal instrumentation.*

Kresowik TF et al. Limitations of electroencephalographic monitoring in the detection of cerebral ischemia accompanying carotid endarterectomy. J Vasc Surg 1991;13:439. *A retrospective review of 458 consecutive patients that does not support the predictive value of intraoperative EEG for CEA.*

Owen JH et al. The clinical application of neurogenic motor evoked potentials to monitor spinal cord function during surgery. Spine 1991;16:S385. *Large clinical series that provides strong evidence for utility of MEPs during spinal surgery.*

Schramm J et al. Surgical and electrophysiologic observations during clipping of 134 aneurysms with evoked potential monitoring. Neurosurgery 1990; 26:61. *Case series describes author's "field" experience in using SSEPs during cerebral aneurysm clipping.*

Shinomiya K, et al. Intraoperative monitoring for tethered cord syndrome. Spine 1991;16:1290. *Important report of ten patients describing author's experience and recommendations for monitoring.*

Yingling CD, Gardi JN. Intraoperative monitoring of facial and cochlear nerves during acoustic neuroma surgery. Otolaryngol Clin North Am 1992; 25:413. *Candid and detailed discussion of neurophysiologic monitoring for acoustic neuroma resection; one chapter is devoted to acoustic neuromas.*

RECOMMENDED READING

Dawson EG et al. Spinal cord monitoring—results of Scoliosis Research Society and the European Spinal Deformity Society Survey. Spine 1991;16:S361.

Evans WE et al. Optimal cerebral monitoring during carotid endarterectomy: Neurologic response under local anesthesia. J Vasc Surg 1985;2:775.

Manninen PH et al. Evoked potential monitoring during posterior fossa aneurysm surgery: A comparison of two modalities. Can J Anesth 1994;41:92.

Riegelman RK. Studying a Study and Testing a Test. Boston: Little, Brown, 1981.

Sackett DL, Haynes RB, Tugwell P. Clinical Epidemiology: A Basic Science for Clinical Medicine (2nd ed). Boston: Little, Brown, 1991.

Sox HC. Probability theory in the use of diagnostic tests. Ann Intern Med 1986; 104:60.

Todd MM. Monitoring in Neuroanesthesia. In LJ Saidman, NT Smith (eds), Monitoring in Anesthesia (3rd ed). Boston: Butterworth-Heinemann, 1993.

21

Intracranial Pressure Monitoring

Wayne K. Marshall, M.D.

This chapter discusses how and why intracranial pressure (ICP) is monitored clinically. Chapters 2 and 3 further discuss the normal and abnormal anatomy and physiology mechanistically contributing to increased ICP.

The most important reason to control ICP is that ischemia secondary to intracranial hypertension is the final common pathway leading to brain or spinal cord cell damage and death after acute injury. Acute ischemia results in oxygen and glucose starvation of cells, leading to anaerobic metabolism, lactic acid production, and a decrease or end to metabolic activity. Measuring ICP to document pathologic increases and effects treatment is of vital interest to the clinician.

CLINICAL RESPONSES TO ELEVATIONS IN INTRACRANIAL PRESSURE
Hemodynamic Responses

The final common pathway causing neuronal damage is tissue ischemia secondary to increases in cerebrospinal fluid (CSF) pressure. Increased CSF pressure decreases cerebral blood flow by decreasing cerebral perfusion pressure (CPP). The concept of CPP is important for understanding the reasons for and mechanisms of action for specific treatment modalities.

The concept of CPP stems from basic circulatory physiology. Blood flows through a capillary bed and perfuses tissues in any organ due to a change in pressure across the capillary bed, such that the pressure at the arterial or inflow side is greater than the pressure at the venous or outflow side. Thus, arterial pressure exceeds venous pressure and blood flows through all capillaries in the body. Conditions that decrease arterial pressure (inflow pressure), and/or increase venous pressure (outflow pressure) tend to decrease capillary flow and therefore perfusion: The tissues get less blood and become ischemic. Within a narrow range of perfusion pressures, all capillary beds exhibit a phenomenon called autoregulation, which in the normal state maintains relatively constant blood flow with changing perfusion pressures (see Figure 3.1).

In the particular case of the spinal cord and brain, this relationship of pressure to flow is particularly well described. The formula for cerebral perfusion pressure in the normal brain:

$$CPP = MAP - ICP$$

where MAP is mean arterial pressure.

ICP is used instead of venous outflow pressure because the brain is encased in a rigid skull. Because the capillary bed resides inside this rigid structure, any increase in pressure inside that structure (ICP) represents resistance to venous blood outflow and therefore decreased CPP. To ensure the accuracy of the CPP measurements, arterial blood pressure must be measured at the level of the external auditory meatus.

Normal CPP is 60–150 mm Hg (see Figure 3.1). This CPP corresponds to a normal global cerebral blood flow (CBF) of 50 ml/100 g/minute, 100% of normal CBF. At CPP below 60 mm Hg, the cerebral vessels are maximally dilated and blood flow is directly proportional to perfusion pressure (see Figure 3.1). Cerebral ischemia, the final common pathway leading to cell death, occurs at a CPP of 45 mm Hg. This value for CPP corresponds to a CBF of 25 ml/100 g/minute, ischemic levels at which electrical abnormalities appear in the electroencephalographic record. As CPP, and therefore CBF, decrease further, electrical silence and irreversible cell damage follow in rapid succession.

Elevated ICP may result in marked hypertension (from uncontrolled sympathetic output) and reflex bradycardia (a reflex response to the hypertension). This Cushing's triad is a sign of significant decompensation in the natural cerebral compensatory mechanisms.

Structural Responses

Rapid increases of ICP may also result in physical changes in the anatomy of the brain. This is again due to the fact that the brain is encased in a rigid skull, with the foramen magnum forming an exit at the base for the spinal cord. There are also several fibrous supports for the brain within the cranial vault: the tentorium cerebelli and the falx. Acute increases in local CSF pressure above these structures may cause the brain to be forced down and through these openings. This in turn causes mechanical damage to the cells from compression and shear forces. Damage to the temporal lobes and to the brain stem itself may result. If severe enough, this type of injury can be rapidly fatal.

CEREBROSPINAL FLUID PRESSURE WAVEFORMS

Normal CSF pressure or ICP is 15 mm Hg or less, measured at the level of the external auditory meatus. The normal CSF pressure waveform is a combination of cardiac and respiratory cyclical waves superimposed over a baseline ICP (Figure 21.1). This characteristic wave is seen when the pressure information is displayed on a display screen or a moving chart recorder. Proper placement and accurate pressure information are deduced from the appropriate appearance of the waves on the trace obtained from the particular monitoring device in use.

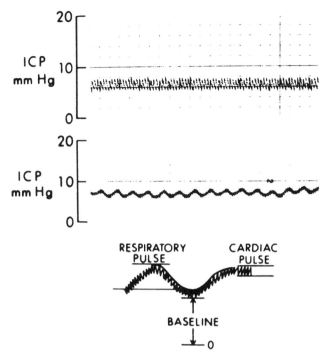

Figure 21.1 Normal ICP (here 5–7 torr) is pulsatile. Cardiac and respiratory cycles are superimposed. The top tracing (faster paper speed) shows the cardiac effect. The middle tracing shows the respiratory effect. The bottom tracing shows the components of an ICP waveform during one breath. *Reprinted with permission from Marmarou A, et al. Intracranial Pressure: Physiology and Pathophysiology. In PR Cooper (ed), Head Injury. Baltimore: Williams & Wilkins, 1982;115–127.*

Abnormal waves become apparent with increased ICP. These waves are usually transient or episodic and are primarily of two types, A waves and B waves (Figure 21.2).

A waves are also known as plateau waves. These are large, high-amplitude (ICP = 50 – 100 torr), sustained (several minutes) waves with rapid descent to baseline levels. They usually denote an extremely grave situation and are associated with a very poor neurologic outcome (see Figure 21.2). B waves are intermediate in severity, being of lower amplitude and shorter duration. There may be rapid stepwise increases to 30–60 mm Hg. A third wave type, the C wave, is found when ICP is elevated. They correspond to arterial pressure waveforms as pulse pressure increases.

INDICATIONS FOR MONITORING

The clinical measurement of ICP logically follows in any circumstance where cerebral perfusion is deemed to be in jeopardy due to an abnormal

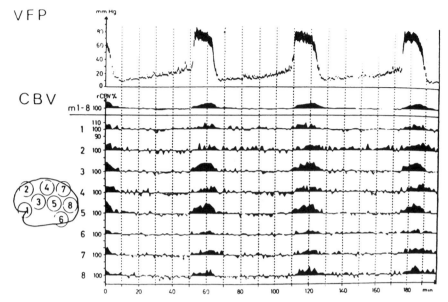

Figure 21.2 Simultaneous tracings of intracranial pressure represented by ventricular fluid pressure (VFP), and cerebral blood volume (CBV) in eight regions of the left cerebral hemisphere. A waves (plateau waves) in the top trace are accompanied by changes in CBV. Mean CBV in the eight regions (M 1–8) are shown in the uppermost curve of the CBV diagram. *Reprinted with permission from J Risberg, N Lundberg, DH Ingvar. Regional cerebral blood volume during acute transient rises of the intracranial pressure (plateau waves). J Neurosurg 1969;31:303.*

intracranial process. The decision to monitor in any particular case is based on clinical judgment and the immediate circumstances. Some of the more common indications include:

1. Head-injured patients, Glasgow score 7 or less
2. Patients with Reye's syndrome
3. Patients with large intracranial tumors
4. Patients with intracranial pathology in whom a neurologic exam cannot be followed
5. Patients undergoing therapy that can adversely affect CPP or ICP

While this list is not exhaustive, it covers the more common indications for ICP monitoring.

TYPES OF INTRACRANIAL PRESSURE MONITORS

Three basic types of ICP monitoring devices are in current use: (1) intraventricular devices, (2) subarachnoid devices, and (3) epidural devices. The different monitors are classified according to invasiveness, location at which the CSF pressure is measured, the physiologic coupling system for each, and the ability to remove CSF with the device. Each is discussed in turn and examples of each are given.

Intraventricular Intracranial Pressure Monitors

Intraventricular devices are the most invasive and the oldest type of monitor in common use. The device is an open-lumen catheter, which is placed into the ventricular system by passing it through brain substance. A burr hole in the skull and a relatively high skill level for safe and successful placement are required. The catheter is filled with preservative-free saline or preservative-free 5% dextrose and water and connected to an external manometer or strain-gauge transducer by fluid-filled tubing; thus the device is fluid-coupled. The transducer can be connected to any modern bedside patient monitor for waveform display and numerical pressure information. Because the catheter is hollow and resides in the ventricular CSF, CSF can be withdrawn and intrathecal drugs administered. It is inexpensive and reliable. This technique is still the standard against which all other intracranial pressure measuring technologies are compared.

Subarachnoid Intracranial Pressure Monitors

Subarachnoid devices are placed into the cranial CSF through a hole in the dura. A burr hole in the skull is necessary for placement, as with the intraventricular catheter. Less skill is required for placement because there is no need to locate the ventricular system. Brain tissue is not usually entered with these devices. Currently there are two such devices in common clinical use, the subarachnoid bolt and the cup catheter.

1. The subarachnoid bolt (Richmond bolt) is, as the name implies, a metal bolt threaded into the skull by means of a small twist-drill hole. The underlying dura is opened surgically before placement. This is known as the Richmond bolt because of the developmental work done at the Medical College of Virginia in Richmond by Becker and his group in the early 1970s. This device is also fluid-coupled to an external transducer, but due to the intimate contact of the tip of the bolt with the surface of the brain, CSF withdrawal is usually not possible.

2. The cup catheter is another subarachnoid device functionally similar to the bolt. It is also placed through a small burr hole and through the opened dura. Like the bolt it is a fluid-coupled device. It is more difficult to place than the bolt because the cup must be placed cup-side down against the surface of the brain at a location somewhat removed from the burr hole.

Epidural Intracranial Pressure Monitors

Epidural devices for ICP monitoring have received the most attention recently. This is due to a concerted effort to develop techniques that avoid the risk of infection inherent to procedures that invade the dura. These devices still require a burr hole in the skull for placement, but the dura remains intact. As a result, no CSF can be withdrawn and no intrathecal drugs can be administered.

The epidural transducer consists of a miniature strain-gauge transducer placed within a metal housing with outside threads similar to but slightly larger than the subarachnoid bolt. The housing is threaded into a small burr hole in such a manner that the surface of the transducer is placed into intimate coplanar-planar contact with the intact dura. Pressure waves in the CSF are transmitted through the dura-transducer interface, and waveforms are displayed on a standard bedside patient monitor. Placement of the transducer is critical because significant error is introduced if the dural surface and the transducer surface are not exactly parallel to each other. There can be no air or fluid between the dura and the transducer. This device is thus not fluid-coupled but direct-coupled.

The epidural catheter tip pressure transducer is a relatively new device that incorporates a direct-deposited, thin-film technology to sense the pressure changes in the CSF. This film is placed in the tip of a very small catheter and covered with a thin membrane. Use of a double lumen in the catheter allows for in vivo calibration and zero determination. The catheter is usually placed epidurally but can also be used subarachnoidally and intraventricularly. The device is designed to interface with any standard bedside patient monitor.

The pneumatic transducer uses air pressure to determine the CSF pressure. A dedicated stand-alone unit is required to monitor ICP. The unit houses the pressure transducer and the pneumatic pump. The catheter houses two lumens and a thin metallic disc, which is in contact with the dura. Gas is pumped into the catheter under pressure. When the pressure or the gas in the inlet port is equal to the pressure on the metallic disc, the disc rises and gas exits the outlet port. The pressure required to allow gas to exit is therefore very close to the ICP in contact with the metallic disc. The sensor catheter is disposable and the measurements reasonably accurate, but the unit is a dedicated machine that can be used on only one patient at a time.

Fiberoptic Intracranial Pressure Monitors

The latest and probably most popular ICP monitor device in clinical use today is the fiberoptic transducer marketed by Camino Laboratories (San Diego, CA). This device uses two fiberoptic light paths and a sensing mirror to measure ICP. The base unit houses the fiberoptic light source and the electronics. The sensor cable assembly houses the two fiber paths and the mirror attached to a moveable membrane in the tip. Light is transmitted at a known intensity through one path to the mirror in the tip of the catheter. This light is reflected back through the other path to a sensor in the base unit. This sensor measures the intensity of the returned light and compares it to the original intensity. The intensity of the returning light is altered by a deflection of the mirror by movement of the membrane in response to ICP pressure waves against the outside surface of the membrane. The difference in the two intensities of light is used to calculate the ICP. This device requires a dedicated monitor and can therefore only be used on one patient at a time. However, the device functions on battery power during transport, which is a significant advantage. In addition, the device has catheters designed for epidural, subdural, and intraventricular use.

TREATMENT OF INTRACRANIAL HYPERTENSION

All therapy for increased ICP is designed to preserve CPP by decreasing ICP without decreasing MAP. Since the brain is enclosed in a rigid cranium, a reduction in ICP is achievable only by reducing the volume of the intracranial contents. Of all the substances contained in the cranial vault, only the volume of CSF and blood can be readily affected by pharmacologic means (Table 21.1). Interstitial fluid and intracellular fluid volumes can be reduced, but less rapidly than blood or CSF. In rare cases, brain substance itself may be surgically removed to create room in the cranial vault for remaining structures.

Blood volume can be reduced by measures that decrease the capacity of the cerebral blood vessels and by measures that facilitate venous drainage from the head. Venous drainage may be facilitated by a head-up posture or position; avoidance of jugular venous compression at the neck; and avoidance of systemic fluid overload.

Cerebral vasoconstriction decreases intracranial blood volume. This can be accomplished by (1) hyperventilation and the associated decrease in arterial PCO_2; (2) administration of barbiturates (it is a direct effect of the drug); (3) avoidance of cerebral vasodilators, such as volatile anesthetic agents (isoflurane) or antihypertensives such as sodium nitroprusside (Nipride); and (4) maintenance of autoregulation by avoiding extreme arterial hypertension.

Cerebrospinal fluid volume can be reduced by drainage through a ventricular catheter. The head-up position also facilitates transference of CSF to the spinal canal.

Interstitial and intracellular fluid volume can be reduced by administration of osmotic (mannitol) or loop (furosemide) diuretics. In acute circumstances, osmotic diuretics pull fluid into the intravascular space. In the longer term, renal excretion removes this fluid from the body. In the event of renal failure, osmotic diuretics may exhibit a biphasic response with tissue fluid increasing later in the course of therapy. Adequate renal function is necessary to elicit a significant response to loop diuretics.

Table 21.1 Drug Effects on Intracranial Pressure

Drug	Primary	Secondary
Potent anesthetic agents		
Halothane	++	0
Enflurane	++	0
Isoflurane	++	0
Desflurane	++	0
Sevoflurane	++	0
Barbiturates		
Thiopental sodium	–	0
Propofol	-	0
Narcotics		
Morphine	0	
Fentanyl citrate	0	+
Alfentanil	±	+
Sufentanil	±	+
Ketamine hydrochloride	+	0
Benzodiazepines		
Diazepam	-	0
Lorazepam	-	0
Midazolam	-	0
Neuromuscular-blocking drugs		
Succinylcholine chloride	+	0
d-tubocurarine	0	+
Pancuronium bromide	0	0
Vecuronium bromide	0	0
Atracurium besylate	0	0
Etomidate	-	0
Diuretics		
Mannitol	-	0
Furosemide	-	0
Vasodilators		
Sodium nitroprusside	+	0
Hydralazine hydrochloride	+	0
Nitroglycerin	+	0
Trimethaphan camsylate	0	+
Calcium channel blocking drugs		
Nimodipine	0	0
Nicardipine	++	0
Propranolol	0	0
Labetalol	0	0
Esmolol	0	0
Nitrous oxide	0	+

++ = major increase: + = moderate increase; ± = minimal, if any change; 0 = no effect:
– = major decrease: - = moderate decrease.
Source: Reprinted with permission from WK Marshall. Intracranial Pressure. In CL Lake (ed),
Clinical Monitoring. Philadelphia: Saunders, 1990;669

KEY REFERENCES

Marshall LF, Bowers SA. Medical Management of Intracranial Pressure. In PR Cooper (ed), Head Injury. Baltimore: Williams & Wilkins, 1982;129–146.

Marshall WK. Intracranial Pressure. In CL Lake (ed), Clinical Monitoring. Philadelphia: Saunders, 1990; 659–686. *These two chapters review ICP monitoring, the physiology of ICP control, and mechanisms of measurement.*

RECOMMENDED READING

Allen R. Intracranial pressure: A review of clinical problems, measurement techniques and monitoring methods. J Med Eng Technol 1986;10:299. *A review of ICP, but from a more technical perspective.*

Barlow P, et al. Clinical evaluation of two methods of subdural pressure monitoring. J Neurosurg 1985;63:578.

Bedford RF, Morris L, Jane IA. Intracranial hypertension during surgery for supratentorial tumor: Correlation with preoperative computed tomography scans. Anesth Analg 1982;61:430.

Chambers IR et al. A clinical evaluation of the Camino subdural screw and ventricular monitoring kits. Neurosurg 1990;26:421.

Crutchfield IS et al. Evaluation of a fiberoptic intracranial pressure monitor. J Neurosurg 1990;72:482.

Friedman WA, Vries JK. Percutaneous tunnel ventriculostomy. J Neurosurg 1980;53:662.

Ghani GA et al. Effects of intravenous nitroglycerin on the intracranial pressure and volume pressure response. J Neurosurg 1983;58:562.

Jennett B, Teasdale G. Management of Head Injuries. Philadelphia: FA Davis, 1981. *ICP viewed from its association with head injuries.*

Jorgensen PB, Riishede J. Comparative Clinical Studies of Epidural and Ventricular Pressure. In M Brock, H Dietz (eds), Intracranial Pressure: Experimental and Clinical Aspects. Berlin: Springer-Verlag, 1972;41–45.

Koster WG, Kuypers MH. Intracranial pressure and its epidural measurement. Med Prog Technol 1980;7:21.

Lassen NA, Ingvar DH. Radioisotopic assessment of regional cerebral blood flow. Prog Nucl Med 1972;1:376.

Marmarou A, Tabaddor K. Intracranial Pressure: Physiology and Pathophysiology. In PR Cooper (ed), Head Injury. Baltimore: Williams & Wilkins, 1982;115–127.

McKay RD, Sundt TM, Michenfelder JD. Internal carotid artery stump pressure and cerebral blood flow during carotid endarterectomy: Modification by halothane, enflurane, and Innovar. Anesthesiology 1976; 45:390.

Mendelow AD, et al. A clinical comparison of subdural screw pressure measurements with ventricular pressure. Neurosurg 1983;58:45.

Michenfelder JD. The Cerebral Circulation. In C Prys-Roberts (ed), The Circulation in Anesthesia. London: Blackwell, 1980;212.

Obrist WD, et al. Regional cerebral blood flow estimated by 133 xenon inhalation. Stroke 1975;6:245.

Ostrup RC et al. Continuous monitoring of intracranial pressure with a miniaturized fiberoptic device. J Neurosurg 1987;67:206.

Risberg I, Lundberg N, Ingvar DH. Regional cerebral blood volume during acute transient rises of the intracranial pressure (plateau waves). J Neurosurg 1969;31:303.

Venes JL, Shaywitz BA, Spender DD. Management of severe cerebral edema in the metabolic encephalopathy of Reye-Johnson syndrome. J Neurosurg 1978;48:903.

Vries JIC, Becker DP, Young HF. A subarachnoid screw for monitoring intracranial pressure. J Neurosurg 1973;39:416.

Wilkinson HA. The intracranial pressure-monitoring cup catheter: Technical note. Neurosurg 1977;1:139.

22

Transcranial Doppler Monitoring

W. Andrew Kofke, M.D.

Transcranial Doppler ultrasonography (TCD) is a relatively new technique that has only recently been examined as a monitor during anesthesia. The interest derives from the unique capacity of TCD to provide real-time cerebral hemodynamic information in a beat-to-beat fashion—something that has heretofore been needed in acute care settings but with no obvious, easily applicable modality. Use of TCD in the operating room has had to await advances regarding appropriate assumptions, clinical applicability of the physics of TCD, and engineering. Many questions regarding its suitability as a clinically relevant tool remain unanswered.

PRINCIPLES OF TRANSCRANIAL DOPPLER ULTRASONOGRAPHY

TCD is based on the Doppler effect described by the physicist Christian Andreas Doppler (1803–1853). This effect results in a sound wave being reflected at a higher or lower frequency depending on the velocity of the reflector. This frequency shift (transmitted-reflected frequency) is directly related to the velocity of blood coursing through an insonated blood vessel. Blood is not a single reflector. The signal received is a mixture of different frequencies produced by many reflectors moving at different velocities. The equipment is designed to detect ultrasound reflections over a linear range at a given depth. Thus, the signal received is produced by a cross-section over a given depth, such that a "cylinder" of tissue reflects the sound waves. This can result in detection of signals in more than one vessel if a bifurcation has been insonated.

The TCD signal is a Fourier transformation of the Doppler signal. The ultrasound is applied through a specific cranial "window," an area of thin bone. The usual windows are in the temporal region and posteriorly through the foramen magnum. The outline of the reflected Doppler signal is quite similar to an intraarterial pressure waveform, thus making it suitable to monitor dynamic physiology (Figure 22.1). Occasionally one can observe overshoot of the systolic value and harmonics. Normal flow velocities from several studies are listed in Table 22.1.

Waveform analysis is currently a subject of research. A straightforward means of characterizing a waveform is with the pulsatility index ([systolic-diastolic] ÷ [mean]) derived from measured velocities. It is thought that an increas-

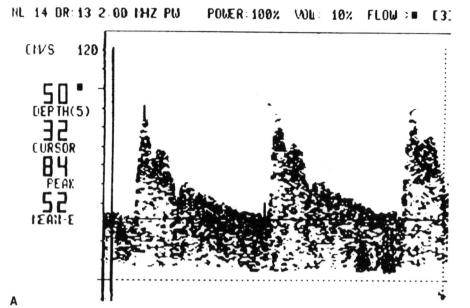

A

Figure 22.1 Rupture of an intracranial aneurysm during induction of anesthesia. The patient was a 56-year-old white female with a ruptured basilar tip aneurysm and rebleeding 12 hours before. Intracranial pressure (ICP) was 10–12 mm Hg; blood pressure was 120 mm Hg. A. Prerupture transcranial Doppler. B. Immediate postrupture transcranial Doppler of the right middle cerebral artery showing an oscillating pattern with retrograde flow during diastole. Ventricular catheter–transduced ICP was 120 mm Hg. C. Transcranial Doppler 15 minutes after rupture. D. Transcranial Doppler 20 minutes after rupture. E. Transcranial Doppler 24 minutes after rupture showing normalization of the waveform and velocity measurements. *Reproduced with permission from CC Eng et al. The diagnosis and management of perianesthetic cerebral aneurysmal rupture aided with transcranial Doppler ultrasonography. Anesthesiology 1993;78:191.*

ing pulsatility index (PI)—that is, a more "spiky" waveform—indicates increased cerebrovascular resistance. Waveforms have been further analyzed by fast Fourier transformation and waveform component analysis.

Assumptions and Caveats

Assumptions and caveats regarding TCD use in other clinical areas also apply in the operating room. First, it is important that the TCD user always be aware that the device monitors velocity, not nutritive cerebral blood flow (CBF). Second, the velocity calculation assumes a constant insonation angle, which is nearly parallel with the insonated blood vessel, and that the blood vessel is predictably oriented from patient to patient. These assumptions may not always be

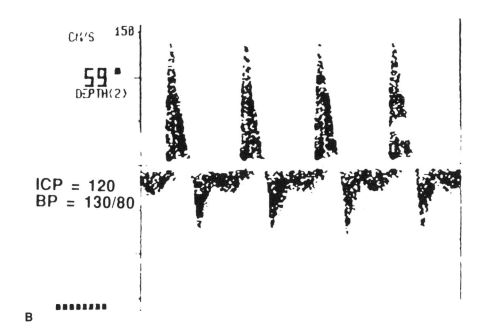

ICP = 120
BP = 130/80

B

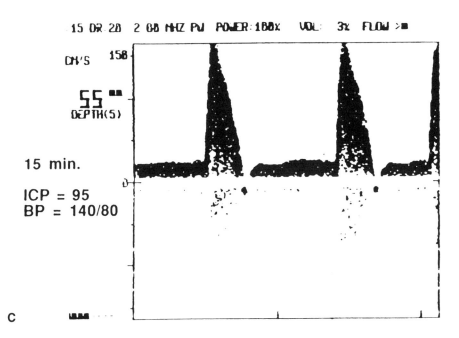

15 min.

ICP = 95
BP = 140/80

C

Figure 22.1 *(continmued)*

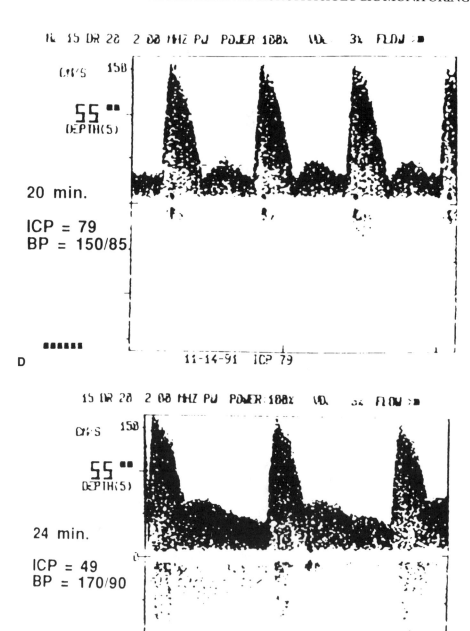

Figure 22.1 *(continmued)*

Table 22.1 Normal Reference Flow Velocities in Various Studies in Adults

n	Age (yr)	Depth (mm)	Velocities ± SD (cm/sec)		
			Mean	Peak Systolic	End Systolic
50	20–65	—	62±12	—	—
20	20–35	—	67±7	—	—
20	49–63	—	58±10	—	—
51	12–81	50	—	90±16	45±10
	<40	50	—	94±18	48±10
	>60	50	—	80±18	36±9
50	20–70	35–45	56±13	82±21	40±9
50	<40	50	58±8	95±14	46±7
	40–60	50	58±12	91±17	44±10
	>60	50	45±11	78±15	32±9
50	<40	45–55	—	104±14	51±9
	40–59	45–55	—	87±18	43±9
	>60	45–55	—	81±20	34±9
35	20–66	—	79±16	—	—
35	20–65	—	79±16	—	—
50	<40	—	51±12	72±14	34±7
51	>60	50–80	—	66±11	23±9
	20–70	50–80	—	71±18	35±10
50	<40	60	50±13	76±17	36±9
50	40–60	60	47±14	86±20	41±7
	>60	60	53±11	73±20	34±9
35	20–66	60	45±14	—	—
	—	63±12	—	—	
50	20–65	—	44±11	—	—
51	<40	—	—	60±13	30±7
	>60	50–80	—	51±8	24±5
50	20–70	50–80	41±9	57±12	28±8
50	<40	60	34±8	53±11	26±7
	40–60	60	37±10	6±21	29±8
	>60	60	30±9	51±12	22±7
	—	60	40±9	56±12	27±7
	20–66	—	47±13	—	—
51	<40	75	—	64±13	32±6
	>60	75	—	51±9	23±6
50	20–70	75	39±9	56±13	27±7
50	<40	75	35±8	56±8	27±5
	40–60	75	36±12	60±17	29±8
	>60	75	30±12	51±19	21±9
51	<40	85	—	64±13	32±6
	>60	85	—	52±9	23±6
50	20–70	75	39±9	56±13	27±7
30	22–79	100	—	59±17	31±9
10	22–79	110	—	60±14	33±10

Source: Reproduced with permission from VL Babikian, LR Wechsler (eds). Transcranial Doppler Ultrasonography. St. Louis: Mosby, 1993;30.

valid. Third, anatomic assumptions are invalid with hydrocephalus, and absolute blood flow velocity (BFV) values are not valid in such situations. That this may also be true in other pathologic situations with distortion of vascular anatomy is a reasonable, but unstudied, speculation that should be considered when assessing BFV in any patient in whom vascular anatomy may be distorted. Fourth, to make clinical and research conclusions about TCD data, it is also important to maintain constancy of position of the TCD probe and insonated vessel.

The validity of the assumption of unchanging proximal intracranial artery caliber has been examined in six human proximal arteries and recorded on videotape during moderate alterations in $PaCO_2$ and blood pressure. The caliber variations were observed to be small and were considered to be insufficient to significantly affect a TCD signal. However, it has been shown that $PaCO_2$ changes over a 25–60 mm Hg increase in basal cerebral artery diameter in subjects more than 10 years old but not those less than 10 years old. Nonetheless, BFV did change with $PaCO_2$ as expected. In children undergoing surgery with hypothermic cardiopulmonary bypass, middle cerebral artery (MCA) diameter did not correlate with blood pressure or temperature. It thus seems that the assumption of constant basal cerebral artery diameter may be open to challenge. Whether such challenges will be found to be of physiologic significance remains to be determined. In general, known CBF effects of anesthetics and interventions have been mirrored by congruent observations with TCD, suggesting that basal artery diameter is constant enough for most clinical purposes.

Equipment and Technical Considerations

TCD has been in clinical use for several years. Nonetheless, even in controlled settings difficulties have been encountered, due in large part to interpatient anatomic differences in temporal window quality. A suitable transtemporal window cannot be identified in approximately 10% of subjects, usually due to hyperostosis related to age, sex, and race.

With the introduction of TCD into the operating room, a variety of equipment considerations had to be solved or still require improvement. The hand-held transducer used for most diagnostic purposes is clearly inadequate for most operating room uses in which temporal trends in BFV are important. A variety of approaches to this problem have been tried, including head straps, surgical clamps, and sewing or gluing the transducer to the skin. Several head strap designs have been introduced. Their use tends to make finding the insonated artery more difficult. In addition, once fixed into position, minor alterations in patient head position can result in major changes in the TCD waveform. Thus, such headstraps are useful only to monitor flow velocity when there is no surgical instrumentation about the head. Accordingly, for surgical procedures they can only be used for induction of anesthesia, posterior fossa procedures, or extracranial procedures.

One promising new device entails using colostomy adhesive to firmly adhere the transducer to the temporal window, thereby decreasing slippage of the transducer across the skin. This should increase the stability of the transducer position with changes in head position. Moreover, this device has several properties that should increase the usefulness of TCD as a monitor. It will enable the clinician to follow trends, average difficult-to-locate signals, detect air or particulate emboli, download data to other computers, automatically intermittently insonate, and set up alarm conditions.

To monitor BFV intraoperatively during most neurosurgical procedures, a sterilized transducer aimed directly at the insonated vessel in the surgical field is required. Presently, this is not commonly done. For posterior fossa work where the temporal windows are not in the surgical field, the hand-held transducer can be secured to a flexible clamp, which can then be secured to the head holder. After the appropriate vessel is found the clamp is tightened down. As the patient's head is previously secured into place, the transducer can in this way be kept in a steady position to monitor BFV throughout the neurosurgical procedure. Despite these efforts, with intraoperative monitoring during craniotomy intracranial air can migrate into the Doppler beam pathway, artifactually attenuating the signal.

Other problems arise when diagnostic equipment is used as a monitor in an acute care setting. Many TCD devices, which are designed as diagnostic instruments, provide excellent static images. However, most available units are not readily amenable to digitizing signals with downloading to computers and do not provide trend analysis, alarms, correlation with other physiologic variables, complex waveform analyses (e.g., fast Fourier transformation), intermittent signal acquisition, or electrocardiogram-gated signal averaging. Moreover, the electrically hostile operating room environment often causes the software to inaccurately identify important waveform characteristics, leading to erroneous digital display of systolic and diastolic velocities and PI. It is anticipated that newly released TCD units, designed as monitors, will circumvent many of these problems.

ANESTHETIC EFFECTS
Anesthetic Effects on Cerebral Blood Flow

Using traditional CBF methodology, the effects of most anesthetics on CBF in humans and other mammals have been determined. Generally, the volatile anesthetics isoflurane, enflurane, halothane, and nitrous oxide produce cerebral vasodilation with increased CBF if systemic blood pressure is maintained. Flow and metabolism become uncoupled with a decrement in cerebral metabolic rate. In contrast, the hypnotic agents thiopental, etomidate, and propofol tend to decrease CBF coupled to CMR. Ketamine, however, increases CBF coupled to increased CMR. Narcotics are generally thought to have little effect on CBF, provided their use is not associated with seizures.

Effects of Anesthetics on Transcranial Doppler Ultrasonography

Most TCD work on anesthetic effects on cerebral artery blood velocity has been via the middle cerebral artery (MCA) windows. Despite a lack of firm information regarding anesthetic effects on basal cerebral artery diameter, TCD effects of anesthetics are generally congruent with those observed with flow determinations. Here we review the data presently available.

Intravenous Anesthetics

Several studies assessing the effects of barbiturates have demonstrated a 20–50% decrease in MCA BFV. Similarly, midazolam, etomidate, and propofol have been reported to also produce 20–50% BFV decrements. Conversely, in normal volunteers ketamine, 0.25 mg/kg, increased BFV and decreased PI with a concomitant increase in blood pressure. Opioids have little effect on BFV.

Volatile Agents

At lower doses the effects of the volatile anesthetics, including halothane, enflurane, isoflurane, and nitrous oxide, are modest, with more significant increases in BFV with higher concentrations. Nitrous oxide also increases BFV, even if added to isoflurane.

Neuromuscular Blockers

Succinylcholine has been reported to increase intracranial pressure (ICP) or to have no effect on ICP. The reasons for this are unclear, but fasciculations, muscle-spindle stimulation, increased CO_2 production, and paraben preservatives have all been suggested. Given to five anesthetized humans with high ICP in (apparently) preservative-free form, succinylcholine was observed to have no effect on MCA BFV. However, for healthy patients, given immediately after thiopental, succinyl-choline with paraben preservative produced a modest increase in BFV.

TRANSCRANIAL DOPPLER ULTRASONOGRAPHY AS AN INTRAOPERATIVE MONITOR

It is expected that TCD may have a use in the operating room and intensive care unit as a dynamic monitor of the cerebral vasculature. However, it has not yet been fully and systematically assessed to ascertain its value as a monitor during anesthesia and surgery. During craniotomy, TCD has been used to identify altered BFV and autoregulation. It was confirmed that TCD could be used as a monitor during craniotomy. Intuitively, TCD should be useful to monitor for dangerous intracranial hypertension, arterial air embolism, adverse effects of abnormal hemodynamic situations, inappropriate perfusion after proximal cerebral arteriotomy, arteriovenous malformation (AVM) resection, or carotid endarterectomy. Moreover, it can provide a means to quickly assess, intraoperatively, cerebrovascular reserve and autoregulatory capacity. The rationale, current clinical experiences, and supporting evidence for many of these suggestions and others are given below. However, whether TCD can be used in any of these situations to alter outcome or costs is unknown.

Table 22.2 Middle Cerebral Artery Blood Flow Velocity with Induction of Anesthesia

	Nontumor				Tumor			
	Awake	Post-induction	Intu-bation	Post intu-bation	Awake	Post-induction	Intu-bation	Post intu-bation
MAP	94	82*	101	90	93	76*	90	81
SD	12	11	16	17	15	11	16	13
p		0.002	0.13	0.39		0.0002	0.46	0.008
MCA BFV	56	46	61	47	98	5	71	59*
SD	14	13	18	14	40	2	24	21
p		0.032	0.35	0.04		0.06	0.02	0.005
PI	0.94	0.96	0.718	0.86	0.85	0.93	0.93	0.89
SD	0.19	0.17	0.17	0.20	0.25	0.22	0.32	0.20
p		0.69	0.004	0.27		0.30	0.90	0.57

*Significant at p<0.005 when compared to awake baseline.
MAP = mean arterial pressure; MCABFV = middle cerebral artery blood flow velocity; PI = pulsatility index; SD = standard deviation; P = significance level.
Source: WA Kofke et al. Transcranial Doppler ultrasonography with induction of anesthesia for neurosurgery. J Neurosurg Anesth 1994;6:89–97.

Effects of Procedures on Transcranial Doppler Ultrasonography
Laryngoscopy and Intubation

Laryngoscopy is a hemodynamic stressor that increases intracranial pressure. In neurosurgical patients (both with and without tumors) undergoing induction of anesthesia, postinduction laryngoscopy was associated with increases in BFV compared to the depressed postthiopental level, although essentially unchanged compared to awake baseline (Table 22.2). Of 196 elective patients, none demonstrated a waveform indicating compromised perfusion. Such data suggest that the ICP rise associated with laryngoscopy may not produce cerebral ischemia. Rather, an element of transient cerebral hyperemia is suggested. This study did not assess patients with severe intracranial hypertension. TCD may have an important role in determining, during anesthetic induction and surgery, whether an ICP rise is compromising cerebral perfusion.

Cardiac Surgery

Cardiac surgery and the associated cardiopulmonary bypass are associated with a 5–10% incidence of postoperative neuropsychiatric deficits. Multiple contributing factors have been implicated, including low CBF, inadequate cannula placement, and cerebral air or particulate emboli. Transcranial Doppler is a useful monitor for these events in this setting.

Arterial Air Embolism Arterial air embolism can be detected by TCD. Cerebral arterial air embolism occurs most commonly during cardiopulmonary bypass with aortotomy or opening of a cardiac chamber. The incidence of cerebral air embolism was shown to be 79% during cardiac valve replacement and 40% during coronary artery bypass graft surgery. This is a major issue as 5–24% of patients undergoing cardiac surgery develop postoperative neurologic (usually neuropsychiatric) deficits. Among other things, air or particulate embolism has been thought to be a major factor in the genesis of this problem. Research is underway to determine methods of quantitating the amount of air entrained to facilitate therapeutic decisions. Thus, TCD will probably become a routine monitor during cardiac surgery. The major research problems now are determining the amount of air that mandates aggressive therapies (e.g., hyperbaric oxygen, barbiturates) to rescue the ischemic brain tissue, and whether it is cost effective.

Optimally, an automatic monitoring system can be used that will detect, recognize, count, and size emboli. A prototype monitor, in addition to producing real-time BFV waveform output, digitally records waveform outlines with facility for playback and computer processing to facilitate interpretation. When used to monitor six carotid endarterectomies and one aortic valve replacement, this device detected embolic rates ranging from 0.15/minute to nearly 3/minute.

Cardiopulmonary bypass (CPB) is associated with large decreases in CBF. Moreover, it is often performed with a nonpulsatile pump. Thus, BFV in adult patients on nonpulsatile bypass is rather low and uniform without pulsatile characteristics of the cardiac pump. Comparisons of CBF and BFV changes that occur in the course of cardiac surgery with hypothermic CPB show a good correlation ($r = 0.77$, $p < 0.0001$). When electroencephalography (EEG) is monitored during CPB, bursts in EEG activity (during burst suppression) transiently increase BFV by 21% from the suppressed level. Infants undergoing hypothermic CPB have been observed to have normal pre-CPB, prehypothermia BFV; but with reperfusion after 48 minutes of hypothermic (15.4°C) circulatory arrest sustained a 43% decrease in BFV. These data agree with [133]Xenon CBF observations of infants in similar circumstances.

Carotid Endarterectomy

TCD can be used during carotid endarterectomy (CEA) to monitor for particulate or air embolism and for adequacy of flow. Sustained low flow may lead to ischemic neurologic injury, so it is essential that critical decreases in flow be identified. EEG has been used, but with an inadequate number of channels the results can be ambiguous. Moreover, insertion of a shunt can produce neurologic side effects, so its use is not a straightforward decision. Kofke et al. described excellent correlation between MCA BFV and stable xenon computer tomography–derived cortical CBF in awake brain tumor patients during balloon occlusion of the internal carotid artery, suggesting that TCD might be useful for drawing inferences about CBF during CEA. In patients monitored during CEA, TCD did not correlate with CBF at high BFV, but at lower velocities and flows the TCD-CBF correlation strengthened. This suggests that TCD is a valuable monitor for detecting low CBF during carotid endarterectomy. There is a significant decrement in MCA

BFV with carotid clamping. In 19 patients studied, three sustained a value of 0 cm/second, and three patients showed an oscillatory positive-negative pattern.

There are difficulties with TCD as a monitor during CEA. Monitored BFV during CEA in 50 awake patients showed a significant decrease in BFV with clamping. However, the patients sustaining neurologic deficits with clamping had a similar BFV decrement, suggesting that use of TCD as a monitor during CEA is not straightforward. When TCD and EEG were used to monitor 89 patients during CEA, there were technical difficulties: No signal could be obtained in 13% and probe position could not be adequately maintained in 27%. In patients with adequate studies TCD failed to provide additional information to alter surgical therapy. Of these patients, one sustained a stroke, which became evident in the recovery room, despite normal stump pressure, EEG, BFV, and duplex scanning or arteriogram.

TCD monitoring can be used to infer flow alterations and may be useful during CEA, but only if changes are interpreted relative to baseline, a concept supported with TCD-three-dimensional xenon CBF correlations in tumor patients undergoing balloon occlusion of the carotid artery. Patients with EEG changes significant enough to warrant shunt placement sustained an 83% decrement in BFV on TCD, contrasted to a 30% decrement in nonshunted patients (p <0.0005). When evaluating the distribution of BFV responses to carotid clamping, EEG showed occasional asymmetry with BFV of less than 60% of baseline and variable asymmetry with BFV of less than 40% of baseline (n = 14). If patients have a definite loss of MCA signal, EEG asymmetry is seen. TCD data may only absolutely indicate need for a shunt when BFV decreases to 0.

Absolute BFV decrements are not useful for using TCD to identify patients with carotid occlusion–induced CBF of less than 20 ml/100 g/minute. Using a clamp-preclamp BFV ratio of less than 0.6 can predict CBF of less than 20 ml/100 g/minute with 89% accuracy; a ratio of less than 0.4 can predict EEG flattening with 98% accuracy. A 70% ipsilateral BFV decrease used as a shunt criterion has a sensitivity of 100% and specificity of 94% for ischemia detection. By comparison, EEG, the "gold standard," was used to predict major stroke with 80% sensitivity and 99% specificity. Introduction of TCD monitoring has been shown to decrease intraoperative stroke rate from 4.8% to 1.5%.

No formal studies of a large number of patients have rigorously assessed the various amounts of decrement in BFV with carotid clamping to conclusively ascertain the "threshold" level (if any) below which a shunt is mandated. However, review of substantial experience suggests a shunt is indicated with a mean MCA BFV reduction of more than 65% (i.e., to below 35% of baseline), the level below which evoked potential abnormalities arise. Also quoted as a threshold value is a mean BFV of 20 cm/second (although such a BFV probably should represent a decrement from a normal baseline).

TCD, in addition to providing absolute BFV and PI data, can easily be used to ascertain cerebral vascular reserve. The response of BFV to $PaCO_2$ alterations provides an index of cerebrovascular autoregulatory reserve: If the vascular bed is fully dilated, as during carotid clamp-induced hypoperfusion, minimal or no increase in BFV is observed with increased $PaCO_2$. In non-CEA acetazolamide studies and during CO_2 inhalation the utility of TCD to evaluate cerebrovascular reserve has been demonstrated. Vasomotor reactivity assessment has also been demonstrated in patients with cerebrovascular disorders.

TCD is also helpful with CEA to identify the occurrence of cerebral arterial emboli after unclamping of the carotid artery. Cerebral arterial emboli due to clotted blood, platelets, atheromatous material, fat, and air produce distinctive patterns on TCD. In CEA, bubble emboli have been noted in 62% and formed-element emboli in 26% of cases. Each embolic type had a distinctive signature. Air emboli were not associated with postoperative stroke, whereas formed-element emboli were implicated when postoperative stroke occurred. Fat and air are thought to produce stronger signals than those produced by whole blood, platelets, or atheromatous material. Thus, TCD should be a valuable modality to monitor for cerebrovascular embolism and might be useful in differentiating the cause of the embolism. This can be most important in making important therapeutic decisions (e.g., embolectomy versus hyperbaric oxygen or other aggressive therapies).

Despite the lack of CBF correlation at higher velocities, extremely elevated flow velocity after endarterectomy may indicate a loss of cerebral autoregulation. Elevated BFV after CEA has been reported in 21% of patients and noted to correlate with higher CBF. Such information can be extremely valuable as an indicator of the importance of avoiding emergence and postoperative hypertension in a given patient. This is made clinically relevant by reports indicating that cerebral hyperemia after carotid endarterectomy represents a subset of patients at high risk of postoperative cerebral hemorrhage, presumably as a consequence of cerebral dysautoregulation.

TCD may be helpful to delineate the etiology of post-CEA stroke. Generally the major differential diagnoses are hemorrhage versus carotid occlusion. TCD detected acute carotid occlusion in three patients. Two of them progressed to sustain an ischemic stroke. With acute carotid occlusion, TCD changed dramatically, with a pronounced decrease in pulsatility and high to normal mean velocity. When comparing patients with carotid occlusion to control neurologic patients without cerebrovascular disease, there is a significant decrease in PI with carotid occlusion. Patients with a decrease in both PI (<.075) and BFV (<40 cm/second) are at higher risk for stroke. Gradual occlusion of the carotid artery has also been detected and isolated MCA occlusion evaluated intraoperatively with TCD.

Resection of Arteriovenous Malformations

Arteriovenous malformations (AVMs) induce an element of baseline abnormality in BFV measurements. Blood vessels distant from the AVM have normal BFV. However, arteries feeding the AVM have elevated mean BFV, decreased PI, and abnormal response to changes in $PaCO_2$. Thus, when using TCD to monitor a patient with an AVM, it is important to be aware of the possibility that the insonated artery may be an AVM feeder artery.

There are reports of cerebral dysautoregulation, hyperemia, and cerebral hemorrhage after AVM resection. Thus, patients with hyperemia after AVM resection are at special risk of hypertension-induced cerebral hemorrhage. Although not vigorously assessed, TCD probably can be used to detect the presence of such a hyperemic condition and to facilitate optimal blood pressure management after resection.

Effects of Physiologic Situations on Transcranial Doppler Ultrasonography

Hypertension

Hypertension can be produced by noxious stimuli in the setting of inadequate anesthesia, fluid overload, or high blood catecholamine levels due to endogenous causes or exogenous administration. Hypertension due to light anesthesia is associated with a marked increase in BFV. TCD effects of hypertension due to catecholamine infusion or fluid overload have not been reported.

Hypothermia

Hypothermia, usually induced via extracorporeal means, has been associated with BFV decreases in infants and adults; cerebral perfusion is reported to become pressure-dependent below 26°C, in agreement with prior reports of cerebral hemodynamic effects of hypothermia. However, when bypass patients' pressure autoregulation is assessed with TCD, pH-stat (temperature-corrected blood gas) management patients exhibit loss of autoregulation whereas alpha-stat (no temperature correction) management patients maintain autoregulation.

Hypotension

Common causes of hypotension in the operating room include relative anesthetic overdose, blood or fluid loss, and vasodilator administration. Less commonly one may see hypotension from heart failure, neurogenic causes, and anaphylaxis. TCD may be a helpful adjunctive monitor in some of these situations. Overdoses of hypnotic anesthetic, such as thiopental, which decreases CBF, can significantly decrease BFV. The TCD effects of volatile agent overdoses are unknown, although 2 MAC isoflurane with hyperventilation may produce zero diastolic flow velocity. Prospective evaluation of patients undergoing cardiac catheterization has shown decreased MCA BFV with lower cardiac index. This is supported by observations of increased BFV in children after transcatheter atrial septal defect closure (with presumed increased cardiac output). The TCD pattern observed in a case of pregnancy-induced orthostatic hypotension was suggestive of the pattern seen with high ICP with zero diastolic (although not end-diastolic) velocity. This report suggests that the patient's blood pressure decreased to approach normal ICP, a concept later supported by experimental and clinical observations. In N_2O-sedated dogs in which hemorrhagic hypotension was induced, absent EEG activity developed at a mean arterial pressure (MAP) of 31 ±7 mm Hg, at which point animals exhibited zero diastolic velocity by TCD (Figure 22.2). This has also been observed in a human with hemorrhage-induced hypotension (personal communication). In both adenosine- and nitroprusside-

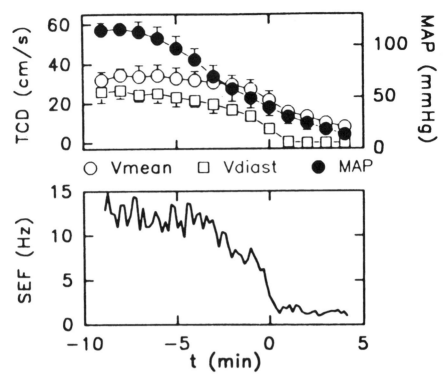

Figure 22.2 Anesthetized dogs underwent hemorrhagic hypotension with monitoring of intraarterial blood pressure, transcranial Doppler, and electroencephalography. Spectral edge frequency decreases precipitously with the onset of zero diastolic velocity. *Reproduced with permission from C Werner et al. Transcranial Doppler sonography indicates critical brain perfusion during hemorrhagic hypotension in dogs. Anesth Analges 1992; 74:S347.*

induced hypotension, a low diastolic velocity and increased PI were produced with a concomitant widening of arterial-jugular venous O_2 content.

Hypoxemia

Decreased PaO_2 increases BFV in normal volunteers. Due to compensatory hypocapnia, actual velocity does not change with decreasing O_2 content (CaO_2) until CaO_2 decreases to less than 70%. When $PaCO_2$ is corrected for, however, a linear relationship is observed: BFV increases with CaO_2 decrement ($r = 0.824$, $p < 0.01$).

Hypercapnea and Hypocapnea

Hypercapnea due to tourniquet release increases BFV in proportion to the increase in end-tidal CO_2 in humans anesthetized with isoflurane, nitrous oxide, and fentanyl. In unanesthetized humans the CO_2-mediated changes in BFV should reflect changes in CBF. During anesthesia in humans with nitrous oxide/halothane, isoflurane, or fentanyl/midazolam, BFV decreased with a decrease in $PaCO_2$ from 35–25 mm Hg. Patients receiving halogenated anesthetics sustain decreased BFV with hyperventilation. However, if 2.4% isoflurane was given for 15 minutes with hyperventilation to end-tidal CO_2 3.47% (25 mm Hg), one-third of patients sustained a zero end-diastolic velocity. This is not observed at lower doses or with low and high enflurane or halothane.

Responsivity of BFV to changes in $PaCO_2$ has been reported to be a useful indicator of autoregulation. This has not been assessed as a clinical monitoring modality intraoperatively.

Antihypertensive Therapy
There have been few systematic studies on the effects of antihypertensive drugs on TCD. Nitroglycerin (NTG) is an arterial and venous vasodilator that at moderate doses has little effect on resistance vessels. Sublingual administration to humans of 1 mg results in no change in CBF with a concomitant 25% decrease in MCA BFV. Such data suggest that NTG dilates the large, basal cerebral arteries by approximately 15% at the 1-mg dose. Nitroprusside and adenosine vasodilators increase PI and decrease diastolic velocity.

Emergence
Monitoring with TCD during craniotomy has resulted in the observation of frequently increased BFV during the preawakening period. In addition, extubation itself is known to be a hemodynamic stressor. With extubation there is a 356% increase in mean BFV with a decrease in PI to 63% of the preemergence value. This is associated with a MAP increase of 79–107 mm Hg and $PETCO_2$ increase of 29.5–41.0 mm Hg.

Effects of Diseases on Transcranial Doppler Ultrasonography
Intracranial Hypertension
Increases in ICP into the 20- to 30-mm Hg range have not been shown to have substantial physiologic significance. As ICP increases, cerebral vasodilation occurs and adequate CBF is maintained. However, as ICP increases, approaching diastolic arterial pressure and infringing on the critical closing pressure of the cerebral microvasculature, BFV becomes discontinuous, decreasing to zero during diastole (Figure 22.3; see also Figure 22.1). This is consistent with suggestions that systolic increase and diastolic decrease in BFV should occur when ICP reaches the "breakpoint" value. The Gosling Pulsatility Index should be a useful indicator of high ICP. In such situations of zero diastolic flow, ICP should be in the 40- to 60-mm Hg range. Indeed, an ICP of 48 mm Hg is the average level at which patients progressing to brain death have been observed initially to sustain a high-ICP, systolic spike pattern, with the oscillating pattern developing at 62.5 mm Hg. The TCD waveform can reflect ICP encroachment on diastolic flow when ICP exceeds diastolic pressure.

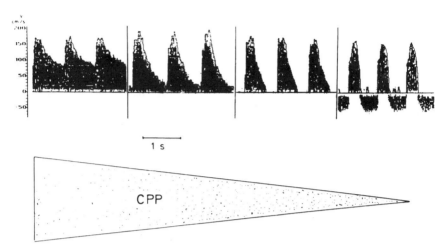

Figure 22.3 Transcranial Doppler reflects cerebral perfusion pressure. Diastolic velocity decreases as cerebral perfusion pressure decreases. As cerebral perfusion pressure continues to decrease blood flow velocity becomes discontinuous, ultimately developing a to-and-fro characteristic as intracranial circulatory arrest arises. (CPP = cerebral perfusion pressure.) *Reproduced with permission from W Hassler, H Steinmetz, J Gawlowski. Transcranial Doppler ultrasonography in raised intracranial pressure and in intracranial circulatory arrest. J Neurosurg 1988;68:745.*

It is of theoretical interest that TCD waveforms might contain information suggesting high ICP that is not high enough to produce zero diastolic velocity. This concept is supported by a reported exponential correlation between ICP and PI. An ICP of 40 mm Hg produced, on average, a PI of about 1.5, the lowest PI at that ICP being approximately 1.3. However, MCA PI has not been correlated with ICP, although a relationship between extracranial carotid flow velocity with ICP can be demonstrated.

When the frequency of this high-ICP waveform was examined with induction of anesthesia in a heterogeneous group of elective neurosurgical patients, none of the patients exhibited the high-ICP waveform with anesthetic induction, suggesting the incidence of dangerous elevations in ICP is less than 1.5% (less than 3.3% in tumor patients). However, there may be a subset of patients (e.g., head trauma patients and those with very large tumors with midline shift, incipient herniation, etc.) in whom such alarming waveforms (zero diastolic velocity) may arise with clinically significant frequency. For routine neurosurgery, TCD probably is not a useful ICP monitor, unless suitable methods are developed to infer moderately increased intracranial pressure (i.e., 20–40 mm Hg).

Despite these observations, there are situations where a high ICP or intracranial circulatory arrest waveform can be falsely positive. TCD pattern in patients with aortic insufficiency can mimic the pattern seen with brain death. Thus, when evaluating TCD waveforms, systemic hemodynamics must be considered.

Head Trauma

Vasospasm was recently detected by TCD in 22% of 30 head-injured patients. Vasospasm was angiographically confirmed and found to correlate with the presence of subarachnoid blood. These data implicate vasospasm as a contributor to low CBF in up to 82% of head trauma patients. Thus, TCD monitoring may be helpful to diagnose the preoperative presence or intraoperative onset of vasospasm and possibly justify or aid in titration of volume-pressor therapy. TCD may also help identify the occurrence of cerebral fat embolism in patients undergoing surgery for orthopedic trauma.

Patients with head injuries occasionally are required to undergo nonneurosurgical procedures when serial neurologic exams are indicated. Transcranial Doppler can be used to supplement other forms of intraoperative neurologic assessments, such as pupil assessment or electrophysiologic monitoring. The development of a high ICP or brain death pattern with progression of a procedure may alter priorities in the care of a patient with multiple trauma. In addition, TCD changes after autoregulatory disruption with head trauma. It may have a role during extracranial surgery in multiply injured head trauma patients. Head trauma patients showed BFV reactivity to changes in $PaCO_2$ of 0–4.63%/mm Hg, with lower reactivity indicating more severe head injury. In this same patient group reactivity to thiopental (5 mg/kg) was also examined. Reactivity to barbiturates (thiopental 5 mg/kg) may also be useful in this patient group in guiding barbiturate treatment of intracranial hypertension; that is, if there is no barbiturate-induced effect there may be no useful role for barbiturate therapy.

TCD ultrasonography has been used for many years as a diagnostic modality outside the acute care setting. However, it has features that make it attractive as a monitor of cerebral hemodynamic function perioperatively. Until very recently there has been a general paucity of information on normal and abnormal BFV responses in anesthetized humans. Technical and knowledge gaps are presently undergoing scrutiny. It is anticipated that with awareness of underlying assumptions, improved TCD monitoring equipment, and increased knowledge, TCD will become a welcome and important added monitor to facilitate care during surgery of patients at risk for cerebrovascular compromise.

KEY REFERENCES

Aaslid R. Transcranial Doppler Sonography. New York: Springer-Verlag, 1986.

Cheng MA et al. The effects of midazolam or sufentanil sedation on middle cerebral artery blood flow velocity in awake patients. J Neurosurg Anesth 1993; 5:232.

Dong M et al. Transcranial Doppler evaluation of anesthetic induction of neurosurgical patients [abstract]. J Neurosurg Anesth 1989,1:153

Eng C et al. The influence of propofol with and without nitrous oxide on cerebral blood flow velocity and CO_2 reactivity in man. Anesth Analg 1992;74:S87.

Halsey JH, McDowell HA, Gelman S. Transcranial Doppler and rCBF compared in carotid endarterectomy. Stroke 1986;17:1206.

Kofke WA et al. Comparison of 3-D Xe CBF, transcranial Doppler, and carotid stump pressure during carotid balloon test occlusion in humans. J Neurosurg Anesth 1991;3:207.

Kofke WA. TCD in Anesthesia. In L Wechsler, V Babikian (eds), Transcranial Doppler Ultrasonography. St. Louis: Mosby, 1992.

Proceedings of the 6th International Symposium and Tutorials on Cerebral Hemodynamics: Transcranial Doppler, Cerebral Blood Flow and Other Modalities. Seattle: The Institute of Applied Physiology and Medicine, 1992.

Shapiro HM. Anesthetic Effects upon Cerebral Blood Flow, Cerebral Metabolism, Electroencephalogram, and Evoked Potentials. In RD Miller (ed), Anesthesia (2nd ed). New York: Churchill Livingstone, 1986;1249–1288.

Steiger HJ. Monitoring for Carotid Surgery. In DW Newell, R Aaslid (eds), Transcranial Doppler. New York: Raven, 1992;197–205.

Wechsler L, Babikian V (eds). Transcranial Doppler Ultrasonography. St. Louis: Mosby, 1992.

Werner C et al. Increase in blood flow velocity in the middle cerebral artery following low-dose ketamine. Anaesth Intens Ther 1989;24:231.

Werner C et al. Sufentanil decreases cerebral blood flow and cerebral blood flow velocity in dogs. J Neurosurg Anesth 1990;2:219.

RECOMMENDED READING

Aggarwal S et al. TCD waveform may predict ICP in patients with fulminant hepatic failure. Stroke 1993;24:508.

Albin MS et al. Intracranail air embolism is detected by transcranial Doppler (TCD) during cardiopulmonary bypass procedures. J Neurosurg Anesth 1990;2:223.

Barzo P et al. Measurements of regional cerebral blood flow and blood flow velocity in experimental intracranial hypertension: Infusion via the cisterna magna in rabbits. Neurosurgery 1991;28:821.

Bass A, et al. Intraoperative transcranial Doppler: Limitations of the method. J Vasc Surg 1989;10:549.

Bernstein EF. Role of transcranial Doppler in carotid surgery. Surg Clin North Am 1990; 70(1):225–234.

Bloom MJ et al. The effects on cerebral blood flow velocity of succinylcholine with and without preservative [abstract]. In Proceedings of the World Congress of Anesthesiologists, 1992.

Dahl A et al. Effect of nitroglycerin on cerebral circulation measured by transcranial Doppler and SPECT. Stroke 1989;20:1733.

Finn JP et al. Impact of vessel distortion on transcranial Doppler velocity measurements: Correlation with magnetic resonance imaging. J Neurosurg 1990;73:572.

Giller CA et al. Cerebral arterial diameters during changes in blood pressure and carbon dioxide during craniotomy. Neurosurgery 1993;32:737.

Giller CA, et al. The transcranial Doppler appearance of acute carotid artery occlusion. Ann Neurol 1992;31:101.

Giller CA. Transcranial Doppler monitoring of cerebral blood flow velocity during craniotomy. Neurosurgery 1989;25:769.

Hillier SC et al. Cerebral hemodynamics in neonates and infants undergoing cardiopulmonary bypass and profound hypothermic circulatory arrest: Assessment by transcranial Doppler sonography. Anesth Analg 1991;72:723.

Kaps M, et al. Transcranial Doppler ultrasound findings in middle cerebral artery occlusion. Stroke 1990;21:532.

Kofke WA et al. Transcranial Doppler ultrasonography with induction of anesthesia for neurosurgery. J Neurosurg Anesth 1994;6:89–97.

Kovarik WD et al. The effect of succinylcholine on intracranial pressure, cerebral blood flow velocity and electroencephalogram in patients with neurologic disorders. J Neurosurg Anesth 1991;3:245.

Lam AM et al. Nitrous oxide is a more potent cerebrovasodilator than isoflurane in humans. J Neurosurg Anesth 1991;3:244.

Lam AM. Change in cerebral blood flow velocity pattern during induced hypotension: A noninvasive indicator of increased intracranial pressure? Br J Anaesth 1992;68:424.

Lewelt W et al. Emergence from anesthesia and cerebral blood flow velocity. J Neurosurg Anesth 1991;3:238.

Lindegaard KF, et al. Evaluation of cerebral AVMs using transcranial Doppler ultrasound. J Neurosurgery 1986;65:335.

Martin NA et al. Posttraumatic cerebral arterial spasm: Transcranial Doppler ultrasound, cerebral blood flow, and angiographic findings. J Neurosurg 1992;77:575.

Minton MD et al. Increases in intracranial pressure from succinylcholine: Prevention by prior nondepolarizing blockade. Anesthesiology 1986;65:165.

Padayachee TS, et al. Monitoring middle cerebral artery blood velocity during carotid endarterectomy. Br J Surg 1986;73:98.

Palmer C et al. Regional cerebral blood flow and glucose utilization during hypothermia in newborn dogs. Anesthesiology 1989;71:730.

Pashayan AG, Mahla ME, Richards RK. Carbon dioxide affects middle cerebral artery blood flow velocity during general anesthesia. Anesthesiology 1991;75:A172.

Piepgras A et al. A simple test to assess cerebrovascular reserve capacity using transcranial Doppler sonography and acetazolamide. Stroke 1990;21:1306.

Piepgras DG et al. Intracerebral hemorrhage after carotid endarterectomy. J Neurosurg 1988;68:532.

Russell GB et al. The hemodynamic effects of extubation in postoperative critical care patients. Anesthesiology 1987;67:A131.

Shaw PJ et al. Early neurological complications of coronary artery bypass surgery. Br Med J 1985;291:1384.

Slee T, et al. Cerebral blood flow velocity following tourniquet release in humans. J Neurosurg Anesth 1990;2:S22.

Spencer MP et al. Detection of middle cerebral artery emboli during carotid endarterectomy using transcranial Doppler ultrasonography. Stroke 1990;21:415.

Spencer MP. Detection of Cerebral Arterial Emboli. In DW Newell, R Aaslid (eds), Transcranial Doppler. New York: Raven, 1992;215–230.

Steiger JH, et al. Results of microsurgical carotid endarterectomy: A prospective study with transcranial Doppler and EEG monitoring, and elective shunting. Acta Neurochir 1989;100:31.

Taylor RH, Burrows FA, Bissonnette B. Cerebral pressure-flow relationship during hypothermic bypass in neonates and infants. Anesth Analg 1992;74:636.

Thiel A et al. Transcranial Doppler sonography: Effects of halothane, enflurane, and isoflurane on blood flow velocity in the middle cerebral artery. Br J Anaesth 1992;68:388.

van der Linden J et al. Cerebral perfusion and metabolism during profound hypothermia in children. A study of middle cerebral artery ultrasonic variables and cerebral extraction of oxygen. J Thorac Cardiovasc Surg 1991;102:103.

Vanelli T, Murkin JM, Lee D. The influence of pH management on mean blood flow velocity in the middle cerebral artery during hypothermic cardiopulmonary bypass [abstract]. Anesthesiology 1991;75:A56.

Young WL et al. The effect of arteriovenous malformation resection on cerebrovascular reactivity to carbon dioxide. Neurosurgery 1990;27:257.

23

Cerebral Oximetry

Jeffry L. Jones, M.D.
Wayne K. Marshall, M.D.

Treatment of brain disorders has become more sophisticated and effective in modern times. Unfortunately, surgical interventions still occur without the ability to fully monitor brain functions. With new developments, we hope to more effectively monitor, diagnose, and treat abnormal cerebral processes. This chapter focuses on one promising technology aimed at cerebral function monitoring—the cerebral oximeter.

CEREBRAL OXIMETRY

Cerebral oximetry has many potential attributes that separate it from other new modalities, such as jugular bulb oximetry and transcranial Doppler. Cerebral oximetry can provide a noninvasive measure of neuronal metabolism. It can be used at the bedside and provides continuous data for more effective patient management. The ability to determine cerebral blood flows and volumes may be developed from this technology as well. By monitoring neuronal metabolic status, appropriate decisions about therapy can be made. Although the technology is not currently available for unrestricted clinical use, this chapter addresses the basic technology involved and how one model was developed.

Neuronal Physiology

To understand the utility of an oximeter, an understanding of neuronal physiology is required. Neurons, like other cell types, rely on oxidative phosphorylation within their mitochondria for energy production. Oxidative phosphorylation accounts for over 95% of the free energy needed to maintain metabolism and impulse formation. Energy is provided in the form of adenosine triphosphate. Neurons rely almost entirely on glucose and oxygen as substrates for energy production. Insufficient supply of either quickly results in neuronal dysfunction and death. Oxygen's primary role is at the end of the electron transport chain. The terminal enzyme in this chain, cytochrome aa3, catalyzes the reaction:

$$O_2 + 4e^- + 4H^+ \rightarrow 2H_2O + \text{free energy} \qquad (1)$$

More than 95% of all oxygen used by the brain is involved in this reaction. Without oxygen, energy is still produced by anaerobic glycolysis. However, this pathway cannot provide sufficient energy to maintain functional neuronal integrity. Therefore, measurement of oxygen availability would give the best indication of brain function by focusing on the cellular metabolic supply and demand.

Technologic Development

Cerebral oximetry, like pulse oximetry, is based on optic spectroscopy. In general, optic spectroscopy involves transmission of light through a medium; components of that medium (chromophores) absorb specific wavelengths of the light. This absorbency can be measured and quantified. However, penetration of light through biologic tissues was a significant problem that previously prevented development of this modality. This problem was solved when near-infrared light was found to penetrate biologic tissues. In 1977, Jobsis applied this technology to cerebral processes specifically. He demonstrated that certain wavelengths within the near-infrared region (range 700–1300 nm) were absorbed by hemoglobin and cytochrome aa3. This exciting discovery opened the door to further development. Initial studies with animals verified that absorption measurements were achievable with near-infrared spectroscopy. As fiberoptic and electronic technology improved, human experiments quickly ensued. From these (human) experiments several algorithms were proposed to transform absorbency spectra into clinically useful, quantifiable data. Three factors determine photon transmission through tissue, on which these algorithms are based: (1) reflectance is mainly a function of the angle at which the photon and tissue meet; (2) absorption is related to the type of chromophores within the medium and varies with wavelength; finally, (3) scattering of photons results in variability of path length, the distance a photon travels from the emitting source to the receiver. Path length determination has become the critical factor in the ability to quantify absorbency.

The Beer-Lambert law relates the absorption of light to specific chromophores and allows them to be quantified. However, it applies only to homogenous mediums that have minimal amounts of scattering. An example of a proposed algorithm based on this law has been provided by Wyatt et al.

$$\text{absorption (O.D.)} = (a \cdot c \cdot L \cdot B) + G \qquad (2)$$

where a = absorption coefficient, c = chromophore concentration, L = distance between entry and exit (path length), B = a path length factor, G = a geometry-dependent factor, and O.D. = optic density. If a, L, and B are measured and G is considered a constant, then the concentration of chromophores can be quantitated from absorption changes by rearranging the equation in the following manner:

$$\Delta[c] = \frac{\Delta O.D.}{(a \cdot L \cdot B)} \qquad (3)$$

Unfortunately, the head is not a homogeneous medium and path length is not easily measured. Therefore, viable quantifications of data have been difficult to achieve. This problem will be addressed later.

OXIMETRIC MODELS

Two basic models of monitors have been developed to provide a basis for near-infrared spectroscopic measurements. The first model performs transcranial measurements. Since near-infrared light can penetrate up to 8 cm, linear transcranial measurements can be made in animals and neonates. Several models of this type have been constructed by researchers. Measurements are usually given in relative amounts of the chromophores. Differences in the various models can involve the source of near-infrared light; the wavelengths used, which affect the mathematic algorithms; and the frequency of light cycling and signal modification.

Despite differences, most transcranial models use similar technology and Beer-Lambert–based algorithms for quantification. Near-infrared light is generated and sent to an emitting source. The source is applied to the skin near the temporal region and transmitted light is detected by a receiver near the contralateral temple. Wyatt and his group constructed a portable device that emits near-infrared light from four laser diodes at wavelengths of 778, 813, 867, and 904 nm. Light detected from the opposite side is transmitted to a photo multiplier tube. This particular oximeter provides quantified measurements based on equation 3. To accomplish this, the path length is assumed to be equal to the distance between the source and the receiver. Concentrations of oxyhemoglobin ($HgbO_2$), reduced hemoglobin (HgbR), and cytochrome (cyt) aa3 are calculated by linear summation with factor multiplication (Figure 23.1). For head diameters greater than 8 cm, the optodes can be positioned orthogonally over the skull in a manner that ensures photon penetration.

The second model of near-infrared–based oximetry has been described by McCormick and his group. This oximeter has several differences distinguishing it from the basic transcranial model. (1) It samples a localized region of the brain. (2) Measurements are provided as regional saturation of the brain. (3) This model can be applied to adults. Somanetics Corp., (Troy, MI) have created a commercial prototype of this oximeter called the INVOS 3100. This oximeter is currently awaiting approval from the Food and Drug Administration (FDA) for nonrestricted clinical use. It measures a regional oxygen saturation (rSO_2) of brain usually taken from the frontal lobe. An incandescent light source is used to generate near-infrared photons. These photons are directed through a lens, which focuses the light through a wavelength filter array. The filter array divides the beam into five discrete wavelength bands at 672, 726, 750, 803, and 840 nm. These bands enter one of three fiberoptic cables. The first is the patient cable, which delivers the bands to the emitter source. The second cable is an auxiliary cable used for research purposes. The third cable is a monitor cable to detect incidental light and assist in system calibration. Light is delivered to each cable simultaneously by microcomputer-controlled timing.

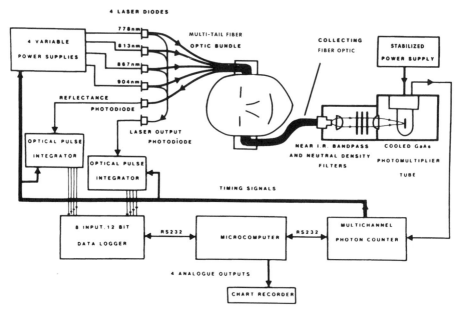

Figure 23.1 The near-infrared spectroscopy system. *Reprinted with permission from DT Delpy et al. Cerebral monitoring in newborn infants by magnetic resonance and near infrared spectroscopy. Scand J Clin Lab Invest 1987; 47(Supp 188):9.*

The monitor cable and receivers are contained in one unit. Source-to-receiver distance is calculated to control the mean path length. From the receiver, the light goes directly to photo detectors, which process the transmitted photons into electronic signals proportional to the detected light intensity. A reference wavelength is used to eliminate the effects of other wavelength attenuations within the system such as interfaces and system gains. The reference wavelength used is the isosbestic point of oxyhemoglobin and reduced hemoglobin—that is, where their optic spectra cross. This occurs at a wavelength of 803 nm (Figure 23.2).

The sampled region is determined by the separation between the source and the receiver. This principle is used to distinguish between superficial and deep structures. Increasing the source-to-receiver distance results in an increase in the path length. Thus, photons penetrate into tissues with more depth and emerge farther from the source. To take advantage of this photon property, two detectors are used, one close to the source and another further away. The close detector samples superficial signals (scalp and skull structures) and the far one samples these as well as those from deeper structures (scalp, skull, and brain). Subtraction of the close detector sample is then made from the far one to give information primarily from brain tissue (Figure 23.3). The separation distances used are 1.0 and 2.7 cm for the close and far detectors, respectively.

The quantification of data measured by this regional oximeter is also different from the techniques used for transcranial oximeters. Instead of

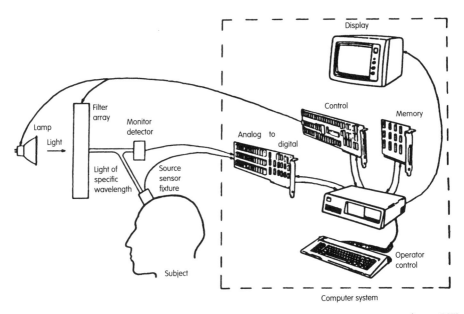

Figure 23.2 The optical spectroscopy unit. *Reprinted with permission from PW McCormick. Noninvasive cerebral spectroscopy for monitoring cerebral oxygen delivery and hemodynamics. Crit Care Med 1991;19:89.*

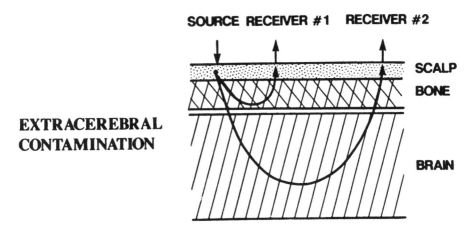

Figure 23.3 The tissue layers propagated by light to reach brain. *Reprinted with permission from PW McCormick, noninvasive cerebral spectroscopy for monitoring cerebral oxygen delivery and hemodynamics. Crit Care Med 1991;19:89.*

attempting to measure definitive values of chromophore concentration, the algorithm relies on a content ratio method of quantification. Content ratios of hemoglobin to oxyhemoglobin are solved from absorption data. These values are proportional to the concentration of the chromophores, but they do not represent actual numbers. When applied over a narrow range of wavelengths, this technique allows path length to be removed from the equations of the Beer-Lambert law and generates quantitative data in the form of hemoglobin oxygen saturation.

Experimental Assessment of Brain Regional Oxygen Saturation Measurement

To test the regional oximeter and the content ratio quantification method, McCormick conducted two studies. In nine neurologically injured, critical care patients, rSO_2 from the oximeter was compared to jugular venous bulb and arterial blood computed saturation measurements. The computed values of the blood samples were obtained with the equation

$$\text{Estimated saturation} = x(SaO_2)+(1-x)(SvO_2) \qquad (4)$$

where x = the percentage of cerebral blood volume that is arterial, SaO_2 = arterial oxygen saturation, and SvO_2 = venous oxygen saturation. Since the exact partitioning of cerebral blood under these conditions is not known, calculations for the extremes of cerebral venous blood percentage (0.72 and 0.82) were made. Sixty-eight simultaneous measurements were taken and the results were correlated with linear regression plots. They found unsatisfactory correlation between the oximeter and computed blood values.

The second experiment was conducted on seven healthy volunteers. Electroencephalographic recordings (19-channel) and rSO_2 measurements from the oximeter were made under hypoxic conditions. The collected data were compared in terms of the time required for each modality to show abnormalities. An abnormal EEG was considered to be onset of theta-delta activity. The first theta-delta burst pattern was marked as the point of EEG-defined hypoxia. The rSO_2 abnormal point was set at 55%. This correlates with an SaO_2 of 90% as calculated from the above equation. The response time of the rSO_2 to hypoxia was significantly shorter when compared to the electroencephalography-based readings.

From the data obtained from the first study, it was apparent to the evaluators that the correlation between the oximeter rSO_2 and the calculated rSO_2 was not close enough to ensure that they were measuring identical phenomena. However, from the hypoxia study, McCormick concluded that this oximeter was at least as sensitive in detecting hypoxia as an EEG. Because of this ability, the oximeter was advocated as a viable clinical tool even if the accuracy is limited. This conclusion was also supported by a study evaluating the response of a similar oximeter mode 1 compared to four-channel EEG during periods of arrhythmia and hypotension in five patients undergoing insertion of an automatic internal cardioversion defibrillator. The oximeter proved to be a more sensitive indicator of reduced cerebral perfusion. Based in part on these findings, development of this oximeter model continued.

POINTS OF CONFLICT

Even though near-infrared spectroscopy has made great strides toward becoming a clinical monitor, persistent problems with this technology may affect future use. More specific concerns regarding the measurement of intracerebral parameters have been raised. These include:

1. Path length. (a) The actual path length of light with near-infrared spectroscopy is difficult to measure and, in most quantitative calculations, is assumed to be equal to the source-to-receiver distance. The path length is a factor required to quantify absorption spectra when the Beer-Lambert principle is applied. An inaccurate path length measurement leads to erroneous quantitative data. (b) In some algorithms it is assumed that the brain is a homogenous scattering medium. In this type of medium, path length can be considered a constant factor. Again, to apply the Beer-Lambert law, this assumption must be made. However, one study suggests that this assumption is incorrect. Piglets were subjected to various physiologic conditions and the rSO_2 and sagittal sinus SO_2 were measured. Path length was measured by phase-modulated spectroscopy to provide an accurate rSO_2. A linear relationship was shown when rSO_2 was plotted against sagittal sinus SO_2, but the slope and intercept varied. In addition, the path length varied among the seven piglets. Therefore, quantification algorithms based on population studies within the same species would be inaccurate.

2. Chromophore sample. Although the ability to measure cytochrome aa3 exists with near-infrared spectroscopy, it is difficult to do because (a) cytochrome aa3 has a broad spectrum that overlaps with hemoglobin's spectra, and (b) hemoglobin has a significantly greater presence than cytochrome aa3. Hemoglobin may account for most of the absorption readings and obscure the effect of cytochrome aa3.

3. Sample size. Both oximeter models sample only portions of the brain. Although this incomplete sampling may be adequate for most situations, cerebral oximetry does not give global cerebral metabolic information, which can be obtained with jugular venous bulb saturation monitoring.

4. Cerebral blood partitioning. The normal partitioning of venous, arterial, and capillary blood is known. However, under abnormal states that disrupt blood vessels and the blood-brain barrier, this may vary. Accurate quantification of rSO_2 may provide data that is difficult to interpret. For example, a normal rSO_2 reading may represent an increased cerebral arterial contribution with inadequate oxygen availability at the neuronal level.

5. Debates about accuracy. Two studies have raised questions about the ability of rSO_2 to accurately measure brain oxygenation. A comparison was made to jugular bulb oximetry in nine patients undergoing elective cardiac

surgery with cardiopulmonary bypass. Both saturations were plotted against jugular bulb venous blood sample saturations taken simultaneously. The rSO_2 was found to be less accurate and precise than the jugular bulb oximeter. Possible explanations given include (a) the regional information provided rSO_2 may be inferior to the global information detected by the jugular bulb oximeter, and (b) the partition ratio of cerebral blood under cardiopulmonary bypass may be altered. If this occurs, the venous component may decrease, leading to a detected saturation that is more reflective of the arterial component.

The optode separation of the regional oximeter may lead to inaccurate brain sampling. Ten patients were evaluated to assess optode separation used for rSO_2 measurement. Cerebral oximetry was compared to middle cerebral artery (MCA) Doppler velocity while pCO_2 increased and a constant oxygen consumption was maintained. As the MCA velocity increased, the rSO_2 did not change significantly. Since the rSO_2 does respond to an increased SaO_2, it was concluded that rSO_2 might be primarily measuring external carotid flow. To verify this conclusion, they used a more powerful oximeter and gradually increased the optode distance. The changes expected in rSO_2 occurred with hypercapnia as the optode separation increased. It was recommended that a wider optode separation and a stronger oximeter were needed for accurate clinical measurements.

Near-infrared spectroscopy is a viable technology for evaluating and monitoring cerebral oxygen utilization. It can provide a noninvasive ability to measure neuronal metabolic demand. Continuous data can be obtained at the bedside to enable clinical decisions to be made more rapidly. The technology has been safely applied to other clinical uses. There is also the potential to determine cerebral flows and volumes. By giving physicians the ability to quickly diagnose and intervene appropriately, cerebral oximetry can lead to improved outcomes.

Before these gains can be made, several problems with this technology must be resolved. For transcranial oximetry we need to have more accurate determination of path length to apply the Beer-Lambert principle. It is uncertain as yet whether the promise of this technology will be realized.

KEY REFERENCES

Brazy JE. Cerebral oxygen monitoring with near–infrared spectroscopy: Clinical application to neonates. J Clin Monit 1991; 7:325. *Reviews near-infrared spectroscopy and its potential application to neonates.*

Harris DNF, Bailey SM. Near-infrared spectroscopy in adults. Anaesthesia 1993;48:694. *A critical assessment suggests that wider optode spacing and more power in the monitor may improve accuracy.*

McCormick PW et al. Noninvasive cerebral optical spectroscopy for monitoring cerebral oxygen delivery and hemodynamics. Crit Care Med 1991;19:89. *Cerebral oximetry demonstrated good in vitro correlation with a reference technique (co-oximeter). The mathematical calculations used are discussed in the appendix.*

RECOMMENDED READING

Brown R, Wright G, Royston D. A comparison of two systems for assessing cerebral venous oxyhemoglobin saturation during cardiopulmonary bypass in humans. Anaesthesia 1993;48:697.

Jobsis FF. Noninvasive, infrared monitoring of cerebral and myocardial oxygen sufficiency and circulatory parameters. Science 1977;198:1264.

Kurth CD et al. Near-infrared monitoring of the cerebral circulation. J Clin Monit 1993;9:163.

McCormick PW et al. Regional cerebrovascular oxygen saturation by optical spectroscopy in humans. Stroke 1991;22:597.

Smith DS et al. Reperfusion hyperoxia in brain after circulatory arrest in humans. Anesthesiology 1990;73:12.

Wyatt JS et al. Quantification of cerebral blood volume in human infants by near-infrared spectroscopy. J Appl Physiol 1990;68:1086.

Wyatt JS et al. Quantification of cerebral oxygenation and hemodynamics in sick newborn infants by near–infrared spectrophotometry. Lancet 1986;2:1063.

24

Arterial-Jugular Oxygen Difference

Terri W. Blackburn, M.D.
Garfield B. Russell, M.D., FRCPC

The brain has an amazing ability to autoregulate its blood flow. The normal brain maintains cerebral blood flow (CBF) at a constant rate, approximately 54 ml/100 g/minute, over wide variations (from 50–150 mm Hg) in mean systemic arterial blood pressure, The normal brain regulates blood to different areas based on the need for metabolic substrates such as oxygen and glucose; that is, there is coupling of CBF and the cerebral metabolic rate of oxygen ($CMRO_2$). Gray matter, which needs more of these substrates, receives 64 ml/100 g/minute, while white matter, which needs fewer substrates, receives 15–20 ml/100 g/minute. Blood flow also varies in different regions of the brain depending on activity or metabolic requirements at a given time. Again, this is coupling of CBF and $CMRO_2$. The $CMRO_2$ for the total brain at rest is 3.4 ml O_2/100 g/minute.

When the brain is traumatized, whether from direct head injury, an intracranial hemorrhage, or tumor invasion, its ability to autoregulate CBF is altered, and in severe head injury resulting in coma, $CMRO_2$ is decreased. In these circumstances one can expect to see one of three responses to the injury: (1) hyperemia, either relative or absolute, (2) retained coupling of CBF and $CMRO_2$, or (3) ischemia. It would be advantageous in the management of these patients if they could be easily classified into a particular type of altered blood flow pattern.

FICK PRINCIPLE

The Fick principle, developed by Adolfo Fick in the last part of the nineteenth century, is a restatement of the law of conservation of mass used in making indirect measurements. Here it is used to describe the relationship between the $CMRO_2$ and CBF based on the cerebral arteriovenous difference of oxygen content ($AVDO_2$)—that is, $AVDO_2 = CMRO_2/CBF$. $AVDO_2$ is also determined by the equation

$$AVDO_2 = \text{hemoglobin concentration} \times 1.39 \times$$
$$(\text{arterial} - \text{jugular venous } O_2 \text{ saturation})$$

The jugular venous O_2 saturation ($SjvO_2$) can be obtained by intermittent sampling of blood from the jugular bulb or, more recently, by continuous $SjvO_2$ monitoring by a fiberoptic catheter inserted into the jugular bulb.

We will first review a technique for placing a fiberoptic catheter for continuous $SjvO_2$ monitoring, then we will examine how $SjvO_2$ and $AVDO_2$ can assist in managing patients with head injury.

JUGULAR BULB CANNULATION
The Fiberoptic Catheter System

Continuous in vivo monitoring of oxyhemoglobin saturation (SO_2) is performed by a catheter using the principle of reflection spectrophotometry. A system to perform this function presently consists of three components: a fiberoptic catheter that contains two plastic optical fibers, an optical module, and a computer. A 40-cm catheter is recommended for $SjvO_2$ monitoring. The optical module transmits light through one of the optical fibers to the blood. Light reflected from the blood is collected by the second optical fiber and transmitted back through the catheter to the optical module. The module then converts the light to electrical signals, amplifies these signals, and transmits these signals to the computer. The computer is then able to calculate SO_2 values based on these electrical signals.

Jugular Bulb Cannulation Technique

Placement of the fiberoptic catheter for continuous $SjvO_2$ monitoring should begin with analysis of the clinical picture and disease process. Typically, the right internal jugular vein (IJ) is larger than the left and is believed to drain most of the blood from the cerebral hemispheres while the left drains most of the blood from the posterior fossa. The jugular bulb is the bulbous dilation of the jugular vein that contains cerebral venous blood just below the base of the skull. In normal brain, the $SjvO_2$ is approximately equal on the right and the left. During a pathologic process, $SjvO_2$ may vary depending on changes in CBF and $CMRO_2$ in diseased areas; therefore, monitoring should be performed, if possible, on the side predominantly draining the injured area. If intracranial pressure (ICP) is being monitored, this can be determined by positioning the patient in a 10- to 15-degree head-up tilt and alternatively occluding each IJ looking for the side with the greatest ICP change with occlusion. If the maximum change in ICP is the same or the ICP is not being monitored, then the catheter can be placed on the side of the predominant lesion as determined by computerized tomography (CT), or in diffuse injury, on the right side. In a patient with a right temporal lobe hemorrhage, for example, the catheter should be placed in the right IJ to evaluate the changes in oxygen supply and demand in this area.

Once the side is chosen, the patient is positioned flat (as long as the ICP is less than 20 mm Hg) with the head turned away from the side to be cannulated

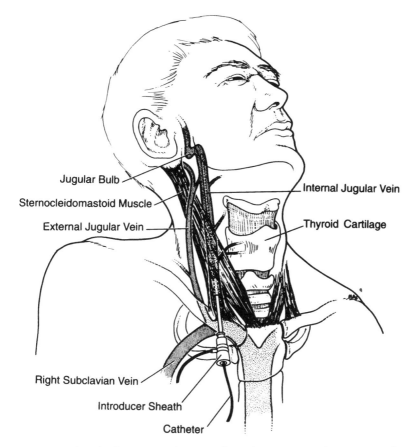

Figure 24.1 Landmarks for retrograde internal jugular vein cannulation. Note the tip of the catheter resting in the jugular bulb after correct placement of the catheter.

(Figure 24.1). The neck is prepped with an antiseptic solution from the level of the mastoid process to the upper thorax. The carotid artery is palpated on the appropriate side medial to the sternocleidomastoid muscle at the level of the inferior border of the thyroid cartilage.

After infiltration with local anesthetic, the IJ is cannulated percutaneously just lateral to the carotid pulsation by advancing a needle from this point toward the external auditory meatus. After cannulation, a 5-French introducer or a 4.5-French peel-away introducer is placed using a Seldinger technique and flushed with saline. A preinsertion calibration of the fiberoptic catheter is performed and the catheter is placed through the introducer into the IJ and threaded until the tip is felt to abut the base of the skull or 15 cm of catheter has been inserted. The introducer is withdrawn or peeled away carefully and the catheter is sutured into place. The position of the catheter is checked radiologically to verify optimal position of the catheter tip in the jugular bulb, above the lower border of the first cervical vertebra (C1), and to detect kinks in the catheter. It is important to position the catheter correctly to minimize contamination from extracranial vessels.

Continuous Jugular Venous Oxygen Saturation Monitoring: Contraindications and Complications

Contraindications to jugular venous bulb cannulation are (1) bleeding diathesis, (2) local infection, (3) local neck trauma, or (4) any significant impairment to cerebral venous drainage. Sepsis and a hypercoagulable state are relative contraindications for catheter placement as the catheter could serve as a focal point for septic or bland thrombus formation. Once the catheter is in position, it is recommended that the system be recalibrated every 12 hours to maintain close agreement between the fiberoptic measurement of $SjvO_2$ and the co-oximeter measurement of $SjvO_2$.

Complications of catheter insertion include (1) carotid cannulation, (2) coiling of the catheter in the jugular vein, (3) decreased cerebral perfusion pressure secondary to increased intracranial pressure from decreased venous return, (4) infection, and (5) bleeding.

JUGULAR VENOUS OXYGEN SATURATION

If arterial blood is fully saturated, then normal $SjvO_2$ is 54–75%. $SjvO_2$ can be used as a rough guide to assess oxygen delivery to the brain. Continuous $SjvO_2$ monitoring is more beneficial than intermittent monitoring because it allows differentiation between rapid fluctuations in $SjvO_2$ caused by routine procedures in anesthesia and intensive care unit care, such as endotracheal tube suctioning, and prolonged desaturations that are more representative of pathophysiologic sequelae. Once a clinically significant desaturation has been detected, the goal is to determine the cause of the desaturation and to reverse the change.

Uses of Jugular Venous Oxygen Saturation

An algorithm for evaluating desaturations in $SjvO_2$ has been previously described and assists in patient evaluation (Figure 24.2). First the accuracy of the $SjvO_2$ change should be ascertained. In one study, almost half of the decreases in $SjvO_2$ recorded were the result of monitoring errors. Since the catheter is positioned facing the flow of blood, it is often pushed against the wall of the vessel or looped in the vessel. Also, movement of the head can cause the catheter to abut the vessel as it exits the cranium. This problem is readily identified by a decrease in the light intensity reading for the catheter. Light intensity is represented by a lighted bar on the display monitor and is updated every 5 seconds. If the light intensity reading is accurate, then a co-oximeter measurement of the $SjvO_2$ is suggested to verify the accuracy of the catheter. This is a quick and easy measurement to obtain and can prevent unnecessary and possibly dangerous therapeutic maneu-

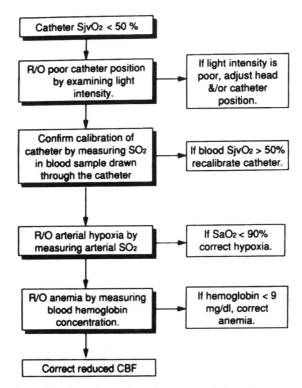

Figure 24.2 Algorithm for diagnosing the cause of jugular venous desaturations. ($SjvO_2$ = jugular venous oxygen saturation; R/O = rule out; SO_2 = oxyhemoglobin saturation; SaO_2 = arterial oxygen saturation; CBF = cerebral blood flow.) *Reprinted with permission from M Sheinberg et al. Continuous monitoring of jugular venous oxygen saturation in head-injured patients. J Neurosurg 1992;76:212.*

vers if it is discovered that an abnormal $SjvO_2$ is the result of a drift in the fiberoptic system causing incorrect readings. Once it is proven that the change in $SjvO_2$ is accurate, the cause must be ascertained. If systemic hypotension exists, then cerebral perfusion pressure (CPP) is probably decreased and the brain, although extracting the same total amount of oxygen, is extracting more oxygen from a given amount of blood. The extraction fraction is increased. If blood pressure is unchanged, an arterial blood gas is obtained. Systemic hypoxemia also causes the $SjvO_2$ to drop, even though the amount of oxygen extracted from the blood is unchanged. Hypocapnia can result in a decrease in $SjvO_2$ by causing vasoconstriction and decreased blood flow to the brain. If neither hypoxemia nor hypocapnia is found, then a blood hemoglobin assessment is needed to look for acute anemia. Anemia also causes a decrease in $SjvO_2$ by causing an increase in the extraction fraction of oxygen in an attempt to maintain oxygen delivery. If all of these measurements are unchanged from before a drop in $SjvO_2$ was detected, then the probable cause of the desaturation is a drop in CBF and measures to increase CBF should be instituted.

Of course, some of the steps of the algorithm can be performed in conjunction with each other, and the order can be changed depending on clinical suspicion. Consider a motor vehicle accident victim with multiple injuries, including head trauma resulting in coma and a splenic laceration being treated conservatively by following serial hematocrits. During routine suctioning of the endotracheal tube, the patient develops a severe coughing spell. Both the systemic arterial saturation (SaO_2) and the $SjvO_2$ decrease; however, 20 minutes later the SaO_2 returns to normal while the $SjvO_2$, which initially returned to baseline, begins to slowly drift downward. The light intensity is quickly evaluated while the trend of systemic blood pressure is reviewed. If these are unchanged then a blood hemoglobin is obtained to look for a sudden drop in hemoglobin secondary to an acute bleed from the splenic laceration.

Limitations of Jugular Venous Oxygen Saturation

There are some shortcomings to monitoring $SjvO_2$. (1) As mentioned above, monitoring errors are very common. The catheter is easily pushed against the wall of the vessel or made to coil back on itself in the vessel by the flow of blood. These problems are usually easily identified by checking the light intensity value of the fiberoptic catheter and by obtaining co-oximeter measurements to verify the readings obtained by the catheter. (2) In the setting of respiratory alkalosis, the $SjvO_2$ may be normal even when tissue oxygen delivery is compromised. The oxyhemoglobin dissociation curve is shifted to the left so that a normal $SjvO_2$ saturation is maintained even though oxygen partial pressure (pO_2) is low. This is detected by obtaining an abnormally low jugular bulb pO_2 (pO_2 less than 27 mm Hg). (3) Inadequate perfusion of the cerebellum, brain stem, or both is usually not detected by $SjvO_2$ monitoring because the posterior circulation blood flow contributes insignificantly to the jugular bulb outflow. Therefore, continuous $SjvO_2$ monitoring would be of little use in a patient with a brain stem hemorrhage. (4) A subpopulation of patients with intracranial hypertension will not demonstrate a decrease in $SjvO_2$ until after neurologic signs of tentorial herniation are observed. A possible reason for this phenomenon is that global CBF is preserved when the brain stem is selectively compressed or that as CBF drops to very low levels, extracerebral contamination of jugular venous blood may increase proportionally and therefore obscure the true saturation of cerebral venous blood. Other measures can be used to help predict the patients in this subpopulation, as discussed next.

ARTERIOVENOUS DIFFERENCE OF OXYGEN CONTENT

As mentioned earlier, $AVDO_2$ is a calculated number obtained using hemoglobin and arterial and jugular venous oxygen saturation, as in $AVDO_2$ = Hb conc $\times$ 1.39 $\times$ (arterial– jugular venous O_2 sat%), and $AVDO_2$ = $CMRO_2$/CBF.

Normal adult $AVDO_2$ is 4–8 ml O_2/100 ml blood. Because $CMRO_2$ is decreased and relatively stable in comatose head trauma patients, $AVDO_2$ is a

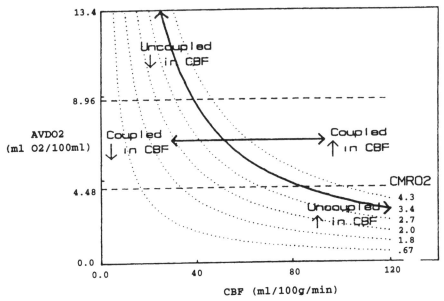

Figure 24.3 Relationship between AVDO$_2$ and CBF. If the CMRO$_2$ and CBF remain coupled, then AVDO$_2$ remains constant and the AVDO$_2$/CBF curve is shifted to the right or left (horizontal arrows). If CMRO$_2$ remains constant, as it does in severe head injury resulting in coma, then changes in AVDO$_2$ reflect uncoupled changes in CBF (curved arrows). Hypoperfusion is demonstrated by a high AVDO$_2$ and low CBF (uncoupled decrease in CBF) except in cases where the hypoperfusion is severe enough to cause ischemia and/or infarction. Then AVDO$_2$ drops and CBF remains low. Hyperemia is demonstrated by a low AVDO$_2$ and high CBF (uncoupled increase in CBF). (AVDO$_2$ = arteriovenous oxygen difference; CBF = cerebral blood flow; CMRO$_2$ = cerebral metabolic rate of oxygen.) *Modified and reprinted with permission from CS Robertson et al. Cerebral arteriovenous oxygen difference as an estimate of cerebral blood flow in comatose patients. J Neurosurg 1989; 70:222.*

good measure of CBF (see Figure 24.3). Therefore, AVDO$_2$ can be used to assess the effects of therapeutic maneuvers such as diuresis, barbiturate therapy, ventilation adjustments, and systemic hypertension on the CBF/CMRO$_2$ ratio.

Use of Arteriovenous Difference of Oxygen Content

Diuresis is almost universally effective in improving the CBF/CMRO$_2$ ratio in the setting of increased ICP. Barbiturate therapy to reduce ICP and improve the CBF/CMRO$_2$ ratio has a variable response. The patients most likely to demonstrate a clinical benefit from barbiturate therapy are those with a low AVDO$_2$ that increases to normal when barbiturates are started. Barbiturates act primarily as a vasoconstrictor to regulate CBF in this setting rather than decreasing metabolic activity. If ventilation is increased in an effort to decrease ICP, vasoconstriction from hypocapnia may be so great as to decrease CBF below what is required to deliver enough oxygen to match or exceed the $CMRO_2$, and $AVDO_2$ increases. (When calculating $AVDO_2$, a 3% increase should be added to the $AVDO_2$ for each mm Hg decrease in $PaCO_2$ in an effort to avoid hyperventilation causing hypocapnia severe enough to cause ischemia.) Systemic hypertension may be used to increase CPP. The appropriateness of this therapy would be indicated by a drop in $AVDO_2$. $AVDO_2$ can assist as well in sorting out the overall clinical effect of combining the above therapeutic maneuvers.

The intraoperative use of $SjvO_2$ and $AVDO_2$ has not been extensively studied. It could be useful for titration of hyperventilation or arterial hypotension with or without ICP monitoring, and also for evaluating the effect of a particular anesthetic technique on the $CBF/CMRO_2$ ratio.

Limitations of Arteriovenous Difference of Oxygen Content

$AVDO_2$ monitoring is not without shortcomings, although many of these are eliminated if the lactate-oxygen index (LOI), discussed next, is monitored. First, since $AVDO_2$ is a global cerebral monitor, it may not reflect small regional flow changes, allowing some ischemic injuries to go undetected. For example, small variations in blood flow around an initial injury may go unnoticed, allowing an increase in the size of the ischemic penumbral zone and thus an increase in secondary brain damage. Second, acute anemia causing ischemia may be missed if the clinician is following $AVDO_2$ measurements only. This problem is alleviated if continuous $SjvO_2$ monitoring is used in conjunction with $AVDO_2$ and the algorithm of evaluating a decrease in $SjvO_2$ is followed.

LACTATE OXYGEN INDEX

The $AVDO_2$ can be misleading if used by itself to detect impending global cerebral ischemia or ischemia prior to neurologic injury. $AVDO_2$ should continue to increase as oxygen demand exceeds oxygen supply in the ischemic pattern; however, it has been demonstrated that the $AVDO_2$ is variable during cerebral ischemia and infarction. As oxygen supply decreases below what is needed to fully meet the demand, anaerobic metabolism and lactate production increase. Ischemia and infarction can be reliably identified if the $AVDO_2$ measurements are supplemented by the LOI.

The LOI is a measure of the ratio of the amount of glucose metabolized anaerobically to the amount metabolized aerobically; that is,

$$LOI = - (arterial - jugular\ venous\ difference\ of\ lactate)/AVDO_2$$

Elevated production of lactate by the brain is indicated by an increase in the LOI. As long as the LOI is less than 0.08, a normal $AVDO_2$ would indicate that CBF is in excess of $CMRO_2$, and an elevated $AVDO_2$ would indicate a decreased CBF. If LOI is greater than or equal to 0.08, then $AVDO_2$ is unreliable as an indicator of the adequacy of CBF, and one should consider methods to

Table 24.1 Classification of Cerebral Blood Flow Abnormalities from Arteriovenous Difference of Oxygen Content and Arterial-Jugular Venous Difference of Lactate

Classification	$AVDO_2$ (ml O_2/100 ml blood)	LOI	CBF (ml/100 g/min)	$CMRO_2$ (ml/100 g/min)
Nonischemic patterns		<0.08		
Hyperemia	<2.9		52.9±18.1	1.95±0.18
Normal CBF	2.9–6.7		41.6±12.4	1.84±0.49
Compensated hypoperfusion	>6.7		23.4±6.9	1.88±0.40
Ischemia-infarction	Variable	≥0.08	33.8±20	1.10±0.67

$AVDO_2$ = arteriovenous oxygen difference; AVDL = arterial jugular venous difference of lactate; LOI = lactate-oxygen index; CBF = cerebral blood flow; $CMRO_2$ = cerebral metabolic rate of oxygen.
Source: Modified from CS Robertson et al. Cerebral arteriovenous oxygen difference as an estimate of cerebral blood flow in comatose patients. J Neurosurg 1989;70:222.

increase CBF in an effort to reverse ischemia. Three nonischemic patterns of CBF and one ischemic or infarction pattern of CBF can be identified using the $AVDO_2$ supplemented by the LOI (Table 24.1).

In nonischemic patterns, LOI is less than 0.08. If CBF is above normal, a state of absolute hyperemia exists and $AVDO_2$ is very low—less than 2.9 ml O_2/100 ml blood. (Almost all comatose head-injured patients have a decreased $CMRO_2$.) Hyperventilation to induce hypocapnia may be most effective in this setting. Barbiturates might also be effective. If CBF is normal but still relatively greater than $CMRO_2$, then a state of relative hyperemia exists and $AVDO_2$ is still low, but not as low, 2.9–6.7 ml O_2/100 ml blood. Again, barbiturates may be an effective therapy. If CBF is reduced to correlate with $CMRO_2$, then a state of compensated hypoperfusion exists and $AVDO_2$ is normal, greater than 6.7 ml O_2/100 ml blood. In the ischemic-infarction pattern, anaerobic metabolism of glucose is present and $AVDO_2$ is variable; the LOI greater than or equal to 0.08 may be the only evidence that ischemia is present.

ILLUSTRATIVE CASE

A 32-year-old previously healthy patient was admitted to the surgical intensive care unit in a coma after falling 30 feet off construction scaffolding. The patient had an oral endotracheal tube placed in the field for airway protection and mechanical ventilation was continued in the hospital. After initial stabilization, he was taken to radiology for a CT scan and found to have a right frontal intraparenchymal hemorrhage and a pelvic fracture. After the patient had been in the unit for 3 hours, his right pupil began to dilate. Mannitol was given and he was immediately taken back to radiology for a repeat CT scan. The repeat scan demonstrated cerebral edema with a midline shift, but no collection of blood or fluid. The patient was returned to the unit, an ICP monitor was placed, and the right jugular bulb was cannulated with a fiberoptic catheter.

Initially, the patient had an ICP of 30 mm Hg, an $SjvO_2$ of 65%, an $AVDO_2$ of 5.23 ml O_2/100 ml blood, an arterial saturation of 98%, and hemoglobin (Hb) of 11.4 g/dL. The LOI was 0.02. Hyperventilation was instituted in an attempt to decrease the relative hyperemia and thereby reduce the ICP and increase the CPP. The patient responded well to hyperventilation and diuretics; his ICP decreased to 12 mm Hg and his right pupil returned to normal. Over the next 2 hours, the $SjvO_2$ slowly decreased to 40%, then abruptly increased to 90%. The $AVDO_2$ now was 1.31 ml O_2/100 ml blood (Hb = 11.8) and the LOI was 0.098. An arterial blood gas assessment revealed a partial pressure of carbon dioxide ($PaCO_2$) of 16 mm Hg. Ventilation was decreased to allow the $PaCO_2$ to rise to 28 mm Hg. With moderate hypocapnia, the $SjvO_2$ returned to 50% with an $AVDO_2$ of 7.87. Since the mean systemic blood pressure was only 70 mm Hg, dopamine was started to increase the CPP by increasing the blood pressure. With a mean blood pressure of 95 mm Hg, the $SjvO_2$ increased to 60% and the $AVDO_2$ decreased to 6.23. Over the next few days, the dopamine was weaned off and the $PaCO_2$ was allowed to normalize. No change was noted in the ICP or $SjvO_2$ with these measures. A repeat CT scan demonstrated significant reduction in the cerebral edema and resolution of the midline shift.

$SjvO_2$ and $AVDO_2$ monitoring have the potential to become very useful modalities in analyzing the relationship between oxygen supply and demand in the brain and allowing sound clinical decisions concerning therapy to be made. However, they both continue to have limitations and, so far, our choice of therapeutic maneuvers has not been expanded. Their usefulness to the anesthesiologist intraoperatively has not been fully evaluated, although this may be a prime area for further research.

KEY REFERENCES

Robertson CS, Narayan RK, Gokaslan ZL et al. Cerebral arteriovenous oxygen difference as an estimate of cerebral blood flow in comatose patients. J Neurosurg 1989;70:222. *This is an excellent study of $AVDO_2$ as an estimate of the $CMRO_2$/CBF ratio in patients with severe head injury resulting in coma. Based on previous studies, $CMRO_2$ is assumed to be constant and decreased in patients with severe head injuries, and therefore, $AVDO_2$ can be used to predict CBF. It also defines situations in which $AVDO_2$ is an unreliable predictor of CBF and explains how AVDL can indicate the presence of ischemia or infarction in those situations.*
Sheinberg M, Kanter MJ, Robertson CS et al. Continuous monitoring of jugular venous oxygen saturation in head-injured patients. J Neurosurg 1992;76:212. *Discusses continuous monitoring of $SjvO_2$ (utilizing a fiberoptic system) to detect jugular venous desaturations. Introduces an algorithm to diagnose the cause of these desaturations so that appropriate therapy can be instituted quickly.*

RECOMMENDED READINGS

Andrews PJD, Dearden NM, Miller JD. Jugular bulb cannulation: Description of a cannulation technique and validation of a new continuous monitor. Br J Anaesth 1991;67:553. *Describes jugular bulb cannulation and compares continuous in vivo* *measurement of oxyhemoglobin using a fiberoptic catheter with intermittent in vitro co-oximeter measurement of hemoglobin saturation. The authors also briefly discuss treatment based on results obtained through continuous SjvO$_2$ monitoring.*

Dearden NM. Jugular bulb venous oxygen saturation in the management of severe head injury. Curr Opin Anaesthesiol 1991;4:279. *This is an excellent review of the use of SjvO$_2$ and AVDO$_2$ as a guide in managing patients with severe head injury.*

Obrist WD, Langfitt TW, Jaggi JL et al. Cerebral blood flow and metabolism in comatose patients with acute head injury. J Neurosurg 1984;61:241. *This study demonstrates that normal coupling of CBF and CMRO$_2$ is retained in only 45% of comatose head-injured patients and that all patients in coma had a significant depression in CMRO$_2$.*

25

A Guide to Intraoperative Neurophysiologic Monitoring: Recommended Techniques and Protocols

Mary C. Schwentker, B.S.

This is a short, user-friendly guide to neurophysiologic monitoring programs for the operating room. This section should be valuable in the development of new programs and modification of practicing programs for the operating room. It should also be quite helpful in troubleshooting. It is important to remember that neuromonitoring for the operating room is a developing field, and state-of-the-art methods and procedures will continue to change. We have found many of these techniques and protocols functional and practical. They are not meant to be all-inclusive or exclusionary in their scope.

AUDITORY EVOKED RESPONSES

Recording Montage

	(+)	(−)
Ch 1	CZ	A1
Ch 2	CZ	A2
Ch 3	A1	A2
Ch 4	CZ	CV1 (CV = cervical vertebrae)

Stimulation

Rate: 11.1–21.1 Hz
Duration: 0.2 ms
Type: alternating click

Intensity: click, 100 db test ear; masking noise, 70 db contralateral ear

Test Parameters

Filters: 100–1,500 Hz
Sweep window: 12 ms
Total number of sweeps: 2,000–3,000

Measure

Waves I, III, and V
Normal latency with ear inserts
Wave I: 2.3–2.5 ms
Wave III: 3.3–3.5 ms
Wave V: 5.5–6 ms
(There is usually a large negative drop after wave V.)

Significant Changes

1. 50% reduction in amplitude
2. More than 1-ms increase in latency compared to baseline

MEDIAN AND ULNAR NERVE SOMATOSENSORY EVOKED POTENTIAL

Recording Montage

	(+)	(−)
Ch 1	FPZ	CP3
Ch 2	FPZ	CP4
Ch 3	FPZ	CV5 (CV = cervical vertebra)
Ch 4	LT ERBs	RT ERBs

Stimulation

Rate: 4.7 Hz
Duration: 0.2 ms
Intensity: 15–25 mA

Test Parameters

Filters: 30–3,000 Hz
Sweep window: 60 ms
Total number of sweeps: 300

Significant Changes

1. A latency increase of more than 10% of baseline
2. A 60% reduction in amplitude from baseline

LOWER-LIMB SOMATOSENSORY EVOKED POTENTIALS

Recording Montage

	(+)	(−)
Ch 1	FPZ	CPZ
Ch 2	CP3	CP4
Ch 3	FPZ	CV7 (CV = cervical vertebra)
Ch 4	LT popliteal fossa (2 electrodes)	
Ch 5	RT popliteal fossa (2 electrodes)	

Stimulation

Stimulation sites:
1. Posterior tibial nerve
2. Common peroneal nerve
3. Sciatic nerve

Rate: 4.7 Hz
Duration: 0.2 ms
Intensity: 15–25 mA

Test Parameters

Filters: 30–3,000 Hz
Sweep window: 80 ms
Total number of sweeps: 500

Significant Changes

1. Increase in latency more than 10% of baseline
2. A 60% reduction in amplitude from baseline

NEUROGENIC MOTOR EVOKED POTENTIALS

Recording Montage

Ch 1   Left popliteal fossa (2 electrodes) distal (+)
Ch 2   Right popliteal fossa (2 electrodes) distal (+)

Stimulation

Stimulating electrodes are placed in two adjacent spinous processes with the anode (+ red) cephalad.

Rate: 4.7 Hz
Duration: 0.3 ms
Intensity: start at 100 V; increase until response is present; do not exceed 400 V.

Test Parameters

Filters: 10–2,000 Hz
Sweep window: 50 ms
Total number of sweeps: less than 100

Significant Changes

1. A latency increase of more than 10% of baseline
2. A 60% reduction in amplitude from baseline

MONITORING FOR TETHERED SPINAL CORD SURGERY

Free-Run Tethered Cord Monitoring

The muscle groups wired depend on which region of the spine the surgeon is working on. The muscles we most commonly monitor are the quadriceps, hamstrings, anterior tibialis, and anal sphincter, typically recording seven channels. Two needle electrodes are placed for each muscle being monitored. These electrodes are plugged into the recording channels of the instrument. One electrode is placed just beneath the skin (+); the other is placed about 4 cm away into the belly of the muscle (–). A commercially available anal sponge electrode is used to monitor the sphincter muscle. A grounding pad is placed on the buttocks.

Test Parameters

Display gain: 50 μV
Display window: 2,000 ms
Filtering: 2–2,000 Hz

The display is set so that the screen is constantly updating a single sweep. There is a speaker attached to every channel, allowing auditory as well as visual feedback.

Significant Changes

After every sweep, the surgeon is informed whether a response was present or not.

PEDICLE SCREW STIMULATION

Free-Run Pedicle Screw Monitoring

The muscle groups monitored are determined by the surgical plan for pedicle screw placement. The muscles monitored are wired with two needle electrodes, one just under the skin (+), the other about 4 cm away inserted into the belly of the muscle. The free-run program uses the same recording parameters as the free-run tethered cord monitoring program. This is run while the hole for the pedicle is being drilled and tapped and while the screw is being placed. Any increase in activity from baseline is reported to the surgeon. Each channel is connected to a speaker, allowing auditory as well as visual feedback.

Stimulated Pedicle Screw Monitoring

This monitoring program is run after the holes for the pedicle screws have been drilled. The surgeon inserts a stimulating pen into each hole and tests for any breaks or weakness in the pedicle wall. The pedicle probe or drill bit can also be used to test the integrity of the hole by holding the stimulating pen against the probe or the drill bit and stimulating. The pedicle screw is tested with the screw in its final position by holding the stimulator against the head of the pedicle screw. The monitoring program is switched back to the free-run program between each step to record any sudden increase in activity from the wired muscle group, indicating a sudden compression of the nerve roots.

The stimulated pedicle screw monitoring program uses the same recording parameters as the tethered cord triggered monitoring program. When using this monitoring program the surgeon has a stimulating pen electrode, which is insulated down to the tip and functions as the cathode. A needle electrode is placed in nearby muscle within the surgical field and acts as the anode. The voltage is increased from zero until a response is recorded, up to 100 V.

Significant Changes

If a response is seen in a muscle below 20 V the pedicle screw is replaced. If a response is seen between 20 and 30 V the pedicle is carefully examined by the surgeon and a decision to replace the screw or not is made.

SELECTIVE DORSAL RHIZOTOMIES

(From Primary Children's Rehabilitation Center, Salt Lake City, Utah)

Intraoperative Monitoring

I. Team approach to intraoperative procedure
Neurosurgeon; anesthesiologist; physiatrist; monitoring, nursing, and scrub technicians; preassessment and follow-up personnel.
  A. Surgery takes place between S1-2 and L2 levels.
  B. Choice of muscle groups to monitor
    1. Presurgery assessment by physiatrist and physical therapist
    2. Levels of nerve roots stimulated
  C. Stimulation occurs at the dorsal or ventral root at exit from spinal cord. Hook-stimulating electrodes are placed approximately 2–4 cm apart directly on the root or rootlet.
  D. Responses are recorded at the appropriate muscle group with electrodes.
II. To cut or not to cut
  A. Physician decision
    1. Physiatrist
    2. Surgeon
  B. Behavioral response
  Response is monitored visually in lower extremities by physiatrist or nurse.
  C. Electrophysiology
    1. Stimulus parameters
      a. 0.05-ms duration pulse
      b. 20-Hz stimulation train
      c. 1-second duration stimulation train
      d. 2-second recording time
      e. 2- to 2,000-Hz filtering
      f. Constant current between 0.2-20 μV
    2. Normal sensory
      a. Higher stimulation threshold than motor
      b. Inhibition at 7–15 pulses/second in normals
    3. Normal motor conduction
      a. Does not exhibit inhibition at rates used
      b. Significantly lower threshold
      c. This.is the "gold standard."
    4. Abnormal sensory

a. Lack of inhibition
b. Spread to other muscle groups—i.e., upper extremities and contralateral side
c. Continued response following stimulation
d. Quality and strength of response
e. Absence of any response

ELECTROENCEPHALOGRAM MONITORING PROGRAMS

Recording Montage

Ch 1	Fp1–F7
Ch 2	F7–T3
Ch 3	T3–T5
Ch 4	T5–01
Ch 5	Fp2–F8
Ch 6	F8–T4
Ch 7	T4–T6
Ch 8	T6–02
Ch 9	Fp1–F3
Ch 10	F3–C3
Ch 11	C3–P3
Ch 12	Fp2–F4
Ch 13	F4–C4
Ch 14	C4–P4

Test Parameters

Paper speed: 10 mm/second
High filter: 70 Hz
Time constant: 1.6 seconds, or longer if necessary
Sensitivity: 70 µV/cm, or higher when necessary
60-Hz notch filter when necessary

FACIAL NERVE MONITORING

Equipment

1. Silverstein Facial Nerve Monitor. Model S8 with muscle movement sensor, remote control probe with tips, grounding pads, and wall-mount battery charger.

2. Brackmann EMG System. Model BR202 with preamplifier BRP118 and wall-mount battery charger.
3. Hilger Stimulator. Model H3 with unipolar probe.
4. Wiegand Monitoring Display. Version 1.0 with W.R. electronics isolation interface model 11W-101 and isolator power supply.
5. Disposable electrocardiogram pads, disposable 0.3-mm electromyography electrodes, specimen cup.

Procedure

1. Attach electrocardiogram electrode for grounding.
2. Slide cheek muscle movement sensor into corner of patient's mouth on surgical side. Tighten the clamp to the point where a gentle tug will not dislodge the sensor. Connect the sensor to the front of Silverstein monitor.
3. Insert electromyograph (EMG) electrodes into orbicularis oculi muscle above the eye with the tips of the electrodes approximately 1 cm apart. Connect these electrodes to channel 1 on preamplifier.
4. Insert EMG electrodes near the mouth into orbicularis oris muscle.
5. To prevent the surgical drapes from interfering with the mouth sensor cut a specimen cup in half and pad the corners. Tape the halved cup securely over the mouth movement sensor.
6. The surgeon is given the unipolar probe to stimulate along the seventh cranial nerve. The current level is selected by the surgeon.

The visual monitor of the computer display will indicate any facial nerve activity. This system is capable of auditory feedback, giving the surgeon a more immediate response. All activity should be discussed with the surgeon.

Index